W0037668

2025
Nelson's Pediatric Antimicrobial Therapy

31st Edition

Debra L. Palazzi, MD, MEd
Editor in Chief

John S. Bradley, MD
Past Editor

John D. Nelson, MD
Emeritus, Founding Editor

John C. Arnold, MD
Elizabeth D. Barnett, MD
Joseph B. Cantey, MD, MPH
David W. Kimberlin, MD
Paul E. Palumbo, MD
Jason Sauberan, PharmD
J. Howard Smart, MD
William J. Steinbach, MD
Contributing Editors

American Academy of Pediatrics

DEDICATED TO THE HEALTH OF ALL CHILDREN®

American Academy of Pediatrics Publishing Staff

Mark Grimes, *Vice President, Publishing*

Jeff Mahony, Senior Director, *Professional and Consumer Publishing*

Cheryl Firestone, *Senior Manager, Digital Publishing*

Soraya Alem, *Digital Production Specialist*

Barrett Winston, Senior Manager, *Publishing Acquisitions and Business Development*

Grace Klooster, *Editor, Professional/Clinical Publishing*

Shannan Martin, *Production Manager, Consumer Publications*

Amanda Helmholz, *Medical Copy Editor*

Mary Louise Carr, MBA, *Marketing Manager, Professional Resources*

Published by the American Academy of Pediatrics

345 Park Blvd

Itasca, IL 60143

Telephone: 630/626-6000

Facsimile: 847/434-8000

www.aap.org

The American Academy of Pediatrics is an organization of 67,000 primary care pediatricians, pediatric medical subspecialists, and pediatric surgical specialists dedicated to the health, safety, and well-being of all infants, children, adolescents, and young adults.

While every effort has been made to ensure the accuracy of this publication, the American Academy of Pediatrics does not guarantee that it is accurate, complete, or without error.

The recommendations in this publication do not indicate an exclusive course of treatment or serve as a standard of medical care. Variations, taking into account individual circumstances, may be appropriate.

Statements and opinions expressed are those of the authors and not necessarily those of the American Academy of Pediatrics.

Any websites, brand names, products, or manufacturers are mentioned for informational and identification purposes only and do not imply an endorsement by the American Academy of Pediatrics (AAP). The AAP is not responsible for the content of external resources. Information was current at the time of publication.

The publishers have made every effort to trace the copyright holders for borrowed materials. If they have inadvertently overlooked any, they will be pleased to make the necessary arrangements at the first opportunity.

This publication has been developed by the American Academy of Pediatrics. The contributors are expert authorities in the field of pediatrics. No commercial involvement of any kind has been solicited or accepted in the development of the content of this publication. Disclosures: Dr Elizabeth Barnett has not disclosed any relationships relevant to the content area she contributed to in this publication. Dr Paul Palumbo has disclosed a data safety monitoring financial relationships with Gilead and Janssen. Any relevant disclosures have been mitigated through a process approved by the AAP Board of Directors.

Every effort has been made to ensure that the drug selection and dosages set forth in this publication are in accordance with current recommendations and practice at the time of publication. We encourage the health care professional to check the package insert of each drug for any change in indications or dosage and for added warnings and precautions as well as to review data published in the medical literature since our current review, for updated data on safety and efficacy.

Please visit www.aap.org/errata for an up-to-date list of any applicable errata for this publication.

Special discounts are available for bulk purchases of this publication. Email Special Sales at nationalaccounts@aap. org for more information.

Printed in the United States of America

9-520/0225   1 2 3 4 5 6 7 8 9 10

MA1185

ISSN: 2164-9278 (print)

ISSN: 2164-9286 (electronic)

ISBN: 978-1-61002-824-0

eBook: 978-1-61002-825-7

Contributing Editors (*continued*)

Paul E. Palumbo, MD

Professor of Pediatrics and Medicine
Geisel School of Medicine at Dartmouth
Director, International Pediatric HIV Program
Dartmouth-Hitchcock Medical Center
Lebanon, NH
Lead editor: Chapters 2, 7, and 8

Jason Sauberan, PharmD

Neonatal Research Institute
Sharp Mary Birch Hospital for Women & Newborns
Rady Children's Hospital San Diego
San Diego, CA
Lead editor: Chapters 2, 3, 13, and 18

J. Howard Smart, MD, FAAP

Chairman, Department of Pediatrics
Sharp Rees-Stealy Medical Group
Assistant Clinical Professor of Pediatrics
University of California, San Diego, School of
    Medicine
San Diego, CA
Lead editor: app development

William J. Steinbach, MD, FAAP

Robert H. Fiser, Jr, MD, Endowed Chair in Pediatrics
Chair, Department of Pediatrics
Associate Dean for Child Health
University of Arkansas for Medical Sciences
Pediatrician in Chief, Arkansas Children's
Little Rock, AR
Lead editor: Chapters 5 and 6

Additional Contributor

Margaret Taylor Danner, MD, FAAP

Assistant Professor of Pediatrics
Division of Pediatric Infectious Diseases
Baylor College of Medicine
Associate Medical Director, Antimicrobial
    Stewardship
Texas Children's Hospital
Houston, TX
Lead editor: Chapter 16

Equity, Diversity, and Inclusion Statement

The American Academy of Pediatrics is committed to principles of equity, diversity, and inclusion in its publishing program. Editorial boards, author selections, and author transitions (publication succession plans) are designed to include diverse voices that reflect society as a whole. Editor and author teams are encouraged to actively seek out diverse authors and reviewers at all stages of the editorial process. Publishing staff are committed to promoting equity, diversity, and inclusion in all aspects of publication writing, review, and production.

Contents

Introduction

It is with *great pleasure* I share the news that the title and responsibility of the editor in chief for this 31st edition, and subsequent editions, is now in the very capable hands of Debra Palazzi, MD, MEd, a professor of pediatric infectious diseases and the division chief of Pediatric Infectious Diseases at the Baylor College of Medicine in Houston, TX. She not only takes regular calls as a pediatric infectious disease doctor at Texas Children's Hospital (973 beds) but also has directed their antimicrobial stewardship program (knows when to use, and when *not* to use, antibiotics). She has been an editor and a course director of the American Academy of Pediatrics (AAP) PREP Infectious Diseases program as well as an associate editor for *JAMA Pediatrics* and is the incoming president of the Pediatric Infectious Diseases Society! Dr Palazzi is an outstanding clinician and teacher (from personal observation), with many awards to her credit…and she is a really nice person.

It has been my honor and privilege to work with all of you and the AAP for the past 25 years (my first edition with John Nelson was the 2000–2001 edition). Readers are likely to see some new (and improved) approaches to infectious diseases in this edition, similar to some that occurred as I started sharing writing responsibility with John Nelson. Our field keeps evolving rapidly, with new antibiotics, new data on antibiotic efficacy and safety from clinical trials, and now molecular diagnostics that can give us the name of a pathogen, but without antimicrobial susceptibilities to guide therapy. Dr Palazzi and our distinguished editors will continue to translate these data into practical suggestions for clinical care and will keep the AAP book *Nelson's* an invaluable print/online/app resource for clinicians for decades to come!

John Bradley
December 10, 2024

Welcome to the 31st edition of *Nelson's Pediatric Antimicrobial Therapy*! It is an incredible honor for me to assume the role of editor in chief of this renowned resource and to work with and learn from such amazing contributors. We are thankful that Dr John Bradley—after serving as editor in chief of *Nelson's* for more than 20 years!—has agreed to continue to share his expertise as a contributing editor for many of the chapters in this edition. We are so fortunate to learn from his extensive knowledge of anti-infective pharmacokinetic and pharmacodynamic principles and his many years of experience treating children with simple and complex infectious diseases.

For the 31st edition of *Nelson's*, we have thoroughly reviewed and updated the chapters by not only referencing the most recent medical literature but also sharing our opinions as practicing clinicians. More than ever, the field of clinical infectious diseases is moving at a tremendous pace, and we have tried to share with you salient updates from clinical trials while filling in evidence gaps with advice about how we would treat.

We are extremely fortunate to have nationally/internationally recognized editors, who are experts in each field, contribute to the *Nelson's* chapters, both the clinical chapters and the mini-educational chapters on why they picked specific agents within a class to use for therapy. We are grateful to Dr Maggie Danner, who updated the chapter on antibiotic allergies.

We continue to work closely with the American Academy of Pediatrics (AAP), and many of us have close connections with the AAP Committee on Infectious Diseases, particularly Dr David Kimberlin, the editor of the *Red Book*. Although *Nelson's* is published by the AAP, it is not actually AAP policy (in contrast to the *Red Book*), so we are able to share personal observations that may not be possible in an AAP publication that requires approval by the AAP Board of Directors.

The *Nelson's* app is a critical part of the success of the *Nelson's* book. We continue to update the searchability of the app, making it an excellent reference for the busy clinician. We welcome comments and feedback to improve this resource; please contact us at nelsonabx@aap.org.

We provide grading of our recommendations—our assessment of how strongly we feel about a recommendation and the strength of the evidence to support our recommendation (noted in the Table). This is not the GRADE (*G*rading of *R*ecommendations *A*ssessment, *D*evelopment, and *E*valuation) method but certainly uses the concepts on which GRADE is based: the strength of recommendation and level of evidence. As with GRADE, we review the literature (and the most important manuscripts are referenced), but importantly, we work within the context of professional society recommendations (eg, the AAP) and our experience.

Strength of Recommendation	Description
A	Strongly recommended
B	Recommended as a good choice
C	One option for therapy that is adequate, perhaps among many other adequate therapies
Level of Evidence	**Description**
I	Based on well-designed, prospective, randomized, and controlled studies in an appropriate population of children
II	Based on data derived from prospectively collected, small comparative trials, or noncomparative prospective trials, or reasonable retrospective data from clinical trials in children, or data from other populations (eg, adults)
III	Based on case reports, case series, consensus statements, or expert opinion for situations in which sound data do not exist

As we state each year, many of the recommendations by the editors for specific situations have not been systematically evaluated in controlled, prospective, comparative clinical trials.

We thank Barrett Winston, senior manager, publishing acquisitions and business development, for doing an impressive job of organizing the editors and being an outstanding advocate for us and the clinician-users of the book. Thank you, Barrett, for working with the *Nelson's* editors to meet our deadlines!

It continues to be a privilege to work with all our friends at AAP Publishing. AAP Publishing shares the book at pediatric meetings as well as personally meets with clinicians and answers questions (or sends them to one of the editors!). Thanks to Mark Grimes, vice president, publishing; to Jeff Mahony, senior director, professional and consumer publishing; and to Mary Louise Carr, marketing manager, professional resources. We are all truly honored that providing better care to children remains our focus in the evolving book and app. We are also very pleased that the AAP is supporting the third edition of *Nelson's Neonatal Antimicrobial Therapy*.

Our molecule of the year is baloxavir, an antiviral approved in 2018 for use in adults and children aged 5 years and older to treat influenza A and B. It is given as a single dose and is most effective if started within 48 hours of symptom onset. Baloxavir can also be used for prophylaxis against influenza.

Thank you for your interest in the *Nelson's* book. The editors love to hear from you about your thoughts on improving this resource. Please contact us at nelsonabx@aap.org.

Warmly,

Deb Palazzi, MD, MEd
November 2024

Abbreviations

3TC, lamivudine

AAAAI, American Academy of Allergy, Asthma and Immunology

AAP, American Academy of Pediatrics

AASLD, American Association for the Study of Liver Diseases

ABLC, amphotericin B lipid complex (Abelcet)

ABPA, allergic bronchopulmonary aspergillosis

ABR, auditory brainstem response

ACOG, American College of Obstetricians and Gynecologists

ADH, antidiuretic hormone

AFB, acid-fast bacilli

AGEP, acute generalized exanthematous pustulosis

AHA, American Heart Association

ALT, alanine aminotransferase

AmB, amphotericin B

AmB-D, amphotericin B deoxycholate

amox/clav, amoxicillin/clavulanate (Augmentin)

amp/sul, ampicillin/sulbactam

AOM, acute otitis media

A/P, atovaquone/proguanil

ARC, augmented renal clearance

ARF, acute rheumatic fever

ART, antiretroviral therapy

ARV, antiretroviral

ASPR, Administration for Strategic Preparedness & Response

AST, aspartate aminotransferase

ASTMH, American Society of Tropical Medicine and Hygiene

ATM/AVI, aztreonam/avibactam

AUC, area under the curve (the mathematically calculated area under the serum concentration-versus-time curve)

BAL, bronchoalveolar lavage

bid, twice daily

BL, β-lactamase

BLI, β-lactamase inhibitor

BMI, body mass index

BPD, bronchopulmonary dysplasia

BSA, body surface area

CABP, community-acquired bacterial pneumonia

CA-MRSA, community-associated methicillin-resistant *Staphylococcus aureus*

cap, capsule

CAP, community-acquired pneumonia

CAZ/AVI, ceftazidime/avibactam

CBC, complete blood cell count

CDC, Centers for Disease Control and Prevention

cephalosporin-R, cephalosporin-resistant

CF, cystic fibrosis

Ch(s), chapter(s)

CLD, chronic lung disease

Cmax, maximal concentration of drug achieved in serum and at the tissue site

CMV, cytomegalovirus

CNS, central nervous system

CPB, cardiopulmonary bypass

CrCl, creatinine clearance

CRGNB, carbapenem-resistant gram-negative bacilli

CRO, carbapenem-resistant organism

CRP, C-reactive protein

CSD, cat-scratch disease

CSF, cerebrospinal fluid

CT, computed tomography

cUTI, complicated urinary tract infection

DAA, direct-acting antiviral

DAT, diphtheria antitoxin

DEC, diethylcarbamazine

div, divided

DOT, directly observed therapy

DR, delayed-release

DRESS, drug rash with eosinophilia and systemic symptoms

DS, double-strength

EBV, Epstein-Barr virus

EBW, expected body weight

ECMO, extracorporeal membrane oxygenation

EM, erythema multiforme

EMR, electronic medical record

EPEC, enteropathogen-producing *Escherichia coli*

ER, extended-release

ESBL, extended-spectrum β-lactamase

ESR, erythrocyte sedimentation rate

ETEC, enterotoxin-producing *Escherichia coli*

EUA, Emergency Use Authorization

FDA, US Food and Drug Administration

FQ, fluoroquinolone

G6PD, glucose-6-phosphate dehydrogenase

GA, gestational age

GBS, group B streptococcus

GC, *Neisseria gonorrhoeae*

G-CSF, granulocyte colony-stimulating factor

gentamicin-S, gentamicin-susceptible

GI, gastrointestinal

GNB, gram-negative bacilli

GNR, gram-negative rod (bacilli)

HAART, highly active antiretroviral therapy

HACEK, *Haemophilus aphrophilus, Aggregatibacter* (formerly *Actinobacillus*) *actinomycetemcomitans, Cardiobacterium hominis, Eikenella corrodens, Kingella* species

HAP, hospital-acquired pneumonia

HAT, human African trypanosomiasis

HBeAg, hepatitis B e antigen

HBV, hepatitis B virus

HCV, hepatitis C virus

HHS, US Department of Health and Human Services

HHV, human herpesvirus

HRSA, Health Resources and Services Administration

hs, bedtime

HSV, herpes simplex virus

HUS, hemolytic uremic syndrome

I&D, incision and drainage

IAI, intra-abdominal infection

IBS-D, irritable bowel syndrome with diarrhea

ID, infectious disease

IDSA, Infectious Diseases Society of America

IFN, interferon

IGRA, interferon-γ release assay

IM, intramuscular(ly)

IMI/REL, imipenem/relebactam

IMP, imipenemase

IND, investigational new drug

INH, isoniazid

IUGR, intrauterine growth restriction

IV, intravenous(ly)

IVesic, intravesical

IVIG, intravenous immune globulin

IVPB, intravenous piggyback (premixed bag)

KPC, *Klebsiella pneumoniae* carbapenemase

L-AmB, liposomal amphotericin B

LD, loading dose

LFT, liver function test

LP, lumbar puncture

LRTI, lower respiratory tract infection

MAC, *Mycobacterium avium* complex

max, maximum

MBL, metallo–β-lactamase

MDR, multidrug resistance/multidrug-resistant

mero/vabor, meropenem/vaborbactam

MF, microfilariae/microfilarial

MIC, minimum inhibitory concentration

MIS-C, multisystem inflammatory syndrome in children

MRI, magnetic resonance image/imaging

MRSA, methicillin-resistant *Staphylococcus aureus*

MRSE, methicillin-resistant *Staphylococcus epidermidis*

MSM, men who have sex with men

MSSA, methicillin-susceptible *Staphylococcus aureus*

MSSE, methicillin-sensitive *Staphylococcus epidermidis*

NA, not applicable

NARMS, National Antimicrobial Resistance Monitoring System for Enteric Bacteria

NDM, New Delhi metallo–β-lactamase

NEC, necrotizing enterocolitis

NICU, neonatal intensive care unit

NNRTI, non-nucleoside reverse transcriptase inhibitor

NRTI, nucleoside reverse transcriptase inhibitor

NS, normal saline (physiologic saline solution)

NVP, nevirapine

oint, ointment

OPC, oropharyngeal candidiasis

ophth, ophthalmic

PAIR, puncture, aspiration, injection, re-aspiration

PBPK, physiologic-based pharmacokinetic

PCP, *Pneumocystis* pneumonia

PCR, polymerase chain reaction

PCV13/20, pneumococcal 13-valent/20-valent conjugate vaccine

PCT, procalcitonin

PD, pharmacodynamic(s)

ped, pediatric

PEG, pegylated

pen-R, penicillin-resistant

pen-S, penicillin-susceptible

PEP, postexposure prophylaxis

PHMB, polyhexamethylene biguanide

PICU, pediatric intensive care unit

PIDS, Pediatric Infectious Diseases Society

PIMS-TS, pediatric inflammatory multisystem syndrome temporally associated with SARS-CoV-2

PIP, piperacillin

PK, pharmacokinetic(s)

PMA, postmenstrual age (weeks of gestation since most recent menstrual period PLUS weeks of chronologic age since birth)

PNA, postnatal age

PO, oral(ly)

PPD, purified protein derivative

PrEP, preexposure prophylaxis

PTLD, posttransplant lymphoproliferative disorder

pwd, powder

PZA, pyrazinamide

q, every

qd, once daily

qhs, every bedtime

qid, 4 times daily

qod, every other day

RAE, retinol activity equivalent

RAL, raltegravir

RIG, rabies immune globulin

RIVUR, Randomized Intervention for Children with Vesicoureteral Reflux

RSV, respiratory syncytial virus

RTI, respiratory tract infection

RT-PCR, real-time polymerase chain reaction

SBL, serine β-lactamase

SCr, serum creatinine

SIADH, syndrome of inappropriate antidiuretic hormone

SJS, Stevens-Johnson syndrome

SMX, sulfamethoxazole

soln, solution

SPAG-2, small particle aerosol generator-2
spp, species
SSLR, serum sickness–like reaction
SSSI, skin and skin-structure infection
staph, staphylococcal
STEC, Shiga toxin–producing *Escherichia coli*
STI, sexually transmitted infection
strep, streptococcal
SUBQ, subcutaneous
susp, suspension
tab, tablet
TAF, tenofovir alafenamide
TAZO, tazobactam
TB, tuberculosis
TBW, total body weight
Td, tetanus, diphtheria
TD, travelers diarrhea
Tdap, tetanus, diphtheria, acellular pertussis
TDM, therapeutic drug monitoring
TEN, toxic epidermal necrolysis
tid, 3 times daily

TIG, tetanus immune globulin
TMP, trimethoprim
TOL/TAZ, ceftolozane/tazobactam
top, topical
UCSF, University of California, San Francisco
ULN, upper limit of normal
URTI, upper respiratory tract infection
UTI, urinary tract infection
vag, vaginal
VCUG, voiding cystourethrogram
VDRL, Venereal Disease Research Laboratories
VIGIV, vaccinia immune globulin intravenous
VIM, Verona integron-encoded metallo–β-lactamase
VSIG, varicella-zoster immune globulin
VZV, varicella-zoster virus
WBC, white blood cell
WHO, World Health Organization
ZDV, zidovudine

Notable Changes to *2025 Nelson's Pediatric Antimicrobial Therapy,* 31st Edition

We are quite grateful to Dr Howard Smart for the continual upgrading of the *Nelson's* app search function. We have linked "similar" terms for each disease entity, based on National Library of Medicine search libraries, so the different terminology used by clinicians better matches the terminology used by an editor (eg, "suppurative lymphadenitis" vs "cervical lymph node abscess").

Bacterial/Mycobacterial Infections and Antibiotics

New Infectious Diseases Society of America/Pediatric Infectious Diseases Society guidelines for treatment of pediatric acute bacterial arthritis were published in 2023 and now recommend as short as 10 to 14 days of total therapy (intravenous [IV] + oral [PO]) for uncomplicated infections without adjacent osteomyelitis.

While pediatric guidance for the treatment of *Clostridioides difficile* infection continues to recommend metronidazole and vancomycin as first-line therapy, adult guidelines recommend fidaxomicin as first-line therapy of initial and recurrent infections. Fidaxomicin can be considered when treating *C difficile* disease in pediatric patients. Additionally, bezlotoxumab (monoclonal antibody directed against the *C difficile* toxin) has been approved for patients who are 1 year or older and should be considered for patients at high risk for recurrence.

Once again, a number of new antibiotics for the treatment of multidrug-resistant gram-negative bacilli are available for adult patients, although only one is approved for children (ceftazidime/avibactam). Some of the new β-lactam/β-lactamase inhibitors for metallo–β-lactamases are now in clinical trials.

Children with an immediate hypersensitivity reaction to penicillin or amoxicillin or a positive skin test result should be offered repeat skin testing in 5 to 10 years; up to 80% of children will outgrow penicillin allergies in 10 years. Antibiotics causing Stevens-Johnson syndrome, toxic epidermal necrolysis, drug rash with eosinophilia and systemic symptoms, or acute generalized exanthematous pustulosis should be avoided permanently. Some allergists will consider PO amoxicillin challenge for children with a history of erythema multiforme minor or serum sickness–like reaction out of concern for infection-mediated reaction (eg, viral, *Mycoplasma*).

Fungal Infections and Antifungal Agents

Revised international clinical practice guidelines for allergic bronchopulmonary aspergillosis reaffirm itraconazole preference.

Viral Infections and Antiviral Agents

Over this past year, developments relating to antiviral agents have centered less on introducing new drugs or new indications for use and more on improving implementation of relatively recent recommendations that were noted in last year's edition of *Nelson's*. Perhaps the most significant of these is the use of nirsevimab for passive immunoprophylaxis to prevent severe respiratory syncytial virus (RSV) disease. Nirsevimab is a long-acting monoclonal antibody that prevents 80% to 90% of the severe outcomes of RSV infection in young infants. It is recommended for universal use as a single dose in all infants younger than 8 months. A second dose is recommended for infants 8 through 19 months with certain risk criteria. Approved just before the 2023–2024 RSV season, nirsevimab was in short supply in much of the country last year. That has been resolved, and now pediatricians and health systems are working on their processes for administering this remarkable drug to every baby in the United States. This is no small task!

Another example is the treatment of infants with congenital cytomegalovirus (CMV) disease. An increasing number of states and localities are implementing universal or targeted testing for CMV in babies, so an increasing number of babies are being identified. With that comes inevitable questions of what to do once a baby is confirmed to have congenital CMV. Recommendations for treatment of congenital CMV infection were liberalized somewhat last year, with 6 *months* of PO valganciclovir continuing to be recommended for infants with moderate to severe symptomatic congenital CMV disease and now 6 *weeks* of PO valganciclovir being recommended for infants with isolated sensorineural hearing loss secondary to congenital CMV infection. Age of initiation of antiviral therapy for the treatment of congenital CMV infection can be up to 13 weeks, whereas previously it needed to be started within the first month after birth.

So, overall, 2025 is likely going to be a year where we catch our breath with antiviral drugs. That said, there are many exciting candidate drugs in differing companies' pipelines, so we anticipate that this pause will be short-lived!

Parasitic Infections and Antiparasitic Agents

We continue to encourage readers faced with diagnosing and treating children with malaria, leishmaniasis, and other uncommon parasitic infections to contact the Centers for Disease Control and Prevention (CDC) for consultation about management and antiparasitic drug availability (770-488-7100). We have not provided detailed treatment recommendations for human African trypanosomiasis and instead encourage readers to check current guidelines and seek expert advice if treating patients with these conditions, as management options are evolving quickly. Availability and sources of drugs to treat parasitic infections change frequently (sodium stibogluconate is no longer available, IV artesunate is no longer provided by the CDC, and fexinidazole has been approved by the US Food and Drug Administration but is unavailable at this time), so clinicians are encouraged to check recent sources of information for the most up-to-date recommendations. Shortages of drugs occur sporadically and unpredictably (mefloquine is one example); checking local availability of drugs and making changes if the drug is unavailable will reduce patient and provider frustration.

1. Antimicrobial Therapy According to Clinical Syndromes

NOTES

- A list of table abbreviations and acronyms can be found at the start of this publication.

- This chapter should be considered guidance for a typical patient. Dosage recommendations (the dose amount, the number of doses per day, and the number of days of treatment) are primarily provided for patients with normal hydration, renal, and hepatic function. Because the dose required is based on the exposure of the antibiotic to the pathogen at the site of infection, higher doses may be necessary if the antibiotic does not penetrate well into the infected tissue (eg, meningitis) or if the child's body eliminates the antibiotic more quickly than average. Higher doses/longer courses may also be needed if the child is immunocompromised, and the immune system cannot help resolve the infection. It is becoming more apparent that the host contributes significantly to microbiologic and clinical cure above and beyond the antimicrobial-attributable effect. Most of the dosages reviewed and approved by the US Food and Drug Administration (FDA) are from the original clinical trials for drug registration, unless a safety issue becomes apparent when the label is modified or in cases in which the original industry sponsor of an antibiotic wishes to pursue approval for additional infection sites ("indications") and conducts new prospective clinical trials to share with the FDA. The original sponsor of the drug may not have studied all pathogens at all sites of infection in neonates, infants, and children. The FDA carefully reviews data presented to it but is not required to review the entire literature on each antibiotic and update the package labels. If the FDA has not reviewed data for a specific indication (eg, ampicillin for group A streptococcal cellulitis), there is usually no opinion about whether the drug may or may not be effective and safe. Ampicillin is not "approved" for skin and soft tissue infections caused by any bacteria. That does not mean that the drug does not work or is unsafe; rather, data on safety and efficacy have not been presented to the FDA to expand the package label. The editors will provide suggestions for clinical situations that may not have been reviewed and approved by the FDA. These recommendations are considered *off-label,* signifying that safety and efficacy data have not been reviewed by the FDA at its high level of rigor.

- Duration of treatment should be individualized. Durations recommended are based on the literature, common practice, and general experience. Critical evaluations of the duration of therapy have been carried out in very few infectious diseases. In general, a more extended period of treatment should be used (1) for tissues in which antibiotic concentrations may be relatively low (eg, undrained abscess, central nervous system [CNS] infection); (2) for tissues in which repair following infection-mediated damage is slow (eg, bone); (3) when the organisms are less susceptible; (4) when a relapse of infection is unacceptable (eg, CNS infections); or (5) when the host is immunocompromised in some way. An assessment after therapy will ensure that your selection of antibiotic, dose, and duration of treatment was appropriate. Until prospective, comparative studies are performed for different durations, we cannot assign a specific increased risk of failure for shorter courses. We support the need for these studies in an outpatient or inpatient controlled clinical research setting.

- Our approach to therapy is continuing to move away from the concept that "one dose fits all." In addition to the dose that provides antibiotic exposure and host immuno-competence, the concept of *target attainment* is being better defined. The severity of illness and the willingness of the practitioner to accept a certain rate of failure need to be considered; hence, broad-spectrum, high-dose treatment is used for a child in florid septic shock (where you need to be right virtually 100% of the time), compared with the child with impetigo (where a treatment that is approximately 70% effective is acceptable, as you can see the child back in the office in a few days and alter the therapy as necessary).

- Combination therapy (eg, adding an aminoglycoside or rifamycin to the primary antimicrobial agent) to improve clinical or microbiologic outcomes in children with serious or disseminated infection caused by enteric bacilli, *Pseudomonas aeruginosa,* or *Staphylococcus aureus* has not been prospectively studied in pediatrics. Retrospective adult data support the use of combination therapy based on outcomes, but data (primarily in adults) also support that the addition of aminoglycosides adds to toxicity. Although a clinical trial to adequately assess the benefits and risks of combination therapy in critically ill children would be difficult to conduct, it is necessary to provide evidence to support recommendations. In this 31st edition of *Nelson's,* combination therapy continues to be recommended for critical illness, but only initially, until antibiotic susceptibility data are known, except for certain infections, like endocarditis, that follow national guidelines or other recommendations for combination therapy.

- Diseases in this chapter are arranged by body systems. Consult Chapter 3 for an alphabetized listing of bacterial and mycobacterial pathogens and uncommon organisms not included in this chapter.

- A more detailed description of treatment options for methicillin-resistant *Staphylococcus aureus* (MRSA) infections and multidrug-resistant gram-negative bacilli (GNB) infections, including a stepwise approach to increasingly broad-spectrum agents for increasingly antibiotic-resistant GNB, is provided in Chapter 12. Although, in the past, vancomycin has been the mainstay of therapy for invasive MRSA, it is nephrotoxic and ototoxic, and it requires monitoring renal function and serum drug concentrations. Its use against organisms with a minimal inhibitory concentration of 2 or greater may not provide adequate exposure for a cure with safe, realistic pediatric doses. Ceftaroline, the first MRSA-active β-lactam antibiotic approved by the FDA for adults in 2010, children in 2016, and neonates in 2019, is as effective for most staphylococcal tissue site infections (no controlled data on CNS infections) as vancomycin, but safer, and may be considered preferred therapy over vancomycin for MRSA.

A. SKIN AND SOFT TISSUE INFECTIONS

NOTE: CA-MRSA (see Ch 12) is prevalent in most areas of the world.[1,2] Recommendations for staph infections are given for these scenarios: standard MSSA and CA-MRSA. Antibiotic recommendations "for CA-MRSA" should be used for (1) empiric therapy in regions with >5%–10% of invasive staph caused by MRSA; (2) clinical suspicion of CA-MRSA; and (3) documented CA-MRSA infections. "Standard recommendations" refers to treatment of MSSA. Oxacillin/nafcillin are considered equivalent agents. For MSSA causing most skin and soft tissue infections and bone/joint infections, 1st-generation cephalosporins (ie, cephalothin, cefazolin, cephalexin) are considered equivalent to oxacillin/methicillin, but for MSSA infections in other tissues (eg, endocarditis), cephalosporins other than 1st generation may not be equivalent (need more high-quality data to know with better certainty). Before using clindamycin for empiric therapy, check your local susceptibility data for S aureus (MSSA and MRSA), as resistance can be as high as 40% in some locations. For MRSA skin infections caused by susceptible organisms, clindamycin and TMP/SMX provide similar clinical cure rates.

Clinical Diagnosis	Therapy (evidence grade)	Comments
Adenitis, acute bacterial[3–7] (S aureus, including CA-MRSA, and group A streptococcus; consider *Bartonella* [CSD] for subacute adenitis.)[8] Also called "suppurative adenitis" or "lymph node abscess"	**Empiric therapy** Standard: oxacillin/nafcillin 150 mg/kg/day IV div q6h OR cefazolin 100 mg/kg/day IV div q8h (AI), OR cephalexin 50–75 mg/kg/day PO div tid CA-MRSA: clindamycin 30 mg/kg/day IV or PO (AI) div q8h OR ceftaroline: 2 mo–<2 y, 24 mg/kg/day IV div q8h; ≥2 y, 36 mg/kg/day IV div q8h (max single dose 400 mg); >33 kg, either 400 mg/dose IV q8h or 600 mg/dose IV q12h (BII), OR vancomycin 40 mg/kg/day IV q8h (BII), OR daptomycin: <6 y, 12 mg/kg IV qd; 7 to ≤11 y, 9 mg/kg IV qd; ≥12 and ≤17 y, 7 mg/kg IV qd; ≥18 y, 6 mg/kg IV qd CSD: azithromycin 10 mg/kg qd (max 500 mg) on day 1, then 5 mg/kg (max 250 mg) for 4 additional days (BII)	May need surgical drainage for staph/strep infection; not usually needed for CSD. Additional antibiotics may not be required after drainage of mild to moderate suppurative adenitis caused by staph/strep. For PO therapy for MSSA: cephalexin or amox/clav. For CA-MRSA: clindamycin, TMP/SMX, or linezolid. For PO therapy for group A streptococcus: amoxicillin or penicillin V. Daptomycin is generally avoided in infants until age 1 y due to potential neurotoxicity. Total therapy (IV + PO) for 7–10 days. For CSD: this is the same high dose of azithromycin that is recommended routinely and FDA approved for strep pharyngitis.

A. SKIN AND SOFT TISSUE INFECTIONS

Clinical Diagnosis	Therapy (evidence grade)	Comments
Adenitis, nontuberculous (atypical) mycobacterial[9-14] Also called "subacute lymphadenitis"	Excision is usually curative (BII); azithromycin PO OR clarithromycin PO for 6–12 wk (with or without rifampin or ethambutol) if susceptible (BII).	Antibiotic susceptibility patterns are quite variable; cultures should guide therapy: excision >97% effective; medical treatment 60%–70% effective. No well-controlled trials are available. With surgical and medical therapy, children usually achieve symptomatic cure within 6 mo.[12] For more resistant organisms, other antibiotics may be active, including TMP/SMX, FQs, doxycycline, or, for parenteral therapy, amikacin, meropenem, or cefoxitin. See Ch 3 for specific mycobacterial pathogens.
Adenitis, tuberculous[15,16] (*Mycobacterium tuberculosis* and *Mycobacterium bovis*)	INH 10–15 mg/kg/day (max 300 mg) PO, IV qd for 6 mo AND rifampin 15–20 mg/kg/day (max 600 mg) PO, IV qd for 6 mo AND PZA 30–40 mg/kg/day PO qd AND ethambutol 15–25 mg/kg/day PO for first 2 mo of therapy (BII); then INH and rifampin daily for drug-susceptible TB INH 20–30 mg/kg/day (max 900 mg) PO AND rifampin 15–20 mg/kg/day (max 600 mg) PO AND PZA 50 mg/kg/day PO qd (max 2 g) (AII)	Surgical excision is not usually indicated because organisms are treatable. Adenitis caused by *M bovis* (unpasteurized dairy product ingestion) is uniformly resistant to PZA. Treat 9–12 mo with INH and rifampin if susceptible (BII). No contraindication to fine-needle aspirate of the node for diagnosis.
Anthrax, cutaneous[17]	Empiric therapy: ciprofloxacin 20–30 mg/kg/day PO div bid OR doxycycline 4.4 mg/kg/day (max 200 mg) PO div bid (regardless of age) (AIII)	If susceptible, amoxicillin or clindamycin (BII). Ciprofloxacin and levofloxacin are FDA approved for inhalational anthrax for children >6 mo and should be effective for skin infection (BII).

Bites, dog and cat[3,18–24] (*Pasteurella multocida*; *S aureus*, including CA-MRSA; *Streptococcus* spp, anaerobes; *Capnocytophaga canimorsus*, particularly in asplenic hosts)	Amox/clav 45 mg/kg/day PO div tid (amox/clav 7:1; see Aminopenicillins in Ch 4) for 5–10 days (AII). For hospitalized children, amp/sul OR, if MRSA suspected, ceftriaxone AND clindamycin or vancomycin (BII).	Amox/clav and amp/sul have good *Pasteurella*, MSSA, and anaerobic coverage but lack MRSA coverage. Ceftriaxone plus clindamycin or vancomycin has good *Pasteurella*, MSSA, MRSA, and anaerobic coverage. For IV therapy options: ceftaroline has good *Pasteurella*, MSSA, and MRSA coverage but lacks *Bacteroides fragilis* anaerobic coverage.[23] Amp/sul, meropenem, and PIP/TAZO lack MRSA coverage. Consider rabies prophylaxis[24] for bites from at-risk animals that were not provoked (observe animal for 10 days, if possible) (AI); state and local public health departments and the CDC can provide advice on risk and management (www.cdc.gov/rabies/hcp/prevention-recommendations/pre-exposure-prophylaxis.html; accessed June 3, 2024); consider tetanus prophylaxis. For penicillin allergy, ciprofloxacin (for *Pasteurella*) plus clindamycin (BIII). Tigecycline or doxycycline may be considered for *Pasteurella* coverage.
Bites, human[3,20,21,25] (*Eikenella corrodens*; *S aureus*, including CA-MRSA; *Streptococcus* spp, anaerobes)	Amox/clav 45 mg/kg/day PO div tid (amox/clav 7:1; see Aminopenicillins in Ch 4) for 5–10 days (AII). For hospitalized children, amp/sul OR, if MRSA suspected, ceftriaxone AND clindamycin or vancomycin (BII).	Human bites have a very high infection rate (do not routinely close open wounds). Amox/clav and amp/sul have good *Eikenella*, MSSA, and anaerobic coverage but lack MRSA coverage. Meropenem lacks MRSA coverage. For penicillin allergy, moxifloxacin can be used.[25]
Bullous impetigo[3,4,6,26] (usually *S aureus*, including CA-MRSA)	Standard: cephalexin 50–75 mg/kg/day PO div tid OR amox/clav 45 mg/kg/day PO div tid (CII) CA-MRSA: clindamycin 30 mg/kg/day PO div tid OR TMP/SMX 8 mg/kg/day of TMP PO div bid; for 5–7 days (CI)	For topical therapy if mild infection: mupirocin or retapamulin oint

A. SKIN AND SOFT TISSUE INFECTIONS

Clinical Diagnosis	Therapy (evidence grade)	Comments
Cellulitis of unknown etiology (usually S aureus, including CA-MRSA, or group A streptococcus)[3,4,26-29]	IV empiric therapy for non-facial cellulitis Standard: oxacillin/nafcillin 150 mg/kg/day IV div q6h OR cefazolin 100 mg/kg/day IV div q8h (BII) CA-MRSA: clindamycin 30 mg/kg/day IV div q8h OR ceftaroline: 2 mo–<2 y, 24 mg/kg/day IV div q8h; ≥2 y, 36 mg/kg/day IV div q8h (max single dose 400 mg); >33 kg, either 400 mg/dose IV q8h or 600 mg/dose IV q12h (BI) OR vancomycin 40 mg/kg/day IV q8h (BII) OR daptomycin: 1–<2 y, 10 mg/kg IV qd; 2–6 y, 9 mg/kg IV qd; 7–11 y, 7 mg/kg qd; 12–17 y, 5 mg/kg qd (BI) For PO therapy for MSSA: cephalexin (AII) OR amox/clav 45 mg/kg/day PO div tid (BII); for CA-MRSA: clindamycin (BII), TMP/SMX (AII), doxycycline (age >7 y), or linezolid (BII)	For periorbital or buccal cellulitis, also consider *Streptococcus pneumoniae* or *Haemophilus influenzae* type b in unimmunized infants. Periorbital swelling that looks like cellulitis may occur with severe sinusitis in older children. Total IV + PO therapy for 7–10 days. Because nonsuppurative cellulitis is most often caused by group A streptococcus, cephalexin alone is usually effective. In adults, a prospective, randomized study of non-purulent cellulitis did not show that the addition of TMP/SMX improved outcomes over cephalexin alone.[28]
Cellulitis, buccal (for unimmunized infants and preschool children, *H influenzae* type b)[30]	Ceftriaxone 50 mg/kg/day (AI) IV, IM q24h, for 2–7 days parenteral therapy before switch to PO (BII)	Rule out meningitis (larger doses may then be needed). For penicillin allergy, levofloxacin IV/PO covers pathogens, but no clinical data available. PO therapy: amoxicillin if BL negative; amox/clav or PO 2nd- or 3rd-generation cephalosporin if BL positive.
Cellulitis, erysipelas (*Streptococcus pyogenes*)[3,4,7,31]	Penicillin G 100,000–200,000 U/kg/day IV div q4–6h (BII) initially, then penicillin V 100 mg/kg/day PO div qid (BIII) OR amoxicillin 50 mg/kg/day PO tid (BIII) for 10 days	Clindamycin is also effective for most strains of group A streptococcus. Few well-designed prospective studies exist to provide evidence for recommendations for cellulitis and erysipelas.[31]
Gas gangrene (See Necrotizing fasciitis later in this table.)		

Impetigo (*S aureus*, including CA-MRSA; occasionally group A streptococcus)[3–7,32]	Mupirocin OR retapamulin topically (BII) to lesions tid; OR, for more extensive lesions, PO therapy Standard: cephalexin 50–75 mg/kg/day PO div tid OR amox/clav 45 mg/kg/day PO tid (AII) CA-MRSA: clindamycin 30 mg/kg/day (CII) PO div tid OR TMP/SMX 8 mg/kg/day of TMP PO div bid (AI); for 5–7 days	A meta-analysis suggests that topical therapy is as effective as PO therapy for mild infection, but many studies did not specify outcomes based on pathogen susceptibilities, and more extensive infection, particularly caused by MRSA, may respond better to PO antibiotic therapy.[32] Controlled data are needed.
Ludwig angina[33] (mixed oral aerobes/anaerobes)	Ceftriaxone 50 mg/kg/day IV PLUS clindamycin 40 mg/kg/day IV div q8h or metronidazole 30–40 mg/kg/day IV div q8h (AIII)	Alternatives: amp/sul; meropenem, imipenem or PIP/TAZO if aerobic GNB also suspected (CIII); high risk of respiratory tract obstruction from inflammatory edema
Lymphadenitis (See Adenitis, acute bacterial, earlier in this table.)		
Lymphangitis (usually group A streptococcus, rarely *S aureus*)[3,4,7]	Penicillin G 200,000 U/kg/day IV div q6h (BII) initially, then penicillin V 100 mg/kg/day PO div qid OR amoxicillin 50 mg/kg/day PO tid for 10 days	Cefazolin IV (for group A strep or MSSA infection) or clindamycin IV (for group A strep, most MSSA and MRSA) or vancomycin For mild disease, penicillin V 50 mg/kg/day PO div qid for 10 days
Myositis, suppurative[34] (*S aureus*, including CA-MRSA; synonyms: "tropical myositis," "pyomyositis," "muscle abscess")	Standard: oxacillin/nafcillin 150 mg/kg/day IV div q6h OR cefazolin 100 mg/kg/day IV div q8h (CII) CA-MRSA: clindamycin 40 mg/kg/day IV div q8h OR ceftaroline: 2 mo–<2 y, 24 mg/kg/day IV div q8h; ≥2 y, 36 mg/kg/day IV div q8h (max single dose 400 mg); >33 kg, either 400 mg/dose IV q8h or 600 mg/dose IV q12h (BI) OR vancomycin 40 mg/kg/day IV q8h (CIII) OR daptomycin: 1–<2 y, 10 mg/kg IV qd; 2–6 y, 9 mg/kg IV qd; 7–11 y, 7 mg/kg qd; 12–17 y, 5 mg/kg qd (BIII)	Surgical debridement is usually necessary. For disseminated MRSA infection, may require aggressive, emergent debridement; consider use of clindamycin to help decrease toxin production (BIII); consider IVIG to bind bacterial toxins for life-threatening disease (CIII); abscesses may develop during therapy.

A. SKIN AND SOFT TISSUE INFECTIONS

Clinical Diagnosis	Therapy (evidence grade)	Comments
Necrotizing fasciitis (Pathogens vary depending on the age of the child and location of infection. Single pathogen: group A streptococcus; *Clostridia* spp, *S aureus* [including CA-MRSA], *P aeruginosa*, *Vibrio* spp, *Aeromonas* spp. Multiple pathogen, mixed aerobic/ anaerobic fasciitis: any organism[s]: above, plus GNB, plus *Bacteroides* spp, and other anaerobes.)[3,35–38]	Empiric therapy: ceftazidime 150 mg/kg/day IV div q8h, or cefepime 150 mg/kg/day IV div q8h AND clindamycin 40 mg/kg/day IV div q8h (BIII); OR meropenem 60 mg/kg/day IV div q8h; OR PIP/ TAZO 400 mg/kg/day PIP component IV div q6h (AIII). ADD vancomycin OR ceftaroline for suspected CA-MRSA, pending culture results (AIII). Mixed aerobic/anaerobic/gram-negative: meropenem or PIP/TAZO (AIII).	Aggressive emergent wound debridement (AII). ADD clindamycin to inhibit synthesis of toxins during the first few days of therapy (AII). Consider IVIG to bind bacterial toxins for life-threatening disease (BIII). Value of hyperbaric oxygen is not well established (CIII).[35,39,40] Focus definitive antimicrobial therapy based on culture results.
Pyoderma, cutaneous abscesses (*S aureus*, including CA-MRSA; group A streptococcus)[4,6,7,26,27,41]	Standard: cephalexin 50–75 mg/kg/day PO div tid OR amox/clav 45 mg/kg/day PO div tid (BII) CA-MRSA: clindamycin 30 mg/kg/day PO div tid (BII) OR TMP/SMX 8 mg/kg/day of TMP PO div bid (AI)	I&D when indicated; IV for serious infections. Approaches to prevention of recurrent MRSA infection include the use of baths with chlorhexidine soap daily or qod (BIII) OR the use of bleach baths twice weekly (½ cup of bleach per full bathtub) (BII). Decolonization with nasal mupirocin in a specific child may also be helpful; decolonization of the entire family may be important in certain situations.[42]
Rat-bite fever (*Streptobacillus moniliformis, Spirillum minus*)[43,44]	Penicillin G 100,000–200,000 U/kg/day IV div q6h (BII) for 7–10 days; for endocarditis, ADD genta-micin for 4–6 wk (CIII). For mild disease, PO therapy with amox/clav (CIII).	Organisms are normal oral flora for rodents. One does not require a bite for infection to develop. High rate of associated endocarditis. Alternatives: doxycycline; 2nd- and 3rd-generation cephalosporins (CIII).
Staphylococcal scalded skin syndrome (*S aureus* [MSSA, occasionally CA-MRSA])[45,46]	Standard: oxacillin 150 mg/kg/day IV div q6h OR cefazolin 100 mg/kg/day IV div q8h (CII) CA-MRSA: clindamycin 30 mg/kg/day IV div q8h (CIII) OR ceftaroline OR daptomycin	Burow or Zephiran compresses for oozing skin and intertriginous areas. Corticosteroids are contraindicated. Surgical debridement should be discouraged.

B. SKELETAL INFECTIONS

Clinical Diagnosis	Therapy (evidence grade)	Comments
	NOTE: Recommendations are given for CA-MRSA and MSSA. Antibiotic recommendations for empiric therapy should include CA-MRSA when suspected or documented, while treatment of MSSA with β-lactam antibiotics is preferred over clindamycin. During the past few years, clindamycin resistance in both MSSA and MRSA has remained stable at 10%–20%, with higher resistance reported by laboratories that report clindamycin-susceptible but D-test–positive strains (methylase-inducible) as resistant. Check your local susceptibility data for *S aureus* before using clindamycin for empiric therapy. For MSSA skeletal infections, oxacillin/nafcillin and cefazolin are considered equivalent. The first PIDS-IDSA guidelines for bacterial osteomyelitis were published in the *Journal of the Pediatric Infectious Diseases Society*, September 2021,[47] and the PIDS-IDSA acute bacterial arthritis guidelines were published in the *Journal of the Pediatric Infectious Diseases Society*, 2023.[48]	
Arthritis, bacterial[47-52]	Switch to appropriate high-dose PO therapy when clinically improved, CRP decreasing (see Ch 14).[50,53,54]	
– Newborns	See Ch 2.	
– Infants (*Kingella kingae*, now recognized as the most common pathogen; *S aureus*, including CA-MRSA; group A streptococcus) – Children (*S aureus*, including CA-MRSA; group A streptococcus; *K kingae*) – Unimmunized or immunocompromised children (pneumococcus, *H influenzae* type b) For Lyme disease and brucellosis, see Table 1L.	Empiric therapy: cefazolin 100 mg/kg/day IV div q8h (in locations where MRSA causes <10% of infections); ADD clindamycin 30 mg/kg/day IV div q8h (to cover CA-MRSA unless clindamycin resistance locally is >10%, then use vancomycin). Ceftaroline can be used for MSSA, MRSA, and *Kingella*. Dexamethasone adjunctive therapy is not routinely recommended[48] (see Comments). For documented CA-MRSA: clindamycin 30 mg/kg/day IV div q8h (AI) OR ceftaroline: 2 mo–<2 y, 24 mg/kg/day IV div q8h; ≥2 y, 36 mg/kg/day IV div q8h (max single dose 400 mg); >33 kg, either 400 mg/dose IV q8h or 600 mg/dose IV q12h (BI) OR vancomycin 40 mg/kg/dose IV q8h (BI). For MSSA: oxacillin/nafcillin 150 mg/kg/day IV div q6h OR cefazolin 100 mg/kg/day IV div q8h (AI). For *Kingella*, BL-negative: cefazolin 100 mg/kg/day IV div q8h OR ampicillin 150 mg/kg/day IV div q6h; OR, for BL-positive, ceftriaxone 50 mg/kg/day IV, IM q24h (All).	Dexamethasone adjunctive therapy (0.15 mg/kg/dose q6h for 4 days in one study) demonstrated significant benefit in decreasing symptoms and earlier hospital discharge (but with some "rebound" symptoms).[55,56] Until additional controlled data are available, dexamethasone is not recommended. **NOTE:** Children with rheumatologic, postinfectious, fungal/mycobacterial infections or malignancy are also likely to improve with steroid therapy. PO step-down therapy options[48]: For CA-MRSA: clindamycin OR linezolid. Little data published on TMP/SMX for invasive MRSA infection, although some experts routinely use TMP/SMX for osteoarticular infections.[57,58] For MSSA: cephalexin OR dicloxacillin caps for older children. For *Kingella*: most penicillins or cephalosporins (but not clindamycin or linezolid).

(Continued on next page)

B. SKELETAL INFECTIONS

Clinical Diagnosis	Therapy (evidence grade)	Comments
– Infants (*Kingella kingae*, now recognized as the most common pathogen; *S aureus*, including CA-MRSA; group A streptococcus) – Children (*S aureus*, including CA-MRSA; group A streptococcus; *K kingae*) – Unimmunized or immunocompromised children (pneumococcus, *H influenzae* type b) For Lyme disease and brucellosis, see Table 1L. *(continued)*	For pen-S pneumococci or group A streptococcus: penicillin G 200,000 U/kg/day IV div q6h (BII). For pen-R pneumococci or *Haemophilus*: ceftriaxone 50–75 mg/kg/day IV, IM q24h (BII). Total therapy (IV + PO) for 14–21 days (AII).[47,48,52]	
– Gonococcal arthritis or tenosynovitis[56,59,60]	Ceftriaxone 50 mg/kg IV, IM (max 1 g) q24h (BII) for 7 days. Consider empiric therapy for *Chlamydia trachomatis*.	Per 2021 CDC guidance, "[w]hen treating for the arthritis-dermatitis syndrome, the provider can switch to an oral agent guided by antimicrobial susceptibility testing 24–48 hours after substantial clinical improvement, for a total treatment course of at least 7 days." Alternative parenteral regimens include cefotaxime (50 mg/kg q8h). www.cdc.gov/std/treatment-guidelines/gonorrhea-adults.htm.
– Other bacteria	See Ch 3 for preferred antibiotics.	
Osteomyelitis[47–59,61–65]	Step down to appropriate high-dose PO therapy when clinically improved (see Ch 14).[47,50,52,53,64]	
– Newborns	See Ch 2.	

– Acute osteomyelitis: usually *S aureus*, including CA-MRSA; group A streptococcus; *K kingae*[47]	Empiric therapy: cefazolin 100 mg/kg/day IV div q8h (in locations where MRSA causes <10% of bone infections), OR clindamycin 30 mg/kg/day IV div q8h (to cover CA-MRSA unless clindamycin resistance is locally >10%; then use ceftaroline or vancomycin). For CA-MRSA: clindamycin 30 mg/kg/day IV div q8h OR ceftaroline: 2 mo–<2 y, 24 mg/kg/day IV div q8h; ≥2 y, 36 mg/kg/day IV div q8h (max single dose 400 mg); >33 kg, either 400 mg/dose IV q8h or 600 mg/dose IV q12h (BI), OR vancomycin 40 mg/kg/day IV q8h (BII). For MSSA: oxacillin/nafcillin 150 mg/kg/day IV div q6h OR cefazolin 100 mg/kg/day IV div q8h (AII). For *Kingella*, BL-negative: cefazolin 100 mg/kg/day IV div q8h OR ampicillin 150 mg/kg/day IV div q6h; OR, for BL-positive, ceftriaxone 50 mg/kg/day IV, IM q24h (AII), or ceftaroline. Total therapy (IV + PO) usually 3–4 wk for uncomplicated MSSA, but may need >4–6 wk for CA-MRSA (BII). Follow closely for clinical response to empiric therapy.	In children with open fractures secondary to trauma, consider adding ceftazidime or cefepime for extended aerobic GNB activity. *Kingella* is resistant to clindamycin, vancomycin, and linezolid. For MSSA (BI) and *Kingella* (BIII), PO step-down therapy with cephalexin 100 mg/kg/day PO div tid. *Kingella* is usually susceptible to amoxicillin. PO step-down therapy options for CA-MRSA include clindamycin and linezolid[66]; some experts routinely use TMP/SMX for osteoarticular infections.[53,58] For prosthetic devices, biofilms may impair microbial eradication, requiring the addition of rifampin or other agents.[65] No prospective, controlled data on the use of antibiotic-containing beads/cement placed at surgery in the site of infection.[47]
– Acute: other organisms	See Ch 3 for preferred antibiotics.	

B. SKELETAL INFECTIONS

Clinical Diagnosis	Therapy (evidence grade)	Comments
– Chronic osteomyelitis (may be a complication of poorly treated acute staph osteomyelitis or the result of trauma-associated infection with multiple potential pathogens), not to be confused with chronic *nonbacterial* osteomyelitis and chronic recurrent multifocal osteomyelitis, which are autoinflammatory diseases	Initial IV therapy, often with cefazolin unless pathogens other than *S aureus* are suspected, as chronically infected bone is surgically debrided (often with multiple procedures). Then prolonged PO step-down therapy may be required for 6–12 mo depending on the success of debridement. For MSSA: cephalexin 100 mg/kg/day PO div qid or tid OR dicloxacillin caps 75–100 mg/kg/day PO div qid for ≥3–6 mo (CIII). For CA-MRSA: clindamycin, linezolid, or TMP/SMX (CIII).	Surgery to debride sequestrum is usually required for cure. For prosthetic joint infection caused by staphylococci, add rifampin (CIII).[65] Osteomyelitis associated with foreign material (spinal rods, prostheses, implanted catheters) may be difficult to cure without removal of the material, but long-term suppression may be undertaken if risks of surgery are high, until some stabilization of the healing infected bone occurs. Watch for β-lactam–associated neutropenia with high-dose, long-term therapy and for linezolid-associated neutropenia/thrombocytopenia with long-term (>2 wk) therapy.[66] PO dicloxacillin is poorly tolerated.
Osteomyelitis of the foot[67] (secondary to penetrating injury to the plantar surface; *S aureus*, including CA-MRSA, with other organisms colonizing foreign bodies) Osteochondritis after a puncture wound through a shoe; *P aeruginosa*	Cefepime 150 mg/kg/day IV div q8h (BIII); ADD vancomycin (enhanced gram-positive coverage) OR gentamicin (enhanced gram-negative coverage), pending culture results.	Surgical debridement with cultures to focus antibiotic therapy. Treatment course is based on pathogen and extent of infection and debridement.

C. EYE INFECTIONS

Clinical Diagnosis	Therapy (evidence grade)	Comments
Cellulitis, orbital[68–71] (cellulitis of the contents of the orbit; may be associated with orbital abscess); usually secondary to sinus infection; caused by respiratory tract flora and S aureus, including CA-MRSA)	Ceftriaxone 50 mg/kg/day IV q24h AND clindamycin 30 mg/kg/day IV div q8h (for S aureus, including CA-MRSA) or vancomycin 40 mg/kg/day IV div q8h or ceftaroline single-drug therapy: 2 mo–<2 y, 24 mg/kg/day IV div q8h; ≥2 y, 36 mg/kg/day IV div q8h (max single dose 400 mg); >33 kg, either 400 mg/dose IV q8h or 600 mg/dose IV q12h (BIII). If MSSA isolated, use oxacillin/nafcillin IV OR cefazolin IV.	Surgical drainage of significant orbital or subperiosteal abscess present by CT scan or MRI. Try medical therapy alone for cellulitis without abscess or with small abscesses (BIII).[72,73] Amp/sul for respiratory flora/anaerobic coverage.[73] Treatment course for 10–14 days after surgical drainage, up to 21 days. CT scan or MRI can confirm cure (BIII). Insufficient evidence about the concurrent use of steroids.[68]
Cellulitis, periorbital[74,75] (preseptal cellulitis)		Periorbital tissues are TENDER with cellulitis. Periorbital edema with sinusitis can look identical but is NOT tender. A multidisciplinary approach with an otolaryngologic, ophthalmologic, and pediatric focus is helpful.[74]
– Cellulitis associated with entry site lesion on skin (S aureus, including CA-MRSA; group A streptococcus) in the fully immunized child	Standard: oxacillin/nafcillin 150 mg/kg/day IV div q6h OR cefazolin 100 mg/kg/day IV div q8h (BII) CA-MRSA: clindamycin 30 mg/kg/day IV div q8h or vancomycin 40 mg/kg/day IV div q8h or ceftaroline: 2 mo–<2 y, 24 mg/kg/day IV div q8h; ≥2 y, 36 mg/kg/day IV div q8h (max single dose 400 mg); >33 kg, either 400 mg/dose IV q8h or 600 mg/dose IV q12h (BII)	PO antistaphylococcal antibiotic (eg, cephalexin or clindamycin) for empiric therapy for less severe infection; treatment course for 7–10 days
– True cellulitis with no associated entry site (in febrile, unimmunized infants; pneumococcal or H influenzae type b	Ceftriaxone 50 mg/kg/day q24h OR cefuroxime 150 mg/kg/day IV div q8h (AII)	Treatment course for 7–10 days; rule out meningitis if bacteremic with H influenzae. Alternative agents for BL-positive strains of H influenzae: other 2nd-, 3rd-, 4th-, or 5th-generation cephalosporins, amp/sul IV or amox/clav PO.

C. EYE INFECTIONS

Clinical Diagnosis	Therapy (evidence grade)	Comments
– Periorbital edema, not true cellulitis; non-tender erythematous swelling. Usually associated with sinusitis; sinus pathogens may *rarely* erode anteriorly, causing cellulitis.	Ceftriaxone 50 mg/kg/day q24h OR cefuroxime 150 mg/kg/day IV div q8h (BIII). For suspected *S aureus*, can use ceftaroline instead of ceftriaxone to cover both sinus pathogens and MSSA/MRSA. For chronic sinusitis, ADD clindamycin (covers anaerobes) to either ceftriaxone or ceftaroline (AIII).	For PO convalescent antibiotic therapy, see Sinusitis, acute, in Table 1D; total treatment course of 14–21 days or 7 days after resolution of symptoms.
Conjunctivitis, acute (Most conjunctivitis is caused by a virus and does not require antibiotic treatment; purulent conjunctivitis is primarily caused by *Haemophilus* and pneumococcus.)[76,77]	Polymyxin/TMP ophth soln OR polymyxin/bacitracin ophth oint OR ciprofloxacin ophth soln (BII), for 7–10 days. For neonatal infection, see Ch 2. Steroid-containing therapy only if HSV ruled out.	Other topical antibiotics (gentamicin, tobramycin, erythromycin, besifloxacin, moxifloxacin, norfloxacin, ofloxacin, levofloxacin) may offer advantages for particular pathogens (CII).
Conjunctivitis, herpetic[78–80] (*may be associated with keratitis*) For neonatal, see Ch 2.	1% trifluridine or 0.15% ganciclovir ophth gel (AII) AND acyclovir PO (80 mg/kg/day div qid; max daily dose: 3,200 mg/day) has been effective in limited studies (BIII). PO valacyclovir (60 mg/kg/day div tid) has superior PK to PO acyclovir and can be considered for systemic treatment. Parenteral (IV) acyclovir if extent of disease is severe (CII).	Consultation with ophthalmologist recommended for assessment and management (eg, concomitant use of topical steroids in certain situations). Recurrences common; corneal scars may form. Long-term suppression (≥1 y) of recurrent infection with PO acyclovir 80 mg/kg/day in 3 div doses (max dose 800 mg) or PO valacyclovir 40 mg/kg/day in 2 div doses (max dose 1,000 mg); decisions to continue suppressive therapy should be revisited annually. The frequency of dosing may need to be increased to qid, or the drug may need to be changed to valacyclovir, if breakthrough ocular infection occurs. Potential risks must balance potential benefits to vision (BIII).

Dacryocystitis[81] (*S aureus* most often, and other skin flora)	No antibiotic usually needed; PO antibiotic therapy for more symptomatic infection, based on Gram stain and culture of pus; topical therapy as for conjunctivitis may be helpful.	Warm compresses; may require surgical probing of nasolacrimal duct
Endophthalmitis[82,83]		
NOTE: This is a medical emergency. Subconjunctival/sub-tenon antibiotics are likely to be required (vancomycin/ceftazidime or clindamycin/gentamicin); steroids commonly used (except for fungal infection); requires anterior chamber or vitreous tap for microbiologic diagnosis. Listed systemic antibiotics to be used in addition to ocular injections.		
– Empiric therapy following open globe injury	Vancomycin 40 mg/kg/day IV div q8h AND cefepime 150 mg/kg/day IV div q8h (AIII)	Consider ceftaroline for empiric MRSA treatment, as it may penetrate the vitreous better than vancomycin (BIII).
– Staphylococcal	Vancomycin 40 mg/kg/day IV div q8h pending susceptibility testing; oxacillin/nafcillin 150 mg/kg/day IV div q6h if susceptible (AIII)	Consider ceftaroline for definitive MRSA treatment, as it may penetrate the vitreous better than vancomycin.
– Pneumococcal, meningococcal, *Haemophilus*	Ceftriaxone 100 mg/kg/day IV q24h; penicillin G 250,000 U/kg/day IV div q4h if susceptible (AIII)	Treatment course for 10–14 days
– Gonococcal	Ceftriaxone 50 mg/kg q24h IV, IM AND azithromycin (AIII)	Treatment course ≥7 days
– *Pseudomonas*	Cefepime 150 mg/kg/day IV div q8h for 10–14 days (AIII) or, if susceptible, levofloxacin[84] (See Ch 3 for dosing.)	Cefepime is preferred over ceftazidime for *Pseudomonas* based on decreased risk of development of resistance during therapy; meropenem IV and imipenem IV are alternatives (no clinical data). Very poor outcomes. PO convalescent therapy with FQs in the adherent child.

C. EYE INFECTIONS

Clinical Diagnosis	Therapy (evidence grade)	Comments
– Candida[85]	Fluconazole (25 mg/kg LD, then 12 mg/kg/day IV), OR voriconazole (9 mg/kg LD, then 8 mg/kg/day IV); for resistant strains, systemic antifungals PLUS intravitreal amphotericin 5–10 mcg/0.1-mL sterile water OR voriconazole 100 mcg/0.1-mL sterile water or physiologic (normal) saline soln (AIII). Duration of therapy is at least 4–6 wk (AIII).	Echinocandins given IV may not be able to achieve adequate antifungal activity in the eye.
Hordeolum (sty) or chalazion[86] – Staphylococcus spp	None usually needed. Topical erythromycin-containing eye oint often used (CIII). If cellulitis develops, may need systemic therapy.	Warm compresses; I&D when necessary
Retinitis		
– Cytomegalovirus[86,87] For congenital, see Ch 2. Predominantly in immunocompromised and transplant patients. For HIV-infected children, see https://clinicalinfo.hiv.gov/en/guidelines/pediatric-opportunistic-infection/cytomegalovirus (accessed September 12, 2024).	See Ch 7. Ganciclovir 10 mg/kg/day IV div q12h for 2 wk (BIII); if needed, continue at 5 mg/kg/day q24h to complete 6 wk total (BIII).	Consultation with an ophthalmologist is recommended for assessment and management. Neutropenia risk increases with duration of therapy. Foscarnet IV and cidofovir IV are alternatives but demonstrate significant toxicities. Letermovir has been approved for prophylaxis of CMV in adult stem cell transplant patients but has not been studied as treatment of CMV retinitis. PO valganciclovir has not been evaluated in HIV-infected children with CMV retinitis but is an option primarily for older children who weigh enough to receive the adult dose of valganciclovir (CIII).

Maribavir is approved for the treatment of adults and pediatric patients (aged ≥12 y and weighing at least 35 kg) with posttransplant CMV infection/disease that is refractory to treatment (with or without genotypic resistance) with ganciclovir, valganciclovir, cidofovir, or foscarnet. However, it should not be used for CMV retinitis, as this was an exclusion criterion in its licensure study.

Intravitreal ganciclovir and combination therapy for non-responding, immunocompromised hosts; however, intravitreal injections may not be practical for most children.

D. EAR AND SINUS INFECTIONS

Clinical Diagnosis	Therapy (evidence grade)	Comments
Bullous myringitis (See Otitis media, acute, later in this table.)		Believed to be a clinical manifestation of acute bacterial otitis media
Mastoiditis, acute [less since introduction of conjugate pneumococcal vaccines]; *S aureus*, including CA-MRSA; group A streptococcus; *Pseudomonas* in adolescents, *Haemophilus* rare)[88–90]	Ceftriaxone 50 mg/kg/day q24h AND clindamycin 40 mg/kg/day IV div q8h (BIII), OR ceftaroline IV For adolescents: cefepime 150 mg/kg/day IV div q8h AND clindamycin 40 mg/kg/day IV div q8h (BIII)	Consider CNS extension (meningitis); surgery as needed for mastoid and middle ear drainage. Step down to appropriate PO therapy after clinical improvement, guided by culture results. Duration of therapy not well-defined; look for evidence of mastoid osteomyelitis or subperiosteal abscess. Based on severity of disease and success of surgical debridement, may need 3–4 wk of therapy.

D. EAR AND SINUS INFECTIONS

Clinical Diagnosis	Therapy (evidence grade)	Comments
Mastoiditis, chronic (See also Otitis, chronic suppurative, below.) (anaerobes; *Pseudomonas; S aureus*, including CA-MRSA)[91]	Antibiotics only for acute superinfections (according to culture of drainage); for *Pseudomonas*: cefepime 150 mg/kg/day IV div q8h Alternatives to enhance anaerobic coverage: meropenem 60 mg/kg/day IV div q8h, OR PIP/TAZO 240 mg/kg/day IV div q4–6h (BIII)	Daily cleansing of ear important; if no response to antibiotics, surgery. Be alert for CA-MRSA.
Otitis, chronic suppurative (*P aeruginosa; S aureus*, including CA-MRSA; and other respiratory tract/skin flora)[91]	Topical antibiotics: FQ (ciprofloxacin, ofloxacin, besifloxacin) with or without steroid (BIII) Cleaning of canal, view of tympanic membrane, for patency; cultures important	Presumed middle ear drainage through open tympanic membrane. Avoid aminoglycoside-containing therapy given risk of ototoxicity.[92] Other topical FQs with/without steroids available.
Otitis externa		
– Bacterial, malignant otitis externa (*P aeruginosa*)[93,94]	Cefepime 150 mg/kg/day IV div q8h (AIII)	Other antipseudomonal antibiotics should also be effective: ceftazidime IV AND tobramycin IV, OR meropenem IV or imipenem IV or PIP/TAZO IV. For more mild infection, ciprofloxacin PO.
– Bacterial, acute otitis externa (*P aeruginosa; S aureus*, including CA-MRSA)[93,94] Also called "swimmer's ear"	Topical antibiotics: FQ (ciprofloxacin or ofloxacin) with steroid, OR neomycin/polymyxin B/hydrocortisone (BII) Irrigating and cleaning canal of detritus important	Wick moistened with Burow (aluminum acetate topical) soln, used for marked swelling of canal; to prevent swimmer's ear, 2% acetic acid to canal after water exposure will restore acid pH.
– Bacterial furuncle of canal (*S aureus*, including CA-MRSA)	Standard: oxacillin/nafcillin 150 mg/kg/day IV div q6h OR cefazolin 100 mg/kg/day IV div q8h (BIII) CA-MRSA: clindamycin, ceftaroline, or vancomycin (BIII)	I&D; antibiotics for cellulitis. PO therapy for mild disease, convalescent therapy. For MSSA: cephalexin. For CA-MRSA: clindamycin, TMP/SMX, OR linezolid (BIII).
– Candida	Fluconazole 6–12 mg/kg/day PO qd for 5–7 days (CIII)	May occur following antibiotic therapy for bacterial external otitis; debride canal.

Otitis media, acute

NOTE: The incidence of AOM and subsequent complications have decreased substantially in the era of conjugate pneumococcal vaccines.[95] With a decrease in disease caused by pen-R pneumococci requiring alternatives to first-line therapy, very few new antibiotics have entered clinical trials within the past few years. Although the risk of antibiotic-resistant pneumococcal otitis has decreased,[96] the percentage of *Haemophilus* responsible for AOM has increased and may continue to increase with widespread use of the new 20-valent conjugate pneumococcal vaccine; therefore, some experts (Ellen Wald) recommend use of amox/clav over amoxicillin as first-line therapy for well-documented AOM.[97] The most current AAP guidelines[98] and meta-analyses[99,100] suggest that the greatest benefit with therapy occurs in children with bilateral AOM who are <2 y; for other children, close observation is also an option. AAP guidelines provide an option for non-severe cases, particularly disease in older children, to provide a prescription to parents but have them fill the prescription only if the child's condition deteriorates.[98] European guidelines are similar, although somewhat more conservative.[101] Although prophylaxis is only rarely indicated, amoxicillin or other antibiotics can be given at the same milligram per kilogram dose as for treatment but less frequently, either qd or bid, to prevent infections (if the benefits outweigh the risks of development of resistant organisms for that child).[98]

– Newborns	See Ch 2.	
– Infants and children (pneumococcus, *H influenzae* non–type b, *Moraxella* most common)[96,97,102]	Amox/clav (90 mg/kg/day amox component PO div bid for unimmunized infants [pneumococcal vaccine] but 45 mg/kg/day amox component PO div bid for immunized infants). Amoxicillin is still a reasonable choice for empiric therapy, but failures will most likely be caused by BL-producing *Haemophilus* (or *Moraxella*). a. For *Haemophilus* strains that are BL positive: amox/clav, cefdinir, cefpodoxime, cefuroxime, ceftriaxone IM, levofloxacin.	See Ch 18 for dosages. Current data suggest that post-PCV13, *H influenzae* is now the most common pathogen, shifting the recommendation for empiric therapy from amoxicillin to amox/clav.[97,98,102] although retrospective review of outcomes suggests that amoxicillin is not inferior to amox/clav.[100] Published data document new but uncommon emergence of penicillin resistance in pneumococci isolated in the post-PCV13 era.[103,104] Return to standard-dosage amoxicillin (45 mg/kg/day) for AOM. Tympanocentesis should be performed in children whose second-line therapy fails.

(Continued on next page)

D. EAR AND SINUS INFECTIONS

Clinical Diagnosis	Therapy (evidence grade)	Comments
– Infants and children (pneumococcus, *H influenzae* non–type b, *Moraxella* most common)[96,97,102] (*continued*)	b. For pen-R pneumococci (much less common in the PCV13/20 era): high-dosage amoxicillin achieves greater middle ear activity than PO cephalosporins. Options include ceftriaxone 50 mg/kg/day IM q24h for 1–3 doses; OR levofloxacin 20 mg/kg/day PO bid for children ≤5 y and 10 mg/kg PO qd for children >5 y; OR a macrolide-class antibiotic: azithromycin PO at 1 of 3 dosages: (1) 10 mg/kg on day 1, followed by 5 mg/kg qd for days 2–5; (2) 10 mg/kg qd for 3 days; or (3) 30 mg/kg once. **Caution:** Up to 40% of pneumococci are macrolide resistant.	
Sinusitis, acute (*H influenzae* non–type b, pneumococcus, group A streptococcus, *Moraxella*)[96,104–107]	Same antibiotic therapy as for AOM, as pathogens are similar: either amox/clav (90 mg/kg/day amox component PO div bid) or amoxicillin alone (90 mg/kg/day PO div bid).[96] Therapy of 14 days may be necessary while mucosal swelling resolves and ventilation is restored. If high-quality evidence for decreased penicillin resistance in the PCV13 era becomes available in the future, the dose of amoxicillin required for treatment may decrease.[105]	IDSA sinusitis guidelines recommend amox/clav as first-line therapy[108]; amoxicillin is still an option.[106] While both represent reasonable and effective therapy, amox/clav provides activity against BL-positive strains of *H influenzae*, which are more likely to be prevalent in both sinusitis and otitis in the PCV13/20 era.[97] There is no controlled evidence to determine whether the use of antihistamines, decongestants, or nasal irrigation is efficacious in children with acute sinusitis.[107]

E. OROPHARYNGEAL INFECTIONS

Clinical Diagnosis	Therapy (evidence grade)	Comments
Dental abscess (mixed aerobic/anaerobic oral flora)[109,110]	Clindamycin 30 mg/kg/day PO, IV, IM div q6–8h OR penicillin G 100,000–200,000 U/kg/day IV div q6h and metronidazole 30–40 mg/kg/day IV div q8h (AIII)	High-quality prospectively collected data on the value of antibiotics have not been published, particularly regarding the need for antibiotics after dental extraction. Recommendations are based on the microbiology of dental abscesses. Amox/clav PO, clindamycin PO are PO options. Metronidazole has excellent anaerobic activity but no aerobic activity. Penicillin failures reported. Other IV options include ceftriaxone and metronidazole, OR meropenem. Tooth extraction usually necessary. Erosion of abscess may occur into facial, sinusitis, deep head, and neck compartments.
Diphtheria pharyngitis[111]	Erythromycin 40–50 mg/kg/day PO div qid for 14 days OR penicillin G 150,000 U/kg/day IV div q6h; PLUS DAT (AIII)	DAT, a horse antiserum, is investigational and available only from the CDC Emergency Operations Center at 770–488–7100; www.cdc.gov/diphtheria/hcp/dat/index.html (accessed September 12, 2024).
Epiglottitis (supraglottitis; *H influenzae* type b in an unimmunized child; rarely pneumococcus, *S aureus*)[112,113]	Ceftriaxone 50 mg/kg/day IV, IM q24h for 7–10 days	Emergency: provide airway. For suspected *S aureus* infection (causes only 5% of epiglottitis), consider adding clindamycin or vancomycin to ceftriaxone or using ceftaroline single-drug therapy.

E. OROPHARYNGEAL INFECTIONS

Clinical Diagnosis	Therapy (evidence grade)	Comments
Gingivostomatitis, herpetic[114–116]	Acyclovir 80 mg/kg/day PO div qid (max dose 800 mg) for 7 days (for severe disease, use IV therapy at 30 mg/kg/day div q8h) (BIII); OR, for infants ≥3 mo, valacyclovir 20 mg/kg/dose PO bid (max dose 1,000 mg; instructions for preparing liquid formulation with 28-day shelf life included in package insert) (CIII)[116]	Early treatment is likely to be the most effective. Start treatment as soon as PO intake is compromised. Valacyclovir is the prodrug of acyclovir that provides improved PO bioavailability compared with PO acyclovir. Extended duration of therapy may be needed for immunocompromised children. The PO acyclovir dose (80 mg/kg/day div into 4 equal doses) provided is safe and effective for varicella, but 75 mg/kg/day div into 5 equal doses has been studied for HSV.[115] Max daily acyclovir dose should not exceed 3,200 mg.
Lemierre syndrome (*Fusobacterium necrophorum* primarily; also reported with MRSA)[117–121] – Pharyngitis with internal jugular vein septic thrombosis; also known as postanginal sepsis, necrobacillosis	Empiric: meropenem 60 mg/kg/day div q8h (or 120 mg/kg/day div q8h for CNS metastatic foci) (AIII) OR ceftriaxone 100 mg/kg/day q24h AND metronidazole 40 mg/kg/day div q8h or clindamycin 40 mg/kg/day div q6h (BIII). ADD empiric vancomycin if MRSA is suspected if clindamycin is not already in the treatment regimen or based on local susceptibility data.	Anecdotal reports suggest that metronidazole may be effective for apparent failures with other agents. Often requires anticoagulation. Metastatic and recurrent abscesses often develop during active, appropriate therapy, requiring multiple debridements and prolonged antibiotic therapy.[121] Treatment duration is often ≥4–6 wk.
Peritonsillar cellulitis or abscess (group A streptococcus with mixed oral flora, including anaerobes, CA-MRSA)[122] See Retropharyngeal; parapharyngeal; lateral pharyngeal cellulitis or abscess later in this table.	Clindamycin 30 mg/kg/day PO, IV, IM div q8h; for preschool infants with consideration of enteric bacilli, ADD ceftriaxone 50 mg/kg/day IV q24h (BIII).	Consider I&D for larger abscess, particularly if no good initial response to medical therapy. Alternatives: meropenem or imipenem or PIP/TAZO. Amox/clav for convalescent PO therapy (BIII). No controlled, prospective data on benefits/risks of steroids.[123]

Pharyngitis (group A streptococcus primarily)[7,124,125]	Amoxicillin 50–75 mg/kg/day PO, qd, bid, or tid for 10 days OR penicillin V 50–75 mg/kg/day PO, qid, bid, or tid, OR benzathine penicillin 600,000 U IM for children <27 kg, 1.2 million U IM if >27 kg, as a single dose (AII) For penicillin-allergic children: erythromycin (estolate) at 20–40 mg/kg/day PO div bid to qid; OR 40 mg/kg/day PO div bid to qid for 10 days; OR azithromycin 12 mg/kg qd for 5 days[a] (AII); OR clindamycin 30 mg/kg/day PO div tid [a] Since 1994 this is the dose investigated and FDA approved for children with strep pharyngitis, and it is higher than the standard dose for other RTIs.	Although penicillin V is the most narrow-spectrum treatment, amoxicillin displays better GI absorption than PO penicillin V; the suspension is better tolerated. These advantages should be balanced by the unnecessary increased spectrum of activity. Once-daily amoxicillin dosage: for children 50 mg/kg (max 1,000–1,200 mg).[7] A 5-day treatment course is FDA approved for azithromycin at 12 mg/kg/day for 5 days, and some PO cephalosporins have been approved (cefdinir, cefpodoxime), with rapid clinical response to treatment that can also be seen with other antibiotics; a 10-day course is preferred for prevention of ARF, particularly in areas where ARF is prevalent, as no data exist on efficacy of 5 days of therapy for prevention of ARF, although data support the treatment of pharyngitis with 5 days of therapy with cephalosporins and penicillin.[7,126,127]
Retropharyngeal; parapharyngeal; lateral pharyngeal cellulitis or abscess (mixed aerobic/anaerobic flora, now including CA-MRSA)[122,128,129]	Clindamycin 40 mg/kg/day IV div q8h or vancomycin 40 mg/kg/day IV div q8h AND ceftriaxone 50 mg/kg/day IV q24h	Consider I&D; possible airway compromise, mediastinitis. Alternatives: meropenem or imipenem (BIII); PIP/TAZO. Can step down to less broad-spectrum coverage based on cultures. Amox/clav for convalescent PO therapy (but no activity for MRSA) (BIII).
Tracheitis, bacterial (S aureus, including CA-MRSA; group A streptococcus; pneumococcus; H influenzae type b, rarely Pseudomonas)[130]	Clindamycin 40 mg/kg/day IV div q8h or vancomycin 40 mg/kg/day IV div q8h AND ceftriaxone 50 mg/kg/day q24h OR ceftaroline single-drug therapy: 2 mo–<2 y, 24 mg/kg/day IV div q8h; ≥2 y, 36 mg/kg/day IV div q8h (max single dose 400 mg); >33 kg, either 400 mg/dose IV q8h or 600 mg/dose IV q12h (BIII)	For susceptible S aureus, oxacillin/nafcillin or cefazolin May represent bacterial superinfection of viral laryngotracheobronchitis, including influenza

F. LOWER RESPIRATORY TRACT INFECTIONS

Clinical Diagnosis	Therapy (evidence grade)	Comments
Abscess, lung		
– Primary (a complication of severe, necrotizing CAP caused by pneumococcus; S aureus, particularly CA-MRSA; group A streptococcus, rarely Mycoplasma pneumoniae)[131,132]	Empiric therapy with ceftriaxone 50–75 mg/kg/day q24h AND clindamycin 40 mg/kg/day div q8h or vancomycin 45 mg/kg/day IV div q8h for ≥14–21 days (AIII) OR (for MRSA) ceftaroline single-drug therapy: 2–<6 mo, 30 mg/kg/day IV div q8h (each dose given over 2 h); ≥6 mo, 45 mg/kg/day IV div q8h (each dose given over 2 h) (max single dose 600 mg) (BII)	For severe CA-MRSA infections, see Chap 12. For presumed Mycoplasma, add FQ (levofloxacin) or macrolide. Bronchoscopy may be necessary if abscess fails to drain; surgical excision is rarely necessary for pneumococcus but may be important for CA-MRSA and MSSA. Focus antibiotic coverage based on culture results. For MSSA: oxacillin/nafcillin or cefazolin.
– Secondary to aspiration (ie, foul smelling; polymicrobial infection with oral aerobes and anaerobes)[133]	Clindamycin 40 mg/kg/day IV div q8h and ceftriaxone 50–75 mg/kg/day q24h or meropenem 60 mg/kg/day IV div q8h for ≥10 days (AIII)	Alternatives: ceftriaxone AND metronidazole OR amp/sul OR imipenem IV OR PIP/TAZO IV (BIII) PO step-down therapy with clindamycin or amox/clav (BIII)
Allergic bronchopulmonary aspergillosis[134]	Prednisone 0.5 mg/kg qd for 1–2 wk and then taper (BII) for mild, acute stage illness AND (for more severe disease) voriconazole[135] 18 mg/kg/day PO div q12h load followed by 16 mg/kg/day div q12h (AIII) OR itraconazole[36] 10 mg/kg/day PO div q12h (BIII). Voriconazole and itraconazole require trough concentration monitoring.	Not all allergic pulmonary disease is associated with true fungal infection. Larger steroid dosages to control inflammation may lead to tissue invasion by Aspergillus. Corticosteroids are the cornerstone of therapy for exacerbations, and itraconazole and voriconazole have a demonstrable corticosteroid-sparing effect.
Aspiration pneumonia (polymicrobial infection with oral aerobes and anaerobes)[133]	Clindamycin 40 mg/kg/day IV div q8h; ADD ceftriaxone 50–75 mg/kg/day q24h for additional Haemophilus activity OR, as a single agent, meropenem 60 mg/kg/day IV div q8h; for ≥10 days (BIII).	Alternatives: ceftriaxone AND metronidazole OR amp/sul IV OR imipenem IV OR PIP/TAZO IV (BIII) PO step-down therapy with clindamycin or amox/clav (BIII)

Atypical pneumonia (See *Mycoplasma pneumoniae* and Legionnaires disease later in this table under Pneumonias of other established etiologies.)

Bronchitis (bronchiolitis), acute[137]	For bronchitis/bronchiolitis in children, no antibiotic needed for most cases, as disease is usually viral	With PCR multiplex diagnosis now widely available, a nonbacterial diagnosis will allow clinicians to avoid use of antibiotics, but viral/bacterial coinfection can still occur.

Community-acquired pneumonia (See Pneumonia, community-acquired, later in this table.)

Cystic fibrosis: Seek advice from experts in acute and chronic management. Larger than standard doses of β-lactam antibiotics have been required in the past to achieve the same blood concentrations as those in children without CF, but in the current era of maximal pulmonary and nutritional support of CF, most antibiotics eliminated by the kidney can be administered at typical doses to achieve adequate blood concentrations. However, we do not know whether the concentrations of antibiotics achieved at the deep sites of infection in the CF lung are adequate, particularly with advanced CF disease. The Cystic Fibrosis Foundation posts guidelines for treatment of pulmonary exacerbation (www.cff.org/medical-professionals/pulmonary-exacerbations-clinical-care-guidelines; reviewed July 2021; accessed September 12, 2024). Dosages of β-lactams should be designed to achieve their PK/PD goals to increase the chance of response.[138,139]

– Acute pulmonary exacerbation (*P aeruginosa* primarily; also *Burkholderia cepacia*, *Stenotrophomonas maltophilia* [and other non-fermenting GNB]; *S aureus* [including CA-MRSA], nontuberculous mycobacteria)[140-145]	Cefepime 150–200 mg/kg/day div q8h or meropenem 120 mg/kg/day div q6h AND tobramycin 6–10 mg/kg/day IM, IV div q6–8h for treatment of acute exacerbation (AII); many alternatives: imipenem IV, ceftazidime IV, or ciprofloxacin 30 mg/kg/day PO, IV div tid For MRSA: ceftaroline 45 mg/kg/day IV div q8h (each dose given over 2 h) (max single dose 600 mg) (BIII) OR vancomycin 60–80 mg/kg/day IV div q8h Duration of therapy not well-defined: 10–14 days (BIII)[141]	Monitor concentrations of aminoglycosides, vancomycin. Insufficient evidence to recommend routine use of inhaled antibiotics for acute exacerbations.[146] Cultures with susceptibility will help select antibiotics, as MDR is common, but synergy testing is not well standardized.[147] Combination therapy may provide synergistic killing and delay the emergence of resistance (BIII). Attempt at early eradication of new-onset *Pseudomonas* may decrease progression of disease.[148] Failure to respond to antibacterials should prompt evaluation for appropriate drug doses and for invasive/allergic fungal disease as well as maximization of pulmonary hygiene.

F. LOWER RESPIRATORY TRACT INFECTIONS

Clinical Diagnosis	Therapy (evidence grade)	Comments
– Chronic inflammation in CF: impact of inhaled antibiotics and azithromycin to minimize long-term damage to lung	Inhaled tobramycin 300 mg bid, cycling 28 days on therapy, 28 days off therapy, is effective adjunctive therapy between exacerbations, with new data suggesting a benefit of alternating inhaled tobramycin with inhaled aztreonam (AI).[149,150] Azithromycin adjunctive chronic therapy, greatest benefit for those colonized with *Pseudomonas* (AII).[151,152]	Other inhaled antibiotics may also be effective[153] (BII). Two newer pwd preparations of inhaled tobramycin are available. Azithromycin does not decrease the benefit of improved pulmonary function with inhaled tobramycin in those with *Pseudomonas* airway colonization.[154]
Pertussis[155,156]	Azithromycin: for those ≥6 mo, 10 mg/kg/day on day 1, then 5 mg/kg/day for days 2–5; for those <6 mo, 10 mg/kg/day for 5 days (recommended dose per CDC); OR clarithromycin 15 mg/kg/day div bid for 7 days; or erythromycin (estolate preferable) 40 mg/kg/day PO div qid for 7–10 days (AII) Alternative: TMP/SMX 8 mg/kg/day of TMP div bid for 14 days (BIII)	Azithromycin and clarithromycin are better tolerated than erythromycin; azithromycin is preferred in young infants to potentially reduce pyloric stenosis risk (see Ch 2). Provide prophylaxis to family members. Unfortunately, no adjunctive therapy has been shown to be beneficial in decreasing the cough.[157]
Pneumonia, community-acquired: empiric therapy for bronchopneumonia, lobar consolidation, or complicated pneumonia with pleural fluid/empyema		
– Mild to moderate "chest cold"– like illness (overwhelmingly viral, especially in preschool children)[158]	No antibiotic therapy unless epidemiologic, clinical, or laboratory reasons to suspect bacterial coinfection, or *Mycoplasma*	Broad-spectrum antibiotics may increase risk of subsequent infection with antibiotic-resistant pathogens.

– Moderate to severe illness (pneumococcus; group A streptococcus; *S aureus*, including CA-MRSA; *M pneumoniae*[129,159,160]; for those with aspiration and underlying comorbidities, *H influenzae*, non-typeable; and for unimmunized children, *H influenzae* type b)

Empiric therapy

For most regions now with high rates of PCV13/20 vaccine use or low rates of pneumococcal resistance to penicillin (fully immunized child): ampicillin 150–200 mg/kg/day div q6h. For milder illness managed completely in the outpatient setting, amoxicillin can be used if *S aureus* is not a significant consideration. Standard-dosage amoxicillin (for pen-S pneumococci) can again be used for empiric therapy (45 mg/kg/day div tid).

For regions with low rates of PCV13/20 vaccine use (or for an unimmunized child), with high rates of pneumococcal resistance to penicillin: ceftriaxone 50–75 mg/kg/day q24h (AI). For PO therapy, high-dosage amoxicillin 80–100 mg/kg/day PO div tid is preferred. For suspected CA-MRSA: ceftaroline: 2–<6 mo, 30 mg/kg/day IV div q8h (each dose given over 2 h); ≥6 mo, 45 mg/kg/day IV div q8h (each dose given over 2 h) (max single dose 600 mg) (BII),[161] OR vancomycin 40–60 mg/kg/day (AIII).[3]

For suspected *Mycoplasma*/atypical pneumonia agents, particularly in school-aged children, ADD azithromycin 10 mg/kg IV, PO on day 1, then 5 mg/kg qd for days 2–5 of treatment (AII).

Consider next-generation sequencing diagnostic tests, tracheal aspirate, or BAL for Gram stain/culture for severe infection in intubated children.

For CA-MRSA: if vancomycin is being used rather than ceftaroline, check vancomycin serum concentrations and renal function, particularly at the higher dosage needed to achieve an AUC:MIC of 400.

Alternatives to azithromycin for atypical pneumonia include erythromycin IV, PO, or clarithromycin PO, or doxycycline IV, PO for children >7 y, or levofloxacin IV, PO.

Benefits of combination empiric therapy with a β-lactam and a macrolide are conflicting and may apply only to certain older pediatric populations.[161,162] Duration of therapy is still not well-defined in prospective, controlled trials in pediatric community-acquired *bacterial* pneumonia. Retrospective data with diagnosis based only on clinical examination and radiograph (eg, lots of viral pneumonia included) suggested that 10 days may be unnecessary for all children (5 days or just 3 days may be sufficient, but most short-course studies do not have a definitive pathogen diagnosis).[163,164] Empiric PO outpatient therapy for less severe illness: standard-dosage amoxicillin may be as effective as high-dosage amoxicillin 80–100 mg/kg/day PO div tid (NOT bid, which is used for otitis) (BII).

F. LOWER RESPIRATORY TRACT INFECTIONS

Clinical Diagnosis	Therapy (evidence grade)	Comments
– **Pleural fluid/empyema** (same pathogens as for community-associated bronchopneumonia) (Based on extent of fluid and symptoms, may benefit from chest tube drainage with fibrinolysis or video-assisted thoracoscopic surgery.)[159,165–169]	Empiric therapy: ceftaroline single-drug therapy: 2–<6 mo, 30 mg/kg/day IV div q8h; ≥6 mo, 45 mg/kg/day IV div q8h (each dose given over 2 h) (max single dose 600 mg) (BII), OR ceftriaxone 50–75 mg/kg/day q24h (BII) AND vancomycin 40–60 mg/kg/day IV div q8h (BIII) or clindamycin 40 mg/kg/day IV div q8h	Initial therapy based on Gram stain of empyema fluid; typically, clinical improvement is slow, with persisting but decreasing "spiking" fever for 2–3 wk. For antibiotic-pretreated children whose cultures are likely to be negative, consider next-generation sequencing tests from blood or BAL to allow the spectrum of antibiotics treatment to be narrowed when test results are available.[170] There are concerns about the effectiveness of vancomycin monotherapy in influenza-associated MRSA pneumonia.[171]
– **Interstitial pneumonia syndrome of early infancy**	If *C trachomatis* suspected, azithromycin 10 mg/kg on day 1, followed by 5 mg/kg/day qd for days 2–5 OR erythromycin 40 mg/kg/day PO qid for 14 days (BII)	Most often respiratory viral pathogens, CMV, or chlamydial; role of *Ureaplasma* uncertain
Pneumonia: definitive therapy for pathogens of CAP		
– **Pneumococcus** (may occur with non-PCV13 serotypes)[131,159–161]		No reported failures of ceftriaxone for pen-R pneumococcus; no need to add vancomycin for this reason (CIII). Levofloxacin is an alternative, particularly for those with severe allergy to β-lactam antibiotics (BII),[172] but due to theoretical cartilage toxicity concerns for humans, may not be first-line therapy.
– Pneumococcal, pen-S	Penicillin G 250,000–400,000 U/kg/day IV div q4–6h for 10 days (BII) OR ampicillin 150–200 mg/kg/day IV div q6h; for outpatient management: amoxicillin 45 mg/kg/day PO div tid	After improvement (decreased fever, no oxygen needed), change to amoxicillin 45 mg/kg/day PO tid OR penicillin V 50–75 mg/kg/day div qid. Treat until patient is clinically asymptomatic and chest radiograph has significantly improved (7–21 days) (BIII).

– Pneumococcal, pen-R	Ceftriaxone 100 mg/kg/day q24h or div q12h for 10–14 days (BIII)	Addition of vancomycin has not been required for treatment of pen-R strains. Ceftaroline is more active against pneumococcus than ceftriaxone, but with no current ceftriaxone resistance, ceftaroline is not required. For PO convalescent therapy, high-dosage amoxicillin (100–150 mg/kg/day PO div tid), OR clindamycin (30 mg/kg/day PO div tid), OR linezolid (30 mg/kg/day PO div tid), OR levofloxacin PO.
– Staphylococcus aureus (including CA-MRSA) is a rare (1%) cause of pediatric CAP.[4,6,131,159,173,174]	For MSSA: oxacillin/nafcillin 150 mg/kg/day IV div q6h or cefazolin 100 mg/kg/day IV div q8h (AII) For suspected CA-MRSA: ceftaroline: 2–<6 mo, 30 mg/kg/day IV div q8h (each dose given over 2 h); ≥6 mo, 45 mg/kg/day IV div q8h (each dose given over 2 h) (max single dose 600 mg) (AII), OR vancomycin 40–60 mg/kg/day (AIII)[3]; may need addition of rifampin, clindamycin, or gentamicin, but no prospective data to validate improved outcomes (AIII) (See Ch 12.)	Check vancomycin serum concentrations and renal function, particularly at the higher dosage designed to attain an AUC:MIC of 400 for invasive CA-MRSA disease. For life-threatening disease, optimal therapy for CA-MRSA has not been studied and remains poorly defined: consider adding gentamicin and/or rifampin for combination therapy (CIII). Linezolid 30 mg/kg/day IV, PO div q8h is another option, more effective in adults than vancomycin for MRSA nosocomial pneumonia[175] (follow platelet and WBC counts weekly). For influenza-associated MRSA pneumonia, vancomycin monotherapy was inferior to combination therapies.[168] Do NOT use daptomycin for pneumonia (inactivated by surfactant). PO convalescent therapy for MSSA: cephalexin PO; for CA-MRSA: clindamycin or linezolid PO. Total course for ≥21 days (AIII).

F. LOWER RESPIRATORY TRACT INFECTIONS

Clinical Diagnosis	Therapy (evidence grade)	Comments
- **Group A streptococcus**	Penicillin G 250,000 U/kg/day IV div q4–6h for 10 days (BII)	Change to amoxicillin 75 mg/kg/day PO div tid or penicillin V 50–75 mg/kg/day div qid to tid after clinical improvement (BIII).

Pneumonia: immunosuppressed, neutropenic host

Clinical Diagnosis	Therapy (evidence grade)	Comments
- **Immunosuppressed, neutropenic host**[176] (*P aeruginosa*, other community-associated or nosocomial GNB, *S aureus*, fungi, AFB, *Pneumocystis*, viral [adenovirus, CMV, EBV, influenza, RSV, others]) For treatment recommendations for fungal pathogens, see Ch 5; for viral pathogens, see Ch 7. In posttransplant patients ≥12 y with CMV disease that is refractory to treatment with ganciclovir, valganciclovir, or foscarnet, maribavir may be considered.	Antibiotic therapy: cefepime 150 mg/kg/day IV div q8h (AII), OR meropenem 60 mg/kg/day div q8h (AII), OR PIP/TAZO 240–300 mg/kg/day div q6h; AND if *S aureus* (including MRSA) is suspected clinically, ADD vancomycin 40–60 mg/kg/day IV div q8h (AIII) OR ceftaroline: 2–<6 mo, 30 mg/kg/day IV div q8h; ≥6 mo, 45 mg/kg/day IV div q8h (max single dose 600 mg) (BIII). Antifungal therapy usually started if no response to antibiotics within 72–96 h (AmB, voriconazole, or caspofungin/micafungin—see Ch 5).	Biopsy/BAL for histology/cultures or serum/BAL for next-generation sequencing testing helps determine need for antifungal, antiviral, and/or antimycobacterial treatment. For septic patients, the addition of tobramycin will increase coverage for most gram-negative pathogens. For those with mucositis, anaerobic coverage may be needed, as provided by carbapenems and PIP/TAZO (or with the addition of clindamycin or metronidazole to other agents). Consider use of 2 active agents for definitive therapy for *Pseudomonas* for neutropenic hosts to assist clearing the pathogen and potentially decrease risk of resistance, but there is no evidence to support better outcomes (BIII).

Pneumonia: nosocomial (health care–associated/ventilator-associated)

– **Nosocomial (health care–associated/ventilator-associated)** (*P aeruginosa*, enteric GNB [*Enterobacter*, *Klebsiella*, *Serratia*, *Escherichia coli*], *Acinetobacter*, *Stenotrophomonas*, and gram-positive organisms including CA-MRSA and *Enterococcus*)[177,178]	Commonly used regimens, but they should be individualized based on the "flora" of the hospital that may colonize (and subsequently infect hospitalized children). Meropenem 60 mg/kg/day div q8h, OR PIP/TAZO 240–300 mg/kg/day div q6–8h, OR cefepime 150 mg/kg/day div q8h; ± gentamicin 6.0–7.5 mg/kg/day div q8h (AIII); ADD vancomycin or ceftaroline for suspected CA-MRSA (AIII).	Pathogens that cause nosocomial pneumonia often have MDR. Cultures are critical. Empiric therapy also based on child's prior colonization/infection. Do not treat colonization, though. For MDR GNB, available IV therapy options include CAZ/AVI (now FDA approved for children), TOL/TAZ, mero/vabor, cefiderocol, plazomicin, or colistin. Aerosol delivery of antibiotics may be required for MDR pathogens, but little high-quality controlled data are available for children.[179]

Pneumonias of other established etiologies (See Ch 3 for treatment by pathogen.)

– *Chlamydophila pneumoniae*,[180] *Chlamydophila psittaci*, or *Chlamydia trachomatis*	Azithromycin 10 mg/kg on day 1, followed by 5 mg/kg/day qd for days 2–5 or erythromycin 40 mg/kg/day PO qid; for 14 days	Doxycycline (patients >7 y). Levofloxacin is also effective.
– Cytomegalovirus (immunocompromised host)[181,182] (See Chs 2 and 7 for CMV infection in newborns and children, respectively.)	See Ch 7. Ganciclovir IV 10 mg/kg/day div q12h for 2 wk (BIII); if needed, continue at 5 mg/kg/day q24h to complete 4–6 wk total (BIII).	Bone marrow transplant recipients with CMV pneumonia whose ganciclovir therapy alone fails may benefit from therapy with IV CMV hyperimmune globulin and ganciclovir given together (BII).[183,184] PO valganciclovir may be used for convalescent therapy (BII). Foscarnet for ganciclovir-resistant isolates. In posttransplant patients ≥12 y with CMV disease that is refractory to treatment with ganciclovir, valganciclovir, or foscarnet, maribavir may be considered.

1

F. LOWER RESPIRATORY TRACT INFECTIONS

Clinical Diagnosis	Therapy (evidence grade)	Comments
– *Enterobacter* spp	Cefepime 100 mg/kg/day div q12h or meropenem 60 mg/kg/day div q8h; OR ceftriaxone 50–75 mg/kg/day q24h AND gentamicin 6.0–7.5 mg/kg/day IM, IV div q8h (AIII)	Addition of aminoglycoside to 3rd-generation cephalosporins (ceftriaxone, ceftazidime) may restrict the emergence of ampC-mediated constitutive high-level resistance, but concern exists for inadequate aminoglycoside concentration in airways; not an issue for ampC-stable β-lactams (cefepime, meropenem, imipenem, or PIP/TAZO).
– *Escherichia coli*	Ceftriaxone 50–75 mg/kg/day q24h (AII)	For cephalosporin-R strains (ESBL producers), use meropenem, imipenem, or ertapenem (AIII). Use ampicillin if susceptible.
– *Francisella tularensis*[185]	Gentamicin 6.0–7.5 mg/kg/day IM, IV div q8h for ≥10 days for more severe disease (AIII); for less severe disease, ciprofloxacin or levofloxacin (AIII)	Other alternative for PO therapy for mild disease: doxycycline PO for 14–21 days (but watch for relapse). See www.cdc.gov/tularemia/about/index.html (accessed September 12, 2024).
– Fungi (See Ch 5.) Community-associated pathogens, which vary by region (eg, *Coccidioides*,[186,187] *Histoplasma*)[188,189] *Aspergillus*; mucormycosis; other mold infections in immunocompromised hosts (See Ch 5.)	For detailed pathogen-specific recommendations, see Ch 5. For suspected endemic fungi or mucormycosis in an *immunocompromised* host,[190] treat empirically with a lipid AmB and not voriconazole; biopsy needed to guide therapy. Posaconazole and isavuconazole[191] have in vitro activity and clinical efficacy data against some *Rhizopus* spp. For suspected invasive aspergillosis, treat with voriconazole (AI) (load 18 mg/kg/day div q12h on day 1, then continue 16 mg/kg/day div q12h).	For immunocompetent hosts, triazoles (fluconazole, itraconazole, voriconazole, posaconazole, and isavuconazole) are better tolerated than AmB and equally effective for many community-associated pathogens (see Ch 6). For dosage, see Ch 5. Check voriconazole trough concentrations; need to be at least >2 mcg/mL. For *Coccidioides* infection refractory to fluconazole therapy, consider increasing the dose, switching to other azoles, or switching to AmB.

– Influenza virus.[192,193] – Recent seasonal influenza A and B strains continue to be resistant to adamantanes.	Empiric therapy, or documented influenza A or B Oseltamivir[193,194] (AII): <12 mo: Full-term infants: 0–8 mo: 3 mg/kg/dose bid 9–11 mo: 3.5 mg/kg/dose bid, although some experts recommend 3 mg/kg/dose bid ≥12 mo: ≤15 kg: 30 mg PO bid >15–23 kg: 45 mg PO bid >23–40 kg: 60 mg PO bid >40 kg: 75 mg PO bid Zanamivir inhaled (AII): for those ≥7 y, 10 mg (two 5-mg inhalations) bid Peramivir (BII): 6 mo–12 y: single IV dose of 12 mg/kg, up to 600 mg max >13 y: single IV dose of 600 mg Baloxavir (BII): ≥5 y: <20 kg: single dose PO of 2 mg/kg 20–79 kg: single dose PO of 40 mg ≥80 kg: single dose PO of 80 mg	New published data continue to confirm the effectiveness of oseltamivir, particularly when started early in the clinical course. Check for antiviral susceptibility each season at www.cdc.gov/flu/hcp/antivirals/index.html (accessed November 6, 2024). For children 12–23 mo, the unit dose of oseltamivir of 30 mg/dose may provide inadequate drug exposure. 3.5 mg/kg/dose PO bid has been studied for PK,[195] but sample sizes were limited. Limited data for oseltamivir in preterm neonates[194]: <38 wk of PMA (gestational plus chronologic age): 1.0 mg/kg/dose PO bid 38–40 wk of PMA: 1.5 mg/kg/dose PO bid The adamantanes (amantadine and rimantadine) had activity against influenza A before the late 1990s, but all circulating A strains of influenza have been resistant for many years. Influenza B is intrinsically resistant to adamantanes. The CDC does not recommend baloxavir for monotherapy for severely immunosuppressed people.
– Klebsiella pneumoniae[195,196]	Ceftriaxone 50–75 mg/kg/day IV, IM q24h (AIII); for ceftriaxone-resistant strains (ESBL and ampC-producing strains), use meropenem 60 mg/kg/day IV div q8h (AIII) or other carbapenem.	For K pneumoniae strains that contain ESBLs or are producing ampC BL, other carbapenems, PIP/TAZO, and FQs are other options. Data in adults suggest that outcomes with PIP/TAZO are inferior to those with carbapenems.[195,196] For KPC-producing strains that are resistant to meropenem, alternatives include CAZ/AVI (FDA approved for adults and children), FQs, and colistin (BIII). See Ch 12.

F. LOWER RESPIRATORY TRACT INFECTIONS

Clinical Diagnosis	Therapy (evidence grade)	Comments
- Legionnaires disease (*Legionella pneumophila*)	Azithromycin 10 mg/kg PO q24h for 5–10 days (AIII)	Alternatives: clarithromycin, erythromycin, ciprofloxacin, levofloxacin, doxycycline Longer durations for non-azithromycin regimens and immunocompromised patients
- Mycobacteria, nontuberculous (MAC most common)[197]	In a normal host with pneumonia that requires therapy, 3 drugs are now recommended: azithromycin PO (or clarithromycin PO) AND ethambutol, AND rifampin, given 3×/wk to prevent macrolide/azalide resistance. Duration of treatment is not well-defined; consider 6–12 wk for susceptible strains but longer, up to 12 mo, for resistant strains. For more extensive cavitary or advanced/severe bronchiectatic disease, ADD amikacin or streptomycin (AIII).	Highly variable susceptibilities of different nontuberculous mycobacterial spp. Culture and susceptibility data are important for success. Check if immunocompromised: HIV or IFN-γ receptor deficiency. Consider consulting an ID physician.
- *Mycobacterium tuberculosis* (See Tuberculosis later in this table.)		
- *Mycoplasma pneumoniae*[159,198]	Azithromycin 10 mg/kg on day 1, followed by 5 mg/kg/day qd for days 2–5, OR clarithromycin 15 mg/kg/day div bid for 7–14 days, OR erythromycin 40 mg/kg/day PO div qid for 14 days	*Mycoplasma* often causes self-limited infection and does not routinely require treatment (AIII). Little prospective, well-controlled data exist for treatment of documented mycoplasma pneumonia, specifically in children.[198] Doxycycline (patients >7 y) or levofloxacin. Macrolide-resistant strains have recently developed worldwide but may respond to doxycycline or levofloxacin.[199] Studies have been difficult without better diagnostic techniques, but respiratory tract PCR testing is now available to assist in early identification of possible infections.

– *Paragonimus westermani*	See Ch 9.
– *Pneumocystis jirovecii*, formerly *carinii*[200], disease in children with immunosuppression or HIV	Severe disease: preferred regimen is TMP/SMX, 15–20 mg/kg/day of TMP IV div q8h for 3 wk (AI). Mild to moderate disease: may start with IV therapy, then, after acute pneumonitis is resolving, TMP/SMX 20 mg/kg/day of TMP PO div qid for 21 days (AII). Use steroid adjunctive treatment for more severe disease (AII).	Alternatives for TMP/SMX intolerant, or clinical failure: pentamidine 3–4 mg IV qd, infused over 60–90 min (AII); TMP AND dapsone; OR primaquine AND clindamycin; OR atovaquone. Prophylaxis: TMP/SMX 5 mg/kg/day of TMP PO, div in 2 doses, q12h, daily or 3×/wk on consecutive days (AI); OR TMP/SMX 5 mg/kg/day of TMP PO as a single dose, qd, 3×/wk on consecutive days (AII); once-weekly regimens have also been successful[201]; OR dapsone 2 mg/kg (max 100 mg) PO qd, or 4 mg/kg (max 200 mg) once weekly; OR atovaquone: 30 mg/kg/day for infants 1–3 mo, 45 mg/kg/day for infants 4–24 mo, and 30 mg/kg/day for children >24 mo.
– *Pseudomonas aeruginosa*[202,203]	Cefepime 150 mg/kg/day IV div q8h ± tobramycin 6.0–7.5 mg/kg/day IM, IV div q8h (AII). Alternatives: meropenem 60 mg/kg/day div q8h, OR PIP/TAZO 240–300 mg/kg/day div q6–8h (AII) ± tobramycin (BIII).	Ciprofloxacin IV, or colistin IV for MDR strains of *Pseudomonas*[203] (See Ch 12.)
– Respiratory syncytial virus infection (bronchiolitis, pneumonia)[204]	For immunocompromised hosts, the only FDA-approved treatment is ribavirin aerosol: 6-g vial (20 mg/mL in sterile water), by SPAG-2, over 18–20 h daily for 3–5 days, although questions remain regarding efficacy.	Treat only for severe disease, immunocompromised, severe underlying cardiopulmonary disease, as aerosol ribavirin provides only a small benefit. Airway reactivity with inhalation precludes routine use. We have not personally used inhaled ribavirin for the past several years. Palivizumab and nirsevimab (Beyfortus) are not effective for treatment of an active RSV infection. RSV antivirals and additional monoclonal antibodies are currently under investigation. Monitor for neutropenia and nephrotoxicity.

F. LOWER RESPIRATORY TRACT INFECTIONS

Clinical Diagnosis	Therapy (evidence grade)	Comments
Tuberculosis		
– Primary pulmonary disease[15,16,205,206]	INH 10–15 mg/kg/day (max 300 mg) PO qd for 6 mo AND rifampin 15–20 mg/kg/day (max 600 mg) PO qd for 6 mo AND PZA 30–40 mg/kg/day (max 2 g) PO qd for first 2 mo of therapy only (AII). Twice-weekly treatment, particularly with DOT, is acceptable.[15] If risk factors present for MDR, ADD ethambutol 20 mg/kg/day PO qd OR streptomycin 30 mg/kg/day IV, IM div q12h initially.	Obtain baseline LFTs. Consider monthly LFTs for at least 3 mo or as needed for symptoms. It is common to have mildly elevated liver transaminase concentrations (2–3 times normal) that do not further increase during the entire treatment interval. Children with obesity may have mild elevation when therapy is started. New recommendations on short-course (4-mo) daily therapy for children with non-severe TB come from the WHO guidelines, March 2022 (www.who.int/publications/i/item/9789240046764; accessed September 12, 2024). Contact TB specialist for therapy for drug-resistant TB.[205] FQs may play a role in treating MDR strains. Bedaquiline, in a new drug class for TB therapy, is approved for adults and children >5 y with MDR TB when used in combination therapy. Delamanid is not approved by the FDA as of September 2024 but is approved in the European Union and many countries in Asia for MDR TB. DOT preferred; after 2 wk of daily therapy, can change to twice-weekly dosing double dosage of INH (max 900 mg). PZA (max 2 g), and ethambutol (max 2.5 g); rifampin remains same dosage (15–20 mg/kg/day, max 600 mg) (AII). LP ± CT of head for children ≤2 y to rule out occult, concurrent CNS infection; consider testing for HIV infection (AIII). *M bovis* infection from unpasteurized dairy products is also called "tuberculosis"; all strains of *M bovis* are PZA resistant. Treat 9–12 mo with INH and rifampin.

– Latent TB infection[15,16,206,207] (skin test conversion; more recently just called "TB disease"[15] in contrast to "TB disease" for symptomatic TB infection)	Many options now
	
	INH/rifapentine:
	Rifampin alone (all ages): 15–20 mg/kg/dose *daily* (max 600 mg) for *4 mo*
	For children 2–11 y: *once-weekly DOT for 12 wk*:
	INH 25 mg/kg/dose (max 900 mg), AND rifapentine:
	  10.0–14.0 kg: 300 mg
	  14.1–25.0 kg: 450 mg
	  25.1–32.0 kg: 600 mg
	  32.1–49.9 kg: 750 mg
	  ≥50.0 kg: 900 mg (max)
	For children 2–11 y: INH 25 mg/kg, rounded up to nearest 50 or 100 mg (max 900 mg). AND rifapentine (See above.)
	INH/rifampin (all ages): INH 10–15 mg/kg/day (max 300 mg)/rifampin 15–20 mg/kg/day (max 600 mg) *daily for 3 mo*
	INH 10–15 mg/kg/day (max 300 mg) PO daily for *6–9 mo (12 mo for immunocompromised patients)* (AIII); treatment with INH at 20–30 mg/kg twice weekly for *9 mo* also effective (AIII)
		Consider LFTs as needed for symptoms. Stop INH/rifapentine if AST or ALT ≥5 times the ULN even in the absence of symptoms or ≥3 times the ULN in the presence of symptoms.
		For children <2 y: INH and rifapentine may be used, but there are less data on safety and efficacy.
		For exposure to known INH-resistant but rifampin-susceptible strains, use rifampin 6 mo (AIII).

– Exposed child <5 y, or immunocompromised patient (at high risk for dissemination)	Prophylaxis for possible infection for 2–3 mo after last exposure, with rifampin 15–20 mg/kg/dose PO qd OR INH 10–15 mg/kg PO qd; for at least 2–3 mo (AIII), with repeat skin test or IGRA test (AIII). Also called "window prophylaxis."	Alternative regimens: INH 10–15 mg/kg PO qd AND rifampin 15–20 mg/kg/dose qd (max 600 mg) for up to 3 mo. If PPD or IGRA test remains negative at 8–10 wk and child appears well, consider stopping empiric therapy. PPD may not be reliable in immunocompromised patients. Not much data to assess reliability of IGRA assays in very young infants or immunocompromised hosts, but not likely to be much better or worse than the PPD skin test.

G. CARDIOVASCULAR INFECTIONS

Clinical Diagnosis	Therapy (evidence grade)	Comments
Bacteremia		
– Occult bacteremia/serious bacterial infection (late-onset neonatal sepsis; fever with focus), infants <1–2 mo (GBS, E coli, Listeria, pneumococcus, meningococcus)[208-213]	In general, hospitalization for late-onset neonatal sepsis in the ill-appearing infant, with cultures of blood, urine, and CSF; start ampicillin for GBS and Listeria at 200 mg/kg/day IV div q6h AND cefepime or ceftazidime for E coli/enteric bacilli; use ceftriaxone for those after the first few weeks following birth (cefotaxime no longer routinely available in the United States); higher dosages if meningitis is documented. In areas with low (<20%) ampicillin resistance in E coli, consider ampicillin and gentamicin (gentamicin will not cover CNS infection following bacteremia caused by ampicillin-resistant E coli when treated with ampicillin and gentamicin).	Current data document the importance of ampicillin-resistant E coli in bacteremia and UTI in infants <90 days.[211-213] For a nontoxic, febrile infant with good access to medical care: blood and urine cultures may be obtained, and we are getting much closer to eliminating LPs in low-risk infants.[208] Risk scores (previously healthy), no skin or soft tissue infection, clinical status, and laboratory tests (urinalysis, WBC count, and, possibly, procalcitonin). Infants may be discharged home without antibiotics and close follow-up if evaluation is negative (Rochester; modified Philadelphia criteria)[209-213] (BII). Standardizing evaluation of these infants by collaborating clinicians can create a local standard of care, as no test or examination has 100% accuracy for these babies.
– Occult bacteremia/serious bacterial infection (fever without focus) in infants from 2–3 to 36 mo of age (H influenzae type b/ pneumococcus in unimmunized patients; meningococcus; pneu-mococcus [non-vaccine strains]; increasingly S aureus)[212]	Empiric therapy: if unimmunized, febrile, mild to moderate toxic: after blood culture: ceftriaxone 50 mg/kg IM (BII). For the fully immunized (H influenzae type b and pneumococcus) and nontoxic infant, routine empiric outpatient therapy for fever with antibiotics is not recommended, but follow closely in case of non-vaccine strain pneumococcal infection, vaccine failure, or meningococcal bacteremia (BIII).[210,212,213]	Conjugated vaccines for H influenzae type b and pneumococcus have virtually eliminated occult bacteremia of infancy by these pathogens. For occult bacteremia, PO convalescent therapy is selected by susceptibility of blood isolate, following response to IM/IV treatment, with CNS and other foci ruled out by examination ± laboratory tests ± imaging. LP is not recommended for routine evaluation of fever but is recommended for bacteremia in younger infants.[208]

– *Haemophilus influenzae* type b, non-CNS infections	Ceftriaxone IM/IV OR, if BL negative, ampicillin IV, followed by PO convalescent therapy (AII)	If BL negative: amoxicillin 75–100 mg/kg/day PO div tid (AII). If positive, consider these options (but there are no data on treatment of bacteremic infection): high-dosage cefixime, ceftibuten, cefdinir PO, or levofloxacin PO (CIII).
– Meningococcus	Ceftriaxone IM/IV or penicillin G IV (if susceptible)	PO convalescent therapy can be considered for occult bacteremia or mild infection (AII).
– Pneumococcus, non-CNS infections	Ceftriaxone IM/IV or penicillin G/ampicillin IV (if pen-S), followed by PO convalescent therapy (AII)	If pen-S or penicillin-intermediate (MIC is ≤2 or lower): amoxicillin 75–100 mg/kg/day PO div tid (AII). If pen-R (MIC is ≥4): continue ceftriaxone IM or switch to clindamycin if susceptible (CIII); linezolid and levofloxacin may also be options (CIII).
– *Staphylococcus aureus*[4,6,214–217] usually associated with focal infection	MSSA: nafcillin or oxacillin/nafcillin IV 150–200 mg/kg/day div q6h ± gentamicin 6 mg/kg/day div q8h (AII). MRSA: ceftaroline: 2 mo–<2 y, 24 mg/kg/day IV div q8h; ≥2 y, 36 mg/kg/day IV div q8h (max single dose 400 mg) (BIII) OR vancomycin[215] 40–60 mg/kg/day (CII) IV div q8h OR daptomycin IV[218] 8–12 mg/kg/day q24h (BII). Treat for 2 wk (IV + PO) from negative blood cultures unless endocarditis/endovascular thrombus is present, which may require up to 6 wk of therapy (BII).	Usually not necessary to add gentamicin or rifampin,[216] although for disseminated MRSA infection, combination therapy is often used but without supporting controlled data (AII). For persisting bacteremia caused by MRSA, consider adding gentamicin or rifampin, or changing from vancomycin (particularly for MRSA with vancomycin MIC of >2 mcg/mL) to daptomycin or ceftaroline (daptomycin will not treat pneumonia). For toxic shock syndrome, clindamycin should be added for the initial 48–72 h of therapy to decrease toxin production (linezolid may also act this way); IVIG may be added to bind circulating toxin; no controlled data exist for these measures. Watch for the development of metastatic foci of infection, including endocarditis. If catheter-related, remove catheter.

G. CARDIOVASCULAR INFECTIONS

Clinical Diagnosis	Therapy (evidence grade)	Comments

Endocarditis: Prospective, controlled data on therapy for endocarditis in neonates, infants, and children are limited, and many recommendations are extrapolated from adult studies, in which some level of evidence exists, or from other invasive bacteremia infection studies. Surgical indications: intractable heart failure; persistent infection; large mobile vegetations; peripheral embolism; and valve dehiscence, perforation, rupture, or fistula, or a large perivalvular abscess.[219-223] Consider community vs nosocomial pathogens based on recent surgeries, prior antibiotic therapy, and possible entry sites for bacteremia (skin, oropharynx and respiratory tract, GI tract). Children with congenital heart disease and those with prosthetic valves/materials are more likely to have more turbulent cardiovascular blood flow, which increases risk for endovascular infection. Catheter-placed bovine jugular valves also seem to increase risk of infection.[222,223] Similar guidelines have been published for both the United States and the European Union.[220,221] Immunocompromised hosts may become bacteremic with a wide range of bacteria, fungi, and mycobacteria.

Clinical Diagnosis	Therapy (evidence grade)	Comments
– **Native valve**[219-221]		
– Empiric therapy for presumed endocarditis (viridans streptococci, *S aureus*, HACEK group)	Ceftriaxone IV 100 mg/kg q24h OR amp/sul 300 mg/kg/day div q4–6h AND gentamicin IV, IM 6 mg/kg/day div q8h (AII). For more acute, severe infection, ADD vancomycin 40–60 mg/kg/day IV div q8h to cover *S aureus* (AIII) (insufficient data to recommend ceftaroline for endocarditis).	Combination (β-lactam + gentamicin) provides bactericidal activity against most strains of viridans streptococci, the most common pathogens in infective endocarditis. Cefepime is recommended for adults,[219] but resistance data in enteric bacilli in children suggest that ceftriaxone remains a reasonable choice. Amp/sul adds extended anaerobic activity and BL stability that is not likely to be needed. May administer gentamicin with a qd regimen (CIII). For β-lactam allergy, use vancomycin 45 mg/kg/day IV div q8h AND gentamicin 6 mg/kg/day IV div q8h.
– Culture-negative native valve endocarditis: treat 4–6 wk (obtain advice from an ID specialist for an appropriate regimen that is based on likely pathogens).[219,220]		
– Viridans streptococci: follow echocardiogram for evidence of worsening vegetation; β-lactam allergy: vancomycin.		

Fully susceptible to penicillin	Ceftriaxone 50 mg/kg IV, IM q24h for 4 wk OR penicillin G 200,000 U/kg/day IV div q4–6h for 4 wk (BII); OR penicillin G or ceftriaxone	The AHA recommends higher dosage of ceftriaxone similar to that of penicillin non-susceptible strains, but for fully susceptible strains, standard-dose ceftriaxone provides the necessary PD exposure.
Relatively resistant to penicillin	Penicillin G 300,000 U/kg/day IV div q4–6h for 4 wk, or ceftriaxone 100 mg/kg IV q24h for 4 wk; AND gentamicin 6 mg/kg/day IM, IV div q8h for the first 2 wk (AIII)	Gentamicin is used for the first 2 wk for a total of 4 wk of therapy for relatively resistant strains. Vancomycin-containing regimens should use at least a 4-wk treatment course, with gentamicin used for the entire course.
– Enterococcus (dosages for native or prosthetic valve infections)		
Ampicillin-susceptible (gentamicin-S)	Ampicillin 300 mg/kg/day IV, IM div q6h or penicillin G 300,000 U/kg/day IV div q4–6h; AND gentamicin 6 mg/kg/day IV div q8h; for 4–6 wk (AII)	Combined treatment with cell wall active antibiotic plus aminoglycoside used to achieve bactericidal activity. Children are not as likely to develop renal toxicity from gentamicin as adults. For β-lactam allergy: vancomycin.
Ampicillin-resistant (gentamicin-S)	Vancomycin 40 mg/kg/day IV div q8h AND gentamicin 6 mg/kg/day IV div q8h; for 6 wk (AIII)	Little data exist in children for daptomycin, ceftaroline, or linezolid.
Vancomycin-resistant (gentamicin-S)	Daptomycin IV if also ampicillin resistant (dose is age dependent; see Ch 18 for doses) ± gentamicin 6 mg/kg/day IV div q8h; for 4–6 wk (AIII)	For gentamicin-resistant strains, use streptomycin or other aminoglycoside if susceptible. If ampicillin-susceptible gentamicin-resistant, can combine ampicillin and ceftriaxone.

G. CARDIOVASCULAR INFECTIONS

Clinical Diagnosis	Therapy (evidence grade)	Comments
- Staphylococci: S aureus, including CA-MRSA; Staphylococcus epidermidis[6,215] Consider continuing therapy at end of 6 wk if vegetations increase on echocardiogram or there is a concern for abscess. Consider septic thrombophlebitis: the risk of persisting organisms is not defined in deep venous thromboses that may be "seed-ed" as a result of bacteremia.	MSSA or MSSE: nafcillin or oxacillin/nafcillin 150–200 mg/kg/day IV div q6h for 4–6 wk AND gentamicin 6 mg/kg/day div q8h for first 14 days. CA-MRSA or MRSE: daptomycin IV[218] 8–12 mg/kg/day q24h (BII), OR vancomycin 40–60 mg/kg/day IV div q8h AND gentamicin for 6 wk; consider for slow response, ADD rifampin 20 mg/kg/day IV div q8–12h. Insufficient data to recommend ceftaroline for MRSA endocarditis.	Surgery may be necessary in acute phase; conflicting data on efficacy of 1st-generation cephalosporins, although more recent data suggest equivalence to penicillins. The AHA suggests gentamicin for only the first 3–5 days for MSSA or MSSE and optional gentamicin for MRSA. Daptomycin dose is age dependent (see Ch 18 for doses).
- Pneumococcus, gonococcus, group A streptococcus	Penicillin G 200,000 U/kg/day IV div q4–6h for 4 wk (BII); alternatives: ceftriaxone or vancomycin	For gonococcal endocarditis: ceftriaxone alone, 1–2 g IV q24h for >4 wk.[59] For penicillin non-susceptible strains of pneumococcus, consult with ID specialist but should be able to use high-dosage penicillin G 300,000 U/kg/day IV div q4–6h or high-dosage ceftriaxone 100 mg/kg IV q12h or q24h for 4 wk, if supported by PD (eg, the time that penicillin or ceftriaxone is above the MIC of the organism, during the dosing interval).
- HACEK (Haemophilus, Aggregatibacter [formerly Actinobacillus], Cardiobacterium, Eikenella, Kingella spp)	Usually susceptible to ceftriaxone 100 mg/kg IV q24h for 4 wk (BII)	Some organisms will be ampicillin susceptible. Usually do not require the addition of gentamicin.

– Enteric GNB	Antibiotics specific to pathogen (usually ceftriaxone plus initial treatment with gentamicin until clinical/microbiologic improvement); duration at least 6 wk (AIII)	For ESBL organisms, carbapenems or β-lactam/BLI combinations, PLUS gentamicin initially, should be effective. See Ch 12. No controlled data on the benefit of gentamicin in combination.
– *Pseudomonas aeruginosa*	Antibiotic specific to susceptibility: cefepime or meropenem PLUS tobramycin	Both cefepime and meropenem are more active against *Pseudomonas* and less likely to allow BL-resistant pathogens to emerge than ceftazidime.
– **Prosthetic valve/material**[219,222,223]	Follow echocardiogram for resolution of vegetation. For β-lactam allergy: vancomycin.	
– Viridans streptococci		
Fully susceptible to penicillin	Ceftriaxone 100 mg/kg IV, IM q24h for 6 wk OR penicillin G 300,000 U/kg/day IV div q4–6h for 6 wk (AII); OR penicillin G or ceftriaxone AND gentamicin 6 mg/kg/day IM, IV div q8h for first 2 wk of 6-wk course (AII)	
Relatively resistant to penicillin	Penicillin G 300,000 U/kg/day IV div q4–6h for 6 wk, or ceftriaxone 100 mg/kg IV q24h for 6 wk; AND gentamicin 6 mg/kg/day IM, IV div q8h for 6 wk (AIII)	Obtain the MIC of the strep spp to the antibiotic used for treatment; based on expected or measured serum antibiotic concentrations, assess PD (ability to achieve the desired time that penicillin [or ceftriaxone] is above the MIC of the organism, during the dosing supported by the interval). See Ch 11. Gentamicin is used for all 6 wk of therapy for prosthetic valve/material endocarditis caused by relatively resistant strains.

– Enterococcus (See dosages earlier in this table under Native Valve.) Treatment course is at least 6 wk, particularly if vancomycin is used.[215,219]

G. CARDIOVASCULAR INFECTIONS

Clinical Diagnosis	Therapy (evidence grade)	Comments
– Staphylococci: *S aureus*, including CA-MRSA; *S epidermidis*[6,219] Consider continuing therapy at end of 6 wk if vegetations persist or increase on echocardiogram.	MSSA or MSSE: nafcillin or oxacillin/nafcillin 150–200 mg/kg/day IV div q6h for ≥6 wk AND gentamicin 6 mg/kg/day div q8h for first 14 days. CA-MRSA or MRSE: daptomycin IV[218] 8–12 mg/kg/day q24h (BII), OR vancomycin 40–60 mg/kg/day IV div q8h AND gentamicin for ≥6 wk; ADD rifampin 20 mg/kg/day IV q8–12h.	Daptomycin dose is age and weight dependent (see Ch 18 for doses). Valve replacement for prosthetic valve endocarditis caused by *S aureus* is preferable in most patients, if not all.
– *Candida*[85,219,220]	AmB lipid formulation, 3–5 mg/kg q24h with/ without flucytosine 100 mg/kg/day div q6h (there is more experience with AmB preparations [no comparative trials against echinocandins]), OR micafungin 2–4 mg/kg/day (BIII). Do not use fluconazole as initial therapy because of inferior fungistatic effect.	Poor prognosis; obtain advice from an ID specialist. Surgery may be required to resect infected valve. Long-term suppressive therapy with fluconazole.

– Culture-negative prosthetic valve endocarditis: treat at least 6 wk.

Endocarditis antibiotic prophylaxis:[220,221,224]. Endocarditis is rarely caused by dental/GI procedures, and antibiotic prophylaxis for procedures prevents an exceedingly small proportion of endocarditis cases; therefore, the risks of antibiotic prophylaxis outweigh the benefits. Highest-risk conditions currently recommended for prophylaxis for children undergoing procedures: (1) prosthetic heart valve (or prosthetic material used to repair a valve); (2) previous endocarditis; (3) cyanotic congenital heart disease that is unrepaired (or palliatively repaired with shunts and conduits); (4) congenital heart disease that is repaired but with defects at the site of repair adjacent to prosthetic material; (5) completely repaired congenital heart disease by using prosthetic material, for the first 6 mo after repair; or (6) cardiac transplant patients with valvulopathy. Routine prophylaxis is no longer required for children with native valve abnormalities. Assessment of recent prophylaxis guidelines does not document an increase in endocarditis.[225]

– In highest-risk patients: dental procedures that involve manipulation of the gingival or periodontal region of teeth	Amoxicillin 50 mg/kg PO 60 min before procedure OR ampicillin or ceftriaxone or cefazolin, all at 50 mg/kg IM/IV 30–60 min before procedure	If penicillin allergy: clindamycin 20 mg/kg PO (60 min before) or IV (30 min before); OR azithromycin 15 mg/kg or clarithromycin 15 mg/kg, 60 min before procedure (little data to support alternative regimens)
– Genitourinary and GI procedures	None	No longer recommended

Lemierre syndrome (*F necrophorum* primarily; also reported with MRSA)[119-121] – Pharyngitis with internal jugular vein septic thrombosis; also known as postanginal sepsis, necrobacillosis	Empiric: meropenem 60 mg/kg/day div q8h (or 120 mg/kg/day div q8h for CNS metastatic foci) (AIII) OR ceftriaxone 100 mg/kg/day q24h AND metronidazole 40 mg/kg/day div q8h or clindamycin 40 mg/kg/day div q6h (BIII). ADD empiric vancomycin if MRSA is suspected if clindamycin is not already in the treatment regimen or local susceptibility data indicate that vancomycin use is preferred.	Anecdotal reports suggest that metronidazole may be effective for apparent failures with other agents. Often requires anticoagulation. Metastatic and recurrent abscesses often develop during active, appropriate therapy, requiring multiple debridements and prolonged antibiotic therapy.[122] Treat until CRP is close to normal (AIII).
Purulent pericarditis		
– Empiric (acute, bacterial: *S aureus* [including MRSA], group A streptococcus, pneumococcus, meningococcus; in unimmunized children, *H influenzae* type b)[226,227]	Ceftaroline: 2–<6 mo, 30 mg/kg/day IV div q8h; ≥6 mo, 45 mg/kg/day IV div q8h (max single dose 600 mg) (BIII), OR vancomycin 40 mg/kg/day IV div q8h and ceftriaxone 50–75 mg/kg/day q24h (AIII)	For presumed staph infection, consider adding gentamicin pending cultures (AIII). Increasingly uncommon with immunization against pneumococcus and *H influenzae* type b.[227] Pericardiocentesis is essential to establish diagnosis. Surgical drainage of pus with pericardial window or pericardiectomy is important to prevent tamponade.
– *Staphylococcus aureus*	For MSSA: oxacillin/nafcillin 150–200 mg/kg/day IV div q6h OR cefazolin 100 mg/kg/day IV div q8h. Treat for 2–3 wk after drainage (BIII). For CA-MRSA: continue ceftaroline or vancomycin. Treat for 3–4 wk after drainage (BIII).	Continue therapy with gentamicin until clinically improved; consider use of rifampin in severe cases due to tissue penetration characteristics.
– *Haemophilus influenzae* type b in unimmunized children	Ceftriaxone 50 mg/kg/day q24h for 10–14 days (AIII)	Ampicillin for BL-negative strains
– Pneumococcus, meningococcus, group A streptococcus	Penicillin G 200,000 U/kg/day IV, IM div q6h for 10–14 days OR ceftriaxone 50 mg/kg qd for 10–14 days (AIII)	Ceftriaxone for penicillin non-susceptible pneumococci

G. CARDIOVASCULAR INFECTIONS

Clinical Diagnosis	Therapy (evidence grade)	Comments
– Coliform bacilli	Ceftriaxone 50–75 mg/kg/day q24h for ≥3 wk (AIII)	Alternative drugs depending on susceptibilities; for *Enterobacter*, *Serratia*, or *Citrobacter*, use cefepime or meropenem. For ESBL *E coli* or *Klebsiella*, use a carbapenem.
– Tuberculous[15,16]	INH 10–15 mg/kg/day (max 300 mg) PO, IV qd for 6 mo AND rifampin 10–20 mg/kg/day (max 600 mg) PO, IV qd for 6 mo. ADD PZA 20–40 mg/kg/day PO qd for first 2 mo of therapy; if suspected MDR, also add ethambutol 20 mg/kg/day PO qd (AIII).	For those at highest risk for restrictive pericarditis, steroids may provide benefit. For children: prednisone 2 mg/kg/day for 4 wk, then 0.5 mg/kg/day for 4 wk, then 0.25 mg/kg/day for 2 wk, then 0.1 mg/kg/day for 1 wk.

H. GASTROINTESTINAL INFECTIONS (See Ch 9 for parasitic infections.)

Clinical Diagnosis	Therapy (evidence grade)	Comments

Diarrhea/Gastroenteritis

Note on *E coli* and diarrheal disease: Antibiotic susceptibility of *E coli* varies considerably from region to region. For mild to moderate disease, TMP/SMX may be started as initial therapy, but for more severe disease and for locations with rates of TMP/SMX resistance >10%–20%, azithromycin, a PO 3rd-generation cephalosporin (eg, cefixime, cefdinir, ceftibuten), or ciprofloxacin should be used (AIII). Diagnostic testing by traditional cultures with antibiotic susceptibility testing is recommended for significant disease (AIII). New molecular tests (particularly multiplex PCR tests) are commercially available and quite helpful to diagnose specific pathogens or presence of enterotoxins, but they do not provide susceptibility information or distinguish between viable and nonviable organisms.

– Empiric therapy for community-associated diarrhea in the United States (E coli [STEC, including O157:H7 strains; ETEC; and EPEC], Salmonella, Campylobacter, and Shigella predominate; Yersinia and parasites cause <5%; viral pathogens are far more common, especially for children <3 y).[228,229]	Azithromycin 10 mg/kg qd for 3 days (BII); OR ciprofloxacin 30 mg/kg/day PO div bid for 3 days; OR cefixime 8 mg/kg/day PO qd (BII). Current recommendation is to avoid treatment of Shiga toxin–containing (STEC O157:H7) strains.[228]	Alternatives: 3rd-generation cephalosporins (eg, ceftriaxone); have been shown effective in uncomplicated Salmonella typhi infections. Rifaximin is a nonabsorbable rifamycin in tab form not to be used for invasive bacterial enteritis: 600 mg/day div tid for 3 days (for nonfebrile, non-bloody diarrhea in children ≥12 y). Most retrospective data support withholding treatment of O157:H7 strains to avoid HUS.[230-232] Antitoxins and immune globulins are under investigation.[233]
– Travelers diarrhea: empiric therapy (E coli, Campylobacter, Salmonella, and Shigella, plus many other pathogens, including protozoa)[234-240] The CDC provides updated advice both pretravel and post-travel at wwwnc.cdc.gov/travel/page/clinician-information-center (reviewed November 3, 2022; accessed September 12, 2024). See 2017 guidelines from International Society of Travel Medicine.[237]	For mild diarrhea, treatment is not recommended.[237] Azithromycin 10 mg/kg qd for 1–3 days (AII); OR rifaximin 200 mg PO tid for 3 days (age ≥12 y) (BII); OR ciprofloxacin 30 mg/kg/day PO div bid for 3 days (BII).	Susceptibility patterns of E coli, Campylobacter, Salmonella, and Shigella vary widely by country, with increasing resistance to commonly used antibiotics; check the CDC and country-specific data for departing or returning travelers. Azithromycin preferable to ciprofloxacin for travelers to Southeast Asia given high prevalence of quinolone-resistant Campylobacter. Rifaximin, not to be used for invasive bacterial enteritis. For adults who travel and take antibiotics (mostly FQs), colonization with ESBL-positive E coli is more frequent on return home.[241] Adjunctive therapy with loperamide (antimotility) is not recommended for children <2 y and should be used only in cases of nonfebrile, non-bloody diarrhea.[235,239,242] May shorten symptomatic illness by about 24 h.

H. GASTROINTESTINAL INFECTIONS (See Ch 9 for parasitic infections.)

Clinical Diagnosis	Therapy (evidence grade)	Comments
– Travelers diarrhea: prophylaxis[234,235,237]	Prophylaxis: early self-treatment with agents listed previously is preferred over long-term prophylaxis, but may use prophylaxis for a short-term (<14 days) visit to very high-risk region: rifaximin (for children ≥12 y), azithromycin (BIII). FQs should not be used for prevention, due to potential cartilage toxicity.	
– Aeromonas hydrophila[243]	Ciprofloxacin 30 mg/kg/day PO div bid for 5 days OR cefixime 8 mg/kg/day PO qd (BIII)	Not all strains produce enterotoxins and diarrhea; role in diarrhea questioned.[243] Resistance to TMP/SMX about 10%–15%. Choose narrowest-spectrum agent based on in vitro susceptibilities.
– Campylobacter jejuni[244,245]	Azithromycin 10 mg/kg/day for 3 days (BII) or erythromycin 40 mg/kg/day PO div qid for 5 days (BII)	Alternatives: doxycycline or ciprofloxacin (high rate of FQ resistance in Thailand, India, and now the United States). Single-dose azithromycin (1 g, once) is effective in adults.
– Cholera[246,247]	Azithromycin 20 mg/kg once; OR erythromycin 50 mg/kg/day PO div qid for 3 days; OR doxycycline 4.4 mg/kg/day (max 200 mg/day) PO div bid, for all ages	Ciprofloxacin or TMP/SMX (if susceptible)
– Clostridioides (formerly Clostridium) difficile (antibiotic-associated colitis)[248-252]	Treatment stratified by severity and recurrence First episode: Mild to moderate illness: metronidazole 30 mg/kg/day PO div qid; OR vancomycin 40 mg/kg/day PO div qid. Severe illness: vancomycin 40 mg/kg/day PO div qid for 7 days. Severe and complicated/systemic: vancomycin PO AND metronidazole IV; consider vancomycin enema (500 mg/100 mL physiologic [normal] saline) soln q8h until improvement.[248,249] For relapsing C difficile enteritis, consider pulse therapy (1 wk on/1 wk off for 3–4 cycles) or prolonged tapering therapy.	Adult guidelines recommend fidaxomicin as first-line therapy, where available; is approved for children down to age 6 mo.[251] Attempt to stop antibiotics that may have caused C difficile infection. Vancomycin is more effective for severe infection.[248,249] Many infants and children aged <2 y may have asymptomatic colonization with C difficile.[249] Higher risk for relapse in children with multiple comorbidities. Fecal microbiota transplant for failure of medical therapy in recurrent enteritis. Bezlotoxumab (IV infusion) is approved for age ≥12 mo to reduce the chance of recurrence in high-risk patients.

– *Escherichia coli*

Enterotoxigenic (etiology of most TD)[235,236]	Azithromycin 10 mg/kg qd for 3 days (AII); OR ciprofloxacin 30 mg/kg/day PO div bid for 3 days (BII); OR cefixime 8 mg/kg/day PO qd for 3 days (CII)	Most illnesses are brief and self-limited and may not require treatment. Alternatives: rifaximin 600 mg/day div tid for 3 days (for nonfebrile, non-bloody diarrhea in children ≥12 y, as rifaximin is not absorbed systemically); OR TMP/SMX. Resistance increasing worldwide; check country-specific rates at the CDC traveler website: wwwnc.cdc.gov/travel/page/clinician-information-center.
Enterohemorrhagic (O157:H7; STEC, etiology of HUS)[228,230–233]	Recommendation to avoid treatment of STEC O157:H7 strains.[228] Most retrospective data support withholding treatment of O157:H7 strains to avoid HUS.[230–232]	Animal model data suggest that some antibiotics (rifamycins) are less likely to increase toxin production than FQs.[253] Injury to colonic mucosa may lead to invasive bacterial colitis that does require antimicrobial therapy.
– Gastritis, peptic ulcer disease (*Helicobacter pylori*)[254–256]	Triple-agent therapy in areas of low clarithromycin resistance (or known clarithromycin susceptibility): clarithromycin 7.5 mg/kg/dose 2–3 times each day, AND amoxicillin 40 mg/kg/dose (max 1 g) PO bid AND omeprazole 0.5 mg/kg/dose PO bid for 14 days (BII). OR if susceptibilities unknown or clarithromycin resistant: quadruple-agent therapy clarithromycin, amoxicillin, omeprazole, AND metronidazole (15 mg/kg/day div bid)[254–257]	Resistance to clarithromycin is as high as 20% in some regions.[254,257] Current use of bismuth in regimens for known or suspected clarithromycin resistance, with bismuth (262 mg qid for those aged <10 y; 524 mg qid ≥10 y), amoxicillin, metronidazole, and omeprazole.[254] Metronidazole resistance reported.[254] Newer, FQ-based treatment combinations used in adults with clarithromycin resistance.[255]

H. GASTROINTESTINAL INFECTIONS (See Ch 9 for parasitic infections.)

Clinical Diagnosis	Therapy (evidence grade)	Comments
- Giardiasis (see Ch 9) (*Giardia intestinalis*, formerly *lamblia*)[258]	Tinidazole[259] (for age ≥3 y) 50 mg/kg/day (max 2 g) for 1 day (BII); OR nitazoxanide PO (take with food), age 12–47 mo, 100 mg/dose bid for 3 days; age 4–11 y, 200 mg/dose bid for 3 days; age ≥12 y, 1 tab (500 mg) bid for 3 days (BII)	If therapy is unsuccessful, another course of the same agent is usually curative. Alternatives: metronidazole 20–30 mg/kg/day PO div tid for 7–10 days (BII); OR paromomycin OR albendazole (CII), OR mebendazole OR furazolidone. Prolonged or combination drug courses may be needed for immunocompromised conditions. Treatment of asymptomatic carriers is controversial but recommended in the United States (per AAP *Red Book*).

- Salmonellosis[260,261] (See Travelers diarrhea: prophylaxis earlier in this section of the table, and Ch 9.)

Non-typhoid strains[260,261]	Usually none for self-limited diarrhea in immunocompetent child (diarrhea is often much improved by the time culture results are available). Treat children with persisting symptomatic infection and all infants <3 mo (greater risk for bacteremia): azithromycin 10 mg/kg PO qd for 3 days (AII); OR ceftriaxone 75 mg/kg/day IV, IM q24h for 5 days (AII); OR cefixime 20–30 mg/kg/day PO for 5–7 days (BII); OR for susceptible strains: TMP/SMX 8 mg/kg/day of TMP PO bid for 14 days (AI).	Alternatives: ciprofloxacin 30 mg/kg/day PO div bid for 5 days (AI). Carriage of strains may be prolonged in treated children, but a current systematic review did not support this earlier observation.[260] For bacteremic infection, ceftriaxone IM/IV may be initially used until secondary sites of infection (bone/joint, liver/spleen, CNS) are ruled out, for a total of 7–10 days.[261]

Typhoid fever[261–265]	Azithromycin 20 mg/kg qd for 5 days (AII); OR ceftriaxone 75 mg/kg/day IV, IM q24h for 5 days (AII); OR cefixime 20–30 mg/kg/day PO div q12h for 14 days (BII); OR for susceptible strains: ampicillin OR TMP/SMX 8 mg/kg/day of TMP PO div bid for 14 days (AI) or ciprofloxacin 30 mg/kg/day div bid	Most strains are FQ resistant. Increasing cephalosporin resistance.[261,266] For newly emergent MDR strains, may require a carbapenem (especially if recent travel to Pakistan). Amoxicillin does not achieve high colonic intraluminal concentrations or high intracellular concentrations. Longer treatment courses for focal invasive disease (eg, osteomyelitis). Corticosteroids may be indicated for severe, life-threatening disease.
– Shigellosis[238,267–269]	Mild episodes do not require treatment. Azithromycin 10 mg/kg/day PO for 3 days (AII); OR ciprofloxacin 30 mg/kg/day PO div bid for 3–5 days (BII); OR cefixime[238] 8 mg/kg/day PO qd for 5 days (AII).	Alternatives for susceptible strains: TMP/SMX 8 mg/kg/day of TMP PO div bid for 5 days; OR ampicillin (not amoxicillin). Ceftriaxone 50 mg/kg/day IM, IV if parenteral therapy necessary, for 2–5 days. Avoid antiperistaltic drugs. Treatment for the improving child is not usually necessary to hasten recovery, but some experts would treat to decrease communicability.
– Yersinia enterocolitica[270–272]	Antimicrobial therapy probably not of value for mild disease in normal hosts. TMP/SMX PO, IV; OR ciprofloxacin PO, IV (BIII). Parenteral therapy for more severe infection: ceftriaxone plus gentamicin.	High rates of resistance to ampicillin. May mimic appendicitis in older children. Limited clinical data exist on PO therapy.

H. GASTROINTESTINAL INFECTIONS (See Ch 9 for parasitic infections.)

Clinical Diagnosis	Therapy (evidence grade)	Comments
Intra-abdominal infection (abscess, peritonitis secondary to bowel/appendix contents)		
– Appendicitis, bowel-associated (enteric GNB, *Bacteroides* spp, *Enterococcus* spp, *Pseudomonas* spp)[273–278]	Source control is critical to curing this infection. Newer data suggest that stratification of cases is important to assess the effect of surgical and medical therapy on outcomes, and using just a one-size-fits-all antibiotic recommendation may not be the best approach.[273–275,276,279] Meropenem 60 mg/kg/day IV div q8h or imipenem 60 mg/kg/day IV div q6h; OR PIP/TAZO 240 mg/kg/day PIP component div q6h; for 4–5 days for patients with adequate source control,[277] ≥7–10 days if suspicion of persisting intra-abdominal abscess (AII). *Pseudomonas* is found consistently in up to 20%–30% of children,[274,277,280] providing evidence to document the need for empiric use of an antipseudomonal drug (preferably one with anaerobic activity), such as a carbapenem or PIP/TAZO, *unless the surgery was highly effective at drainage/source control* (gentamicin is not active in an abscess), which may explain successful outcomes in retrospective studies that did not include antipseudomonal coverage.[278,279,281–283]	Many other regimens may be effective. Because reported retrospective data are published from different centers, be aware that the patient populations, extent of disease, and surgical approach to treatment are not standardized across hospitals, so antibiotic(s) that work in institution A may not be as effective in institution B.[274,275] Options include ampicillin 150 mg/kg/day div q8h AND gentamicin 6.0–7.5 mg/kg/day IV, IM div q8h AND metronidazole 40 mg/kg/day IV div q8h; OR ceftriaxone 50 mg/kg q24h AND metronidazole 40 mg/kg/day IV div q8h. Narrow the spectrum of antibiotics as soon as susceptibility data are available; susceptibility data are particularly useful for PO step-down therapy if appropriate for the child. Data support IV outpatient therapy or PO step-down therapy[278,280,284] when clinically improved, particularly when PO therapy can be focused on the most prominent, invasive cultured pathogens. Publications on outcomes of antibiotic therapy regimens (IV or PO) without culture data cannot be accurately interpreted.
– Tuberculosis, abdominal (*M bovis*, from unpasteurized dairy products in the United States,[5,16,285] and in parts of the world as a complication of systemic TB caused by *M tuberculosis*)[286]	INH 10–15 mg/kg/day (max 300 mg) PO qd for 6–9 mo AND rifampin 10–20 mg/kg/day (max 600 mg) PO qd for 6–9 mo (AII) AND, for abdominal infection caused by *M tuberculosis*, ADD PZA 30–40 mg/kg/day (max 2 g) PO qd for first 2 mo of therapy only. *M bovis* is naturally resistant to PZA.	Corticosteroids have been routinely used as adjunctive therapy to decrease morbidity from inflammation.[286,287] DOT preferred; after 2+ wk of daily therapy, can change to twice-weekly dosing double dosage of INH (max 900 mg); rifampin remains same dosage (10–20 mg/kg/day, max 600 mg) (AII).

	Some experts recommend routine empiric use of ethambutol, based on local resistance data. If risk factors are present for MDR, ADD ethambutol 20 mg/kg/day PO qd OR an FQ (moxifloxacin or levofloxacin).	LP ± CT of head for children ≤2 y with active disease to rule out occult, concurrent CNS infection (AIII). No published prospective comparative data on a 6-mo vs 9-mo treatment course in children.
Perirectal abscess (*Bacteroides* spp, other anaerobes, enteric bacilli)[288]	Ceftriaxone or ciprofloxacin AND metronidazole (BIII). In high-risk or health care–associated infection, PIP/TAZO OR cefepime AND metronidazole.	Surgical drainage alone may be curative. Obtaining cultures and susceptibilities is increasingly important with rising resistance to cephalosporins in community *E coli* isolates. May represent inflammatory bowel disease.
Peritonitis		
– Peritoneal dialysis indwelling catheter infection (staphylococci; enteric GNB; yeast)[289,290]	Antibiotic added to dialysate in concentrations approximating those attained in serum for systemic disease (eg, 4 mcg/mL for gentamicin, 25 mcg/mL for vancomycin, 125 mcg/mL for cefazolin, 25 mcg/mL for ciprofloxacin) after a larger LD (AII)[290]	Selection of antibiotic based on organism isolated from peritoneal fluid; systemic antibiotics if there is accompanying systemic signs of infection, including bacteremia/fungemia
– Primary spontaneous bacterial peritonitis (pneumococcus or group A streptococcus)[291] – Also a complication in children with cirrhosis, with a wide range of pathogens, many of which can be MDR	Ceftriaxone 50 mg/kg/day q24h; if pen-S, then penicillin G 150,000 U/kg/day IV div q6h; for 7–10 days (AII)	Other antibiotics according to culture and susceptibility tests. Spontaneous pneumococcal peritonitis now infrequent in PCV13/20-immunized children.

I. GENITAL AND SEXUALLY TRANSMITTED INFECTIONS

Clinical Diagnosis	Therapy (evidence grade)	Comments
Consider testing for HIV and other STIs in a child with one documented STI; consider sexual abuse in prepubertal children. The recommendations below focus on adult and adolescent infections as per the CDC STI treatment guidelines (2021),[59] which are posted online at www.cdc.gov/std/treatment-guidelines/STI-Guidelines-2021.pdf (accessed September 12, 2024), with supplemental data published in 2022.[56] Neonatal and child recommendations can be found on the same web page.		
Chancroid (*Haemophilus ducreyi*)[59]	Azithromycin 1 g PO as single dose OR ceftriaxone 250 mg IM as single dose	Alternative: erythromycin 1.5 g/day PO div tid for 7 days; OR ciprofloxacin 1,000 mg PO qd, div bid for 3 days
Chlamydia trachomatis (cervicitis, urethritis)[59]	Doxycycline (patients >7 y) 4.4 mg/kg/day (max 200 mg/day) PO div bid for 7 days; OR azithromycin 20 mg/kg (max 1 g) PO for 1 dose	Alternatives: levofloxacin 500 mg PO q24h for 7 days
Epididymitis (associated with positive urine cultures and STIs)[59,292]	Ceftriaxone 50 mg/kg/day q24h for 7–10 days AND (for older children) doxycycline 200 mg/day div bid for 10 days	Microbiology not well studied in children; in infants, also associated with urogenital tract anomalies. Postviral inflammation may be one etiology of epididymitis in boys.[292] Treat infants for *S aureus* and *E coli*; may resolve spontaneously; in STI, treat for *Chlamydia* and gonococcus.
Gonorrhea[59,293,294]	Antibiotic resistance is an ongoing problem, with new data suggesting the emergence of global azithromycin resistance.[56,293,294]	
– Newborns	See Ch 2.	

– Genital infections (uncomplicated vulvovaginitis, cervicitis, urethritis, or proctitis) and pharyngitis[56,59,293,294]	2021 CDC guidelines for uncomplicated GC[59]: ceftriaxone 25–50 mg/kg IV/IM in a single dose, not to exceed 250 mg in children ≤45 kg or 500 mg in those >45 kg. For adults, the CDC no longer recommends azithromycin (1 g PO for 1 dose). Doxycycline 200 mg/day div q12h for 7 days if chlamydia has not been excluded.	Increased dose of ceftriaxone to reflect small decreases in documented in vitro susceptibility for GC; azithromycin no longer recommended, with 4% of strains overall with resistance, but highest resistance rates found in isolates from MSM. If ceftriaxone is unavailable, give gentamicin 240 mg IM as a single dose plus azithromycin 2 g PO as a single dose OR cefixime 800 mg PO as a single dose.[59] FQs are not recommended due to resistance.
– Conjunctivitis[59]	Ceftriaxone 1g IM for 1 dose	Lavage the eye with saline.
– Disseminated gonococcal infection[59]	Ceftriaxone 50 mg/kg/day IM, IV q24h (max 1 g) AND azithromycin 1 g PO for 1 dose; total course for 7 days	No studies in children: increase dosage for meningitis.
Granuloma inguinale (donovanosis; *Klebsiella* [formerly *Calymmatobacterium granulomatis*])[59]	Azithromycin 1 g PO once weekly or 500 mg qd for at least 3 wk and until all lesions have completely healed	Primarily in tropical regions of India, Pacific, and Africa. Options: doxycycline 4.4 mg/kg/day div bid (max 200 mg/day) PO for at least 3 wk OR erythromycin base 500 mg PO qid for at least 3 wk OR TMP/SMX 1 DS (160-mg/800-mg) tab PO bid for at least 3 wk; all regimens continue until all lesions have completely healed.
Herpes simplex virus, genital infection (first episode)[59,295,296]	Acyclovir 20 mg/kg/dose (max 400 mg) PO tid for 7–10 days (first episode) (AI); OR valacyclovir 20 mg/kg/dose (directions for extemporaneous suspension on package label), max 1 g PO bid for 7–10 days (first episode) (AI); OR famciclovir 250 mg PO tid for 7–10 days (AI); for more severe infection: acyclovir 15 mg/kg/day IV div q8h as 1-h infusion for 7–10 days (AII)	For recurrent episodes: treat with acyclovir PO, valacyclovir PO, or famciclovir PO, immediately when symptoms begin, for 5 days. For suppression: acyclovir 20 mg/kg/dose (max 400 mg) PO bid; OR valacyclovir 20 mg/kg/dose PO qd (max 500 mg to start, or 1 g for difficult to suppress). Important issues for HSV in pregnancy for the fetus/ newborn.[295] Prophylaxis is recommended by ACOG in pregnant women.[296]

I. GENITAL AND SEXUALLY TRANSMITTED INFECTIONS

Clinical Diagnosis	Therapy (evidence grade)	Comments
Lymphogranuloma venereum (*C trachomatis*)[59]	Doxycycline 4.4 mg/kg/day (max 200 mg/day) PO (patients >7 y) div bid for 21 days	Alternatives: erythromycin 2 g/day PO div qid for 21 days; OR azithromycin 1 g PO once weekly for 3 wk
Pelvic inflammatory disease (*Chlamydia* or gonococcus, plus anaerobes)[59,297]	Ceftriaxone 250 mg IM for 1 dose AND both doxycycline 200 mg/day PO div bid and metronidazole 1 g/day PO div bid for 14 days OR cefotetan 2 g IV q12h AND doxycycline 100 mg PO or IV q12h	Optional regimen: cefoxitin 2 g IV q6h; AND doxycycline 200 mg/day PO or IV div bid; OR clindamycin 900 mg IV q8h AND gentamicin 1.5 mg/kg IV, IM q8h, OR amp/sul (3 g IV q6h) AND doxycycline (100 mg bid). After clinical improvement with parenteral therapy, transition to PO therapy with doxycycline 100 mg 2 times/day and metronidazole 500 mg 2 times/day is recommended to complete 14 days of therapy. Initial IM + PO therapy (similar to above) can be considered for mild to moderate disease.
Syphilis[59,298] (Test for HIV.)	Penicillin G regimens provided below are preferred.[59]	
– Congenital	See Ch 2.	
– Neurosyphilis (positive CSF VDRL or CSF pleocytosis with serologic diagnosis of syphilis)	Penicillin G crystalline 200,000–300,000 U/kg/day (max 24 million U/day) div q6h for 10–14 days (AIII)	For adults: penicillin G procaine 2.4 million U IM daily PLUS probenecid 500 mg PO qid, for 10 to 14 days OR ceftriaxone 2 g IV daily for 10 to 14 days
– Primary, secondary	Penicillin G benzathine 50,000 U/kg (max 2.4 million U) IM as a single dose (AIII); do not use benzathine-procaine penicillin mixtures.	Follow-up serologic tests at 6, 12, and 24 mo; 15% may remain seropositive despite adequate treatment. Alternatives if penicillin-allergic: doxycycline (patients >7 y) 4.4 mg/kg/day (max 200 mg) PO div bid for 14 days, OR ceftriaxone 1 g daily for 10 days. CSF examination should be performed for children being treated for primary or secondary syphilis to rule out asymptomatic neurosyphilis. Test for HIV.

– Syphilis lasting for ≤1 y, without clinical symptoms (early latent syphilis)	Penicillin G benzathine 50,000 U/kg (max 2.4 million U) IM ×1 (AIII)
	Alternative if allergy (nonpregnant) to penicillin: doxycycline (patients >7 y) 4.4 mg/kg/day (max 200 mg/day) PO bid for 14 days
– Syphilis lasting for >1 y, without clinical symptoms (late latent syphilis) or syphilis lasting for unknown duration	Penicillin G benzathine 50,000 U/kg (max 2.4 million U) IM weekly for 3 doses (AIII)
	Alternative if allergy (nonpregnant) to penicillin: doxycycline (patients >7 y) 4.4 mg/kg/day (max 200 mg/day) PO bid for 28 days. Look for neurologic, eye, and aortic complications of tertiary syphilis.
Trichomoniasis[59]	Tinidazole 50 mg/kg (max 2 g) PO for 1 dose (BII) OR metronidazole 500 mg PO bid for 7 days (preferred for women) OR metronidazole 2 g PO for 1 dose (BII)	
Urethritis, nongonococcal (See Gonorrhea earlier in this table for gonorrhea therapy.)[59,299]	Azithromycin 20 mg/kg (max 1 g) PO for 1 dose, OR doxycycline (patients >7 y) 4.4 mg/kg/day (max 200 mg/day) PO bid for 7 days (AII)	Erythromycin, levofloxacin, or ofloxacin Increasing resistance noted in *Mycoplasma genitalium*[299]
Vaginitis[60]		
– Bacterial vaginosis[59,300]	Metronidazole 500 mg PO bid for 7 days OR metronidazole vaginal gel (0.75%) qd for 5 days, OR clindamycin vaginal cream for 7 days	Alternative: tinidazole 1 g PO qd for 5 days, OR clindamycin 300 mg PO bid for 7 days Recurrence common; new approaches to prevention of new infections under study[300] Caused by synergy of *Gardnerella* with anaerobes
– Candidiasis, vulvovaginal[59,301]	Topical vaginal cream/tabs/suppositories (alphabetic order): butoconazole, clotrimazole, econazole, fenticonazole, miconazole, sertaconazole, terconazole, or tioconazole for 3–7 days (AII); OR fluconazole 10 mg/kg (max 150 mg) as a single dose (AII)	For uncomplicated vulvovaginal candidiasis, no topical agent is clearly superior. For severe acute *Candida* vulvovaginitis, fluconazole (max 150 mg) given q72h for a total of 2 or 3 doses. Avoid azoles during pregnancy. For recurring disease,[301] consider 10–14 days of induction with topical agent or fluconazole, followed by fluconazole once weekly for 6 mo (AI).

I. GENITAL AND SEXUALLY TRANSMITTED INFECTIONS

Clinical Diagnosis	Therapy (evidence grade)	Comments
– Prepubertal vaginitis[302,303]	No prospective studies	Cultures from symptomatic prepubertal girls are statistically more likely to yield *E coli*, enterococcus, coagulase-negative staphylococci, and streptococci (viridans streptococcus and group A streptococcus), but these organisms may also be present in asymptomatic girls. Consider the presence of a foreign body.
– *Streptococcus*, group A[304]	Penicillin V 50–75 mg/kg/day PO div tid for 10 days	Amoxicillin 50–75 mg/kg/day PO div tid

J. CENTRAL NERVOUS SYSTEM INFECTIONS

Clinical Diagnosis	Therapy (evidence grade)	Comments
Abscess, brain (respiratory tract flora, skin flora, or bowel flora, depending on the pathogenesis of infection [direct extension or bacteremia]; rarely parasitic)[305,306]	Until etiology is established, use empiric therapy for presumed mixed-flora infection with origins from the respiratory tract, skin, and/or bowel, based on individual patient evaluation and risk for brain abscess. Initial coverage should include respiratory tract flora (including anaerobes), skin flora (including MSSA/MRSA), and bowel flora (gram-positive, gram-negative, anaerobes), particularly for children with structural heart disease with right-to-left intracardiac shunting. Many antibiotic combinations will be effective, particularly for antibiotics used to treat meningitis.	Surgery for abscesses ≥2 cm in diameter. For single pathogen abscess, use a single agent in doses that will achieve effective CNS exposure. The blood-brain barrier is not intact in brain abscesses. If CA-MRSA suspected, ADD vancomycin 60 mg/kg/day IV div q6–8h ± rifampin 20 mg/kg/day IV div q12h, pending culture results. We have successfully treated MRSA intracranial infections with ceftaroline, but no prospective data exist. If secondary to chronic otitis, include meropenem or cefepime in regimen for anti-*Pseudomonas* activity. For enteric GNB, consider ESBL-producing *E coli* and *Klebsiella* that are resistant to ceftriaxone and require meropenem.

Meropenem 120 mg/kg/day div q8h (AIII); OR nafcillin 150–200 mg/kg/day IV div q6h AND ceftriaxone 100 mg/kg/day IV q24h AND metronidazole 30 mg/kg/day IV div q8h (BIII); for 2–3 wk after successful drainage (depending on pathogen, size of abscess, and response to therapy); longer course if no surgery (3–6 wk) (BIII). Follow resolution by imaging.

Seizure potential is less for meropenem than imipenem.

Encephalitis[307] (may be infectious or immune-complex mediated, not distinguishable clinically[308])

– Amebic (*Naegleria fowleri*, *Balamuthia mandrillaris*, and *Acanthamoeba*)	See Amebiasis in Table 9B.	
– Cytomegalovirus	See Cytomegalovirus in Ch 7. Not well studied in children. Consider ganciclovir 10 mg/kg/day IV div q12h; for severe immunocompromised, ADD foscarnet 180 mg/kg/day IV div q8h for 3 wk.	Follow quantitative PCR in CSF for CMV DNA. Reduce dose for renal insufficiency. Monitor for neutropenia.
– Enterovirus	Supportive therapy; no antivirals currently FDA approved	Pocapavir and pleconaril[309] have not been approved by the FDA as of August 2024. Pocapavir can be used under an expanded access IND, but pleconaril is not available for compassionate use.
– Epstein-Barr virus[310]	Not studied in a controlled comparative trial. Consider ganciclovir 10 mg/kg/day IV div q12h or acyclovir 60 mg/kg/day IV div q8h for 3 wk.	Follow quantitative PCR in CSF for EBV DNA. Efficacy of antiviral therapy not well-defined.

J. CENTRAL NERVOUS SYSTEM INFECTIONS

Clinical Diagnosis	Therapy (evidence grade)	Comments
– Herpes simplex virus[311] (See Ch 2 for neonatal infection.)	Acyclovir 60 mg/kg/day IV as 1- to 2-h infusion div q8h for 21 days for ≤4 mo; for those >4 mo, 45 mg/kg/day IV for 21 days (AIII)	Ongoing study (NCT03084783) to assess the risks/benefits of dexamethasone. Perform CSF HSV PCR near end of 21 days of therapy, and continue acyclovir until PCR negative. Safety of high-dosage acyclovir (60 mg/kg/day) not well-defined beyond the neonatal period; can be used, but monitor for neurotoxicity and nephrotoxicity; the FDA has approved acyclovir at this dosage for encephalitis for children up to 12 y. Monitor for neutropenia and nephrotoxicity.
– *Toxoplasma* (See Ch 9 for neonatal congenital infection.)	See Ch 9.	
– Arbovirus (flavivirus—Japanese encephalitis, Zika, West Nile, St Louis encephalitis, tick-borne encephalitis; togavirus—western equine encephalitis, eastern equine encephalitis; bunyavirus—La Crosse encephalitis, California encephalitis)[307,312,313]	Supportive therapy	Investigational only (antiviral, interferon, immune globulins). No specific antiviral agents are yet commercially available for any of the arboviruses, including Zika or West Nile.

Meningitis, bacterial, community-associated

NOTES

– Pediatric community-associated bacterial meningitis is quite uncommon in the era of conjugate vaccines. Rare cases caused by non-vaccine strains of pneumococcus, or occurring in immunocompromised children, may still occur. The incidence of highly resistant pneumococci in invasive pediatric infections is so low that vancomycin is no longer needed for empiric therapy (toxicity of exposure is no longer justified). Ceftriaxone resistance is not a public health issue at this time.

– Dexamethasone 0.6 mg/kg/day IV div q6h for 2 days as an adjunct to antibiotic therapy decreases hearing deficits and other neurologic sequelae in adults and children (for *Haemophilus*; unproven benefit for pneumococcus; not prospectively studied in children for meningococcus or *E coli*). The first dose of dexamethasone is given before or concurrent with the first dose of antibiotic; probably little benefit if given ≥1 h after the antibiotic.[314]

– Empiric therapy[315]	Ceftriaxone 100 mg/kg/day IV q24h (AII)	Vancomycin may not be needed for empiric treatment of possible pen-R pneumococcus given current, exceedingly high ceftriaxone susceptibility in North America.[316] The blood barrier is not competent early in the antibiotic treatment course, allowing increased penetration as culture/susceptibility results are pending. The first case of ceftriaxone treatment failure 30 y ago initially responded to our treatment with ceftriaxone.[317]
– *Haemophilus influenzae* type b[315] in unimmunized children	Ceftriaxone 100 mg/kg/day IV q24h; for 10 days (AI)	Alternative: ampicillin 200–400 mg/kg/day IV q6h (for BL-negative strains). Add dexamethasone (0.6 mg/kg/day IV div q6h) before or with first dose of antibiotics.
– Meningococcus (*Neisseria meningitidis*)[315]	Penicillin G 250,000 U/kg/day IV div q4h; or ceftriaxone 100 mg/kg/day IV q24h, or cefotaxime 200 mg/kg/day IV div q6h; treatment course for 7 days (AI)	Meningococcal prophylaxis: rifampin 10 mg/kg PO q12h for 4 doses OR ceftriaxone 125–250 mg IM once OR ciprofloxacin 500 mg PO once (adolescents and adults)
– Neonatal	See Ch 2.	
– Pneumococcus (*S pneumoniae*)[315,316]	For pen-S and cephalosporin-susceptible strains: penicillin G 250,000 U/kg/day IV div q4–6h, OR ceftriaxone 100 mg/kg/day IV q24h; for 10 days (AI). For pen-R pneumococci (assuming ceftriaxone susceptibility): continue ceftriaxone IV for total course (AIII).	Some pneumococci may be resistant to penicillin but still be susceptible to ceftriaxone and may be treated with the cephalosporin alone. In parts of the world without widespread use of conjugate pneumococcal vaccines, with widespread penicillin- and ceftriaxone-resistant strains, add vancomycin to ceftriaxone pending cultures and susceptibilities. With the efficacy of current pneumococcal conjugate vaccines, primary bacterial meningitis is uncommon, and penicillin resistance for all invasive pneumococcal infections has decreased substantially.

J. CENTRAL NERVOUS SYSTEM INFECTIONS

Clinical Diagnosis	Therapy (evidence grade)	Comments
Meningitis, TB (*M tuberculosis; M bovis*)[16]	For non-immunocompromised children: INH 15 mg/kg/day PO, IV div q12–24h AND rifampin 20–30 mg/kg/day PO, IV div q12–24h for 12 mo AND PZA 30 mg/kg/day PO div q12–24h for first 2 mo of therapy, AND streptomycin 30 mg/kg/day IV, IM div q12h or ethionamide or moxifloxacin/levofloxacin for first 4–8 wk of therapy; followed by INH and rifampin combination therapy to complete at least 12 mo for the total course. Streptomycin or ethionamide is used instead of ethambutol in children, primarily infants, who have this infection.	*M bovis* strains are intrinsically resistant to PZA. Instead of streptomycin, amikacin or kanamycin can be used. Aminoglycosides are rapidly bactericidal for mycobacteria. Ethionamide is used to ensure multidrug coverage and can be stopped if strain is fully susceptible to usual therapy. Hyponatremia from inappropriate ADH secretion is common; ventricular drainage may be necessary for obstructive hydrocephalus. Administer corticosteroids (can use same dexamethasone dose as for bacterial meningitis, 0.6 mg/kg/day IV div q6h) for 4 wk until neurologically stable, then taper dose for 1–3 mo to decrease neurologic complications and improve prognosis by decreasing incidence of infarction.[318] Watch for rebound CNS inflammation during taper; if present, then increase dose to previously effective level, then taper more slowly. For recommendations for drug-resistant strains and treatment of TB in HIV-infected patients, visit the CDC website for TB: www.cdc.gov/tb (accessed September 12, 2024).

Shunt infections: The use of antibiotic-impregnated shunts has decreased the frequency of this infection.[319] Shunt removal is usually necessary for cure, with placement of a new external ventricular drain; intraventricular injection of antibiotics should be considered in children responding poorly to systemic antibiotic therapy. Duration of therapy varies by pathogen and response to treatment.[315]

– Empiric therapy pending Gram stain and culture[315,320]	Vancomycin 60 mg/kg/day IV div q8h, AND cefepime 50 mg/kg IV q8h (AII)	If Gram stain shows only gram-positive cocci, can start with vancomycin alone. For ESBL-containing GNB, meropenem should be used as the preferred carbapenem for CNS infection.
– *Staphylococcus epidermidis* or *Staphylococcus aureus*[315,320]	Vancomycin (for *S epidermidis* and CA-MRSA) 60 mg/kg/day IV div q8h; OR nafcillin (if organisms susceptible) 150–200 mg/kg/day AND rifampin; for 10–14 days (AIII)	For children who cannot tolerate vancomycin, ceftaroline has anecdotally been successful: ceftaroline[320]: 2–<6 mo, 30 mg/kg/day IV div q8h (each dose given over 2 h); ≥6 mo, 45 mg/kg/day IV div q8h (each dose given over 2 h) (max single dose 600 mg) (BIII). Linezolid, daptomycin, and TMP/SMX are other untested options.
– Gram-negative bacilli[315]	Empiric therapy with meropenem 120 mg/kg/day IV div q8h OR cefepime 150 mg/kg/day IV div q8h (AIII) For *E coli* (without ESBLs): ceftriaxone 100 mg/kg/day IV q12h for at least 14 days but preferably 21 days	Remove shunt. Select appropriate therapy based on in vitro susceptibilities. Meropenem, ceftriaxone, and cefepime have all been studied in pediatric meningitis. Systemic gentamicin as combination therapy is not routinely recommended with carbapenems and cefepime. Intrathecal therapy with aminoglycosides not routinely necessary with highly active β-lactam therapy and shunt removal. See Ch 12.

K. URINARY TRACT INFECTIONS

Clinical Diagnosis	Therapy (evidence grade)	Comments

NOTE: Antibiotic susceptibility profiles of *E coli*, the most common cause of UTI, vary considerably. Check your local microbiology laboratory for susceptibilities from urinary tract isolates in your clinic (community-acquired) and your hospital (nosocomially acquired). For mild disease, TMP/SMX may be initial empiric therapy if local susceptibility is ≥80%, and up to a 20% failure rate is acceptable. Amoxicillin resistance in most communities is >50%. For moderate to severe disease (possible pyelonephritis), obtain cultures and begin a PO 2nd- or 3rd-generation cephalosporin (cefuroxime, cefaclor, cefprozil, cefixime, ceftibuten, cefdinir, cefpodoxime), ciprofloxacin PO, or ceftriaxone IM. Given the high urine concentrations achievable by β-lactam antibiotics (penicillins, cephalosporins, carbapenems), and the fact that susceptibility reporting from the microbiology laboratory may be based on achievable *serum* concentrations, not *urine* concentrations, situations may exist for which an antibiotic that is reported as R (resistant) will actually be effective therapy and easily achieve concentrations in *urine* (100-fold higher than serum) that can inhibit pathogens to cure an infection.[321] Although we are reluctant to recommend an antibiotic that the laboratory reports as R, if your patient is improving on your empiric treatment, it is reasonable to continue that treatment and follow the progress closely. In that context, cephalexin may be more effective against *E coli* for UTI than one might expect from the hospital antibiogram report based on serum concentrations. Antibiotic susceptibility testing will help direct you to the most narrow-spectrum agent.

Cystitis, acute (*E coli*)[322,323]	For mild to moderate disease: TMP/SMX 8 mg/kg/day of TMP PO bid for 3 days (see NOTE above about resistance rates to TMP/SMX), OR cephalexin 50–75 mg/kg/day div q8–12h. In children with moderate to severe disease, it is often difficult to distinguish between upper tract and lower tract infections: cefixime 8 mg/kg/day PO qd; OR ceftriaxone 50 mg/kg IM q24h for 3–5 days (with normal anatomy) (BIII); but narrow the spectrum of antibiotic, if possible, based on urine culture data. For children who do not respond to treatment, obtain follow-up culture after 36–48 h. Routine follow-up cultures of urine are not needed for the child who responds to treatment.	Alternative: amoxicillin 30–45 mg/kg/day PO div tid OR amox/clav PO if susceptible (BII); ciprofloxacin 20–30 mg/kg/day PO div bid for suspected or documented resistant (including ESBL-producing) organisms for both cystitis and complicated UTI.[324] Ciprofloxacin is approved for complicated UTIs for children ≥12 mo. Gentamicin is another option with excellent activity against community strains of *E coli*, but it is only IM or IV and is nephrotoxic.

Nephronia, lobar *Escherichia coli* and other enteric rods (also called "focal bacterial nephritis")[325,326]	Ceftriaxone 50 mg/kg/day IV, IM q24h. Duration depends on resolution of renal cellulitis vs development of abscess (10–21 days) (AIII). For ESBL-positive *E coli*, carbapenems and FQs are often active agents.	Nephronia, a complication of pyelonephritis, is an invasive, consolidative parenchymal infection; it can evolve into renal abscess. Step-down therapy with PO cephalosporins once cellulitis/abscess has initially responded to therapy.
Pyelonephritis, acute (*E coli*)[196,322–324,327–331]	Ceftriaxone 50 mg/kg/day IV, IM q24h OR gentamicin 5–6 mg/kg/day IV, IM q24h (yes, qd). For documented or suspected ceftriaxone-resistant ESBL-positive strains, use meropenem IV, imipenem IV, or ertapenem IV[196,328,329], OR gentamicin IV/IM OR TOL/TAZ. Switch to PO therapy following clinical response (BII). If organism resistant to amoxicillin and TMP/SMX, use a PO 1st-, 2nd-, or 3rd-generation cephalosporin (BIII); if cephalosporin-R or for *Pseudomonas*, can use ciprofloxacin PO 30 mg/kg/day div q12h (up to 40 mg/kg/day)[324] (BIII); for 7–14 days total (depending on response to therapy). See Ch 12.	For mild to moderate infection, shorter courses and PO therapy are likely to be as effective as IV/IM therapy for a standard duration of 7–14 days, for susceptible strains, down to 3 mo of age.[327,328,330] In children, it is often difficult to distinguish between upper tract and lower tract infections. If bacteremia documented and infant <2–3 mo, rule out meningitis and treat 10–14 days IV + PO (AIII). Aminoglycosides at any dose are more nephrotoxic than β-lactams but represent effective therapy (AI). For dosing of gentamicin, qd is preferred to tid.[327] The duration of treatment is a function of the extent of infection (with potential renal abscess formation in severe pyelonephritis); no prospective data collection has addressed the extent of infection at the time of diagnosis. Early renal cellulitis should respond to 5–7 days of therapy; renal abscesses may take ≥14 days to resolve.[328]

K. URINARY TRACT INFECTIONS

Clinical Diagnosis	Therapy (evidence grade)	Comments
Recurrent UTI, prophylaxis[322,330,332–335]	Only for those with grade III–V reflux or with recurrent febrile UTI: TMP/SMX 2 mg/kg/dose of TMP PO qd OR nitrofurantoin 1–2 mg/kg PO qhs; more rapid resistance may develop by using β-lactams (BII).	Prophylaxis is not recommended for patients with grade I–II reflux and no evidence of renal damage (although the RIVUR study[334] included these children, and they may also benefit), but early treatment of new infection is recommended for these children. Cranberries can prevent UTI.[333] *Resistance eventually develops to every antibiotic;* follow resistance patterns for each patient. The use of periodic urine cultures is controversial, as there are no comparative data to guide management of asymptomatic bacteriuria in a child at high risk for recurrent UTI. Although one can prevent febrile UTIs, it is not clear that one can prevent renal scar formation.[336]

L. MISCELLANEOUS SYSTEMIC INFECTIONS

Clinical Diagnosis	Therapy (evidence grade)	Comments
Actinomycosis[337–339]	Penicillin G 250,000 U/kg/day IV div q6h, OR ampicillin 150 mg/kg/day IV div q8h until improved (often up to 6 wk for extensive infection); then long-term convalescent therapy with penicillin V 100 mg/kg/day (up to 4 g/day) PO for 6–12 mo (AII)	Surgery with debridement as indicated. Alternatives: amoxicillin, doxycycline (for children >7 y), clarithromycin, erythromycin, ceftriaxone IM/IV, or meropenem IV. Long-term therapy is needed to prevent relapse.
Anaplasmosis[340,341] (human granulocytotropic anaplasmosis, *Anaplasma phagocytophilum*)	Doxycycline 4.4 mg/kg/day IV, PO (max 200 mg/day) div bid for 7–10 days (regardless of age) (AIII)	No contraindication for doxycycline treatment in ANY age-group. For mild disease, consider rifampin 20 mg/kg/day PO bid for 7–10 days (BII).

Anthrax, sepsis/pneumonia, community vs bioterror exposure (inhalation, GI, cutaneous, meningoencephalitis)[17]	For community-associated anthrax infection, amoxicillin 75 mg/kg/day div q8h OR doxycycline for children >7 y For bioterror-associated exposure (regardless of age): ciprofloxacin 20–30 mg/kg/day IV div q12h, OR levofloxacin 16 mg/kg/day IV div q12h not to exceed 250 mg/dose (AIII); OR doxycycline 4.4 mg/kg/day PO (max 200 mg/day) div bid	For invasive infection after bioterror exposure, 2 or 3 antibiotics may be required.[17] For PO step-down therapy, can use PO ciprofloxacin or doxycycline; if susceptible, can use penicillin, amoxicillin, or clindamycin. May require long-term PEP after bioterror event due to inhalation of spores that have not yet germinated and to ongoing exposure to spores in the environment that was exposed.
Appendicitis (See Appendicitis, bowel-associated, in Table 1H under Intra-abdominal infection.)		
Brucellosis[342,343]	Doxycycline 4.4 mg/kg/day PO (max 200 mg/day) div bid (for children >7 y) AND rifampin (15–20 mg/kg/day div q12h) (BIII); OR for children <8 y: TMP/SMX 10 mg/kg/day of TMP IV, PO div q12h AND rifampin 15–20 mg/kg/day div q12h (BIII); for at least 6 wk	Combination therapy with rifampin will decrease the risk of relapse. For more serious infections, ADD gentamicin 6.0–7.5 mg/kg/day IV, IM div q8h for the first 1–2 wk of therapy to further decrease risk of relapse (BIII), particularly for endocarditis, osteomyelitis, or meningitis. Prolonged treatment for 4–6 mo and surgical debridement may be necessary for deep infections (AIII).
Cat-scratch disease (*Bartonella henselae*)[344–346]	Supportive care for adenopathy (I&D of infected lymph node); azithromycin 12 mg/kg/day PO qd for 5 days shortens the duration of adenopathy (AIII). No prospective data exist for invasive CSD: gentamicin (for 14 days) AND TMP/SMX AND rifampin for hepatosplenic disease and osteomyelitis (AIII). For CNS infection, use ceftriaxone AND gentamicin ± TMP/SMX (AIII).	This dosage of azithromycin has been documented to be safe and effective for strep pharyngitis and may offer greater deep tissue exposure than the dosage used in early studies[8] and used for otitis media. Alternatives: ciprofloxacin, doxycycline.
Chickenpox/shingles (VZV)	See Varicella-zoster virus in Ch 7.	
COVID-19 (acute SARS-CoV-2 infection)	See Coronavirus (SARS-CoV-2) in Table 7C.	

L. MISCELLANEOUS SYSTEMIC INFECTIONS

Clinical Diagnosis	Therapy (evidence grade)	Comments
Ehrlichiosis (human monocytic ehrlichiosis, caused by *Ehrlichia chaffeensis*, and *Ehrlichia ewingii*)[340,341,347,348]	Doxycycline 4.4 mg/kg/day IV, PO div bid (max 100 mg/dose) for 7–10 days (regardless of age) (AIII)	For mild disease, consider rifampin 20 mg/kg/day PO div bid (max 300 mg/dose) for 7–10 days (BIII).
Febrile, neutropenic patient (empiric therapy for invasive infection: *Pseudomonas*, enteric GNB, staphylococci, streptococci, yeast, fungi)[176,349–352]	Cefepime 150 mg/kg/day div q8h (AI); OR meropenem 60 mg/kg/day div q8h (AIII); OR PIP/TAZO (300 mg/kg/day PIP component div q8h for infants/children >9 mo; 240 mg/kg/day div q8h for infants 2–9 mo); OR ceftazidime 150 mg/kg/day IV div q8h AND tobramycin 6 mg/kg/day IV q8h (AII). ADD vancomycin 40 mg/kg/day IV div q8h if clinically unstable, or MRSA or coagulase-negative staph infection suspected (eg, central catheter infection) (AIII). ADD metronidazole to ceftazidime or cefepime if colitis, head/neck space infection, or other deep anaerobic infection suspected (AIII).	Alternatives: other anti-*Pseudomonas* β-lactams (imipenem) AND antistaphylococcal antibiotics, including ceftaroline for MRSA. If no response within 72–96 h and no alternative etiology demonstrated, begin additional empiric therapy with antifungals (BII)[176]; dosages and formulations outlined in Ch 5. Increasingly resistant pathogens (ESBL *E coli* and KPC *Klebsiella*) will require alternative empiric therapy if MDR organisms are colonizing the patient, caused a previous infection in the child, or present on the child's hospital unit. For *low-risk* patients with negative cultures and close follow-up, alternative management strategies have been explored: PO therapy with amox/clav and ciprofloxacin may be used, with cautious discontinuation of antibiotics (even in those without marrow recovery).[176,353]
HIV infection	See Ch 7.	
Infant botulism[354]	Botulism immune globulin for infants (BabyBIG) 50 mg/kg IV for 1 dose (AI); BabyBIG can be obtained from the California Department of Public Health at www.infantbotulism.org, through your state health department.	See www.infantbotulism.org for information for physicians and parents. Website organized by the California Department of Public Health (accessed September 12, 2024). Aminoglycosides should be avoided because they potentiate the neuromuscular effect of botulinum toxin.

Kawasaki syndrome[355–358]	No antibiotics; IVIG 2 g/kg as a single dose (AI)[359], may need to repeat dose in up to 15% of children for persisting fever that lasts 24 h after completion of the IVIG infusion (AII). Corticosteroids as primary adjunctive therapy in the acute phase of Kawasaki syndrome can be associated with reduced coronary artery abnormalities, reduced inflammatory markers, and shorter duration of hospital stay when compared to no corticosteroids.[356,357] Consult an ID physician, a rheumatologist, or a pediatric cardiologist. Adjunctive therapy with corticosteroids for those at high risk for the development of aneurysms.[356,357]	Aspirin 80–100 mg/kg/day qid in acute febrile phase; once afebrile for 24–48 h, high-dose aspirin may no longer add benefit, but dose is changed to low-dose antiplatelet therapy. Role of corticosteroids, anakinra, infliximab, etanercept, calcineurin inhibitors, and antithrombotic therapy, as well as methotrexate, for IVIG-resistant Kawasaki syndrome is under investigation, and some interventions are likely to improve outcome in severe cases.[357–360] Infliximab may decrease acute symptoms in patients whose IVIG fails but may not decrease the risk for coronary artery abnormalities. Similar findings were noted with another tumor necrosis factor inhibitor, etanercept, in the overall population, although subsets of children within the study may have benefited.
Leprosy (Hansen disease)[361]	Dapsone 1 mg/kg/day PO qd AND rifampin 10 mg/kg/day PO qd; ADD (for multibacillary disease) clofazimine 1 mg/kg/day PO qd; for 12 mo for paucibacillary disease; for 24 mo for multibacillary disease (AII).	Consult the HRSA National Hansen's Disease (Leprosy) Program at www.hrsa.gov/hansens-disease (reviewed August 2024; accessed September 12, 2024) for advice about treatment and free antibiotics: 800-642-2477.
Leptospirosis[362,363]	Penicillin G 250,000 U/kg/day IV div q6h, OR ceftriaxone 50 mg/kg/day IV, IM q24h; for 7 days (BII) For mild disease in all age-groups, doxycycline (>7 y) 4.4 mg/kg/day (max 200 mg/day) PO div bid for 7–10 days (BII)	Alternative: for those with mild disease, intolerant of doxycycline, azithromycin 20 mg/kg on day 1, 10 mg/kg for days 2 and 3, or amoxicillin
Lyme disease (*Borrelia burgdorferi*)[364,365]	Neurologic evaluation, including LP, if there is clinical suspicion of CNS involvement	
– Early localized disease (erythema migrans, single or multiple) (any age)	Doxycycline 4.4 mg/kg/day (max 200 mg/day) PO div bid for 10 days for all ages (AII) OR amoxicillin 50 mg/kg/day (max 1.5 g/day) PO div tid for 14 days (AII)	Alternative: cefuroxime, 30 mg/kg/day PO, in 2 divs doses for 14 days OR 1,000 mg/day) PO, in 2 divs doses for 14 days OR azithromycin 10 mg/kg/day PO qd for 7 days

L. MISCELLANEOUS SYSTEMIC INFECTIONS

Clinical Diagnosis	Therapy (evidence grade)	Comments
– Arthritis (no CNS disease)	PO therapy as outlined in early localized disease but for 28 days (AIII)	Persistent or recurrent joint swelling after treatment: repeat a 4-wk course of PO antibiotics or give ceftriaxone 50–75 mg/kg IV q24h for 14–28 days. For persisting arthritis after 2 defined antibiotic treatment courses, use symptomatic therapy.
– Isolated facial (Bell) palsy	Doxycycline as outlined in early localized disease, for 14 days (AIII); efficacy of amoxicillin unknown	LP is not routinely required unless CNS symptoms develop. Treatment to prevent late sequelae; will not provide a quick response for palsy.
– Carditis	PO therapy as outlined in early localized disease, for 14 days (range 14–21 days) OR ceftriaxone 50–75 mg/kg IV q24h for 14 days (range 14–21 days) (AIII)	
– Neuroborreliosis	Doxycycline 4.4 mg/kg/day (max 200 mg/day) PO div bid for 14–21 days (AIII) OR ceftriaxone 50–75 mg/kg IV q24h OR penicillin G 300,000 U/kg/day IV div q4h; for 14–21 days (AIII)	
Melioidosis (*Burkholderia pseudomallei*)[366,367]	Acute sepsis: meropenem 75 mg/kg/day div q8h; OR ceftazidime 150 mg/kg/day IV div q8h; followed by TMP/SMX (10 mg/kg/day of TMP) PO div for 3–6 mo	Alternative convalescent therapy: amox/clav (90 mg/kg/day of amox div tid, not bid) for children ≤7 y, or doxycycline for children >7 y; for 20 wk (AII). MDR strains may be susceptible to cefiderocol IV.

Mycobacteria, nontuberculous[9,11,12,197]

– Adenitis in normal host (See Adenitis entries in Table 1A.)	Excision usually curative (BIII); azithromycin PO OR clarithromycin PO for 6–12 wk (with or without rifampin or ethambutol) if susceptible (BII)	Antibiotic susceptibility patterns are quite variable; cultures should guide therapy; medical therapy is 60%–70% effective. Data suggest that toxicity of antimicrobials may not be worth the small clinical benefit. For more resistant organisms, other antibiotics may be active, including TMP/SMX, FQs, doxycycline, or, for parenteral therapy, amikacin, meropenem, or cefoxitin. See Ch 3 for specific mycobacterial pathogens.
– Pneumonia or disseminated infection in normal or compromised hosts (HIV, IFN-γ receptor deficiency, CF)[11,197,368,369]	The more severe the infection, the more aggressive the treatment: usually treated with 3 or 4 active drugs (eg, clarithromycin OR azithromycin, AND ethambutol, AND amikacin, cefoxitin, or meropenem). Also test for ciprofloxacin, TMP/SMX, rifampin, linezolid, clofazimine, and doxycycline (BII).	Outcomes particularly poor for *Mycobacterium abscessus*.[369,370] See Ch 18 for dosages; cultures are essential, as the susceptibility patterns of nontuberculous mycobacteria are varied.
Nocardiosis (*Nocardia asteroides* and *Nocardia brasiliensis*)[371,372]	TMP/SMX 8 mg/kg/day of TMP div bid or sulfisoxazole 120–150 mg/kg/day PO div qid for ≥6–12 wk. For severe infection, particularly in immunocompromised hosts, IN ADDITION to TMP/SMX, use amikacin 15–20 mg/kg/day IM, IV div q8h OR imipenem or meropenem (not ertapenem) (AIII). For susceptible strains, ceftriaxone.	Wide spectrum of disease, from skin lesions to brain abscess. Surgery when indicated. Alternatives: doxycycline (for children >7 y), amox/clav, or linezolid. Immunocompromised children may require months of therapy.

L. MISCELLANEOUS SYSTEMIC INFECTIONS

Clinical Diagnosis	Therapy (evidence grade)	Comments
Plague (*Yersinia pestis*)[373–375]	Gentamicin 7.5 mg/kg/day IV div q8h (AII) OR doxycycline 4.4 mg/kg/day (max 200 mg/day) PO div bid OR ciprofloxacin 30 mg/kg/day PO div bid. Gentamicin is poorly active in abscesses; consider alternatives for bubonic plague.	A complete listing of treatment options and doses for children is provided on the CDC website (www.cdc.gov/plague/about/index.html; accessed September 12, 2024).
Q fever (*Coxiella burnetii*)[376,377]	Acute stage: doxycycline 4.4 mg/kg/day (max 200 mg/day) PO div bid for 14 days (AII) for children of any age. Endocarditis and chronic disease (ongoing symptoms for 6–12 mo): doxycycline for children >7 y AND hydroxychloroquine for 18–36 mo (AIII). Seek advice from pediatric ID specialist for children ≤7 y; may require TMP/SMX 8–10 mg/kg/day of TMP div q12h with doxycycline; OR levofloxacin with rifampin for 18 mo.	Follow doxycycline and hydroxychloroquine serum concentrations during endocarditis/chronic disease therapy. CNS: use FQ (no prospective data) (BII). Clarithromycin may be an alternative based on limited data (CIII).
Rocky Mountain spotted fever (fever, petechial rash with centripetal spread; *Rickettsia rickettsii*)[378,379]	Doxycycline 4.4 mg/kg/day (max 200 mg/day) PO div bid for 7–10 days (AI) for children of any age	Start empiric therapy early.
Tetanus (*Clostridium tetani*)[380,381]	Metronidazole 30 mg/kg/day IV, PO div q8h OR penicillin G 100,000 U/kg/day IV div q6h for 10–14 days; AND TIG 500 U IM (AII)	Wound debridement essential; may infiltrate wound with a portion of TIG dose, but not well studied; IVIG may provide antibody to toxin if TIG not available. Immunize with Td or Tdap. See Ch 15 for prophylaxis recommendations.

Toxic shock syndrome (toxin-producing strains of *S aureus*, including MRSA, or group A streptococcus)[3,6,7,382,383]	Empiric: oxacillin/nafcillin 150 mg/kg/day IV div q6h AND vancomycin 45 mg/kg/day IV div q8h (for MRSA); OR ceftaroline single-drug therapy (MSSA/MRSA); 2 mo–<2 y, 24 mg/kg/day IV div q8h; ≥2 y, 36 mg/kg/day IV div q8h (max single dose 400 mg); >33 kg, either 400 mg/dose IV q8h or 600 mg/dose IV q12h (BI) AND clindamycin 30–40 mg/kg/day div q8h (to decrease toxin production) for 7–10 days (AII)	Clindamycin added for the initial 48–72 h of therapy to decrease toxin production. Ceftaroline is an option for MRSA treatment, particularly with renal injury from shock and vancomycin (BII). IVIG may provide additional benefit by binding circulating toxin (CIII). For MSSA: oxacillin/nafcillin AND clindamycin ± gentamicin. For CA-MRSA: ceftaroline (or vancomycin) AND clindamycin ± gentamicin. For group A streptococcus: penicillin G AND clindamycin.
Tularemia (*F tularensis*)[185,384]	Gentamicin 6.0–7.5 mg/kg/day IM, IV div q8h; for 10–14 days (AII) Alternative for mild disease: ciprofloxacin (for 10 days)	Doxycycline as an alternative, although relapse rates may be higher than with other antibiotics. See www.cdc.gov/tularemia/hcp/clinical-care/index.html (accessed October 14, 2024).

2. Antimicrobial Therapy for Neonates

NOTES

- A list of table abbreviations and acronyms can be found at the start of this publication.

- Prospectively collected neonatal antimicrobial pharmacokinetic (PK), safety, and efficacy data continue to become available, thanks in large part to federal legislation (especially the US Food and Drug Administration [FDA] Safety and Innovation Act of 2012 that mandates neonatal studies). In situations of inadequate data, suggested doses in this chapter are based on efficacy, safety, and pharmacologic data from older children or adults. These may not account for the effect of developmental changes (effect of ontogeny) on drug metabolism and, hence, are not optimal, particularly for the unstable preterm neonate.[1]

- For those drugs with an intramuscular (IM) route, an assumption is being made that the IM absorption in neonates is similar to that in older children or adults in whom that route has been better studied. The IM and intravenous (IV) routes are not equivalent. The IM route is reasonable as post-initial IV therapy in hemodynamically stable neonates with difficult-to-maintain IV access whose infection has been microbiologically controlled and who are clinically recovering.

  Oral (PO) convalescent therapy for neonatal infections has not been well studied but may be used cautiously in non–life-threatening infections in adherent families with ready access to medical care.[2,3]

- **Substitution for cefotaxime in neonates and very young infants:** Since 2018, US pharmaceutical companies have discontinued manufacturing and marketing cefotaxime. The FDA is allowing importation of cefotaxime from a Canadian distributor (877-404-3338). For centers without cefotaxime readily available, we are recommending the following 3 agents as substitutes:

Ceftazidime has evidence supporting use and is FDA approved for neonates. The FDA-approved dosage differs from what we are recommending in Table 2B.

Cefepime has been FDA approved for infants 2 months and older and for children since 1999. Although neonatal PK and safety studies have been published, the original manufacturer did not seek approval from the FDA for neonates and infants younger than 2 months, so the FDA has not evaluated data or approved cefepime for neonates. Both cefepime and ceftazidime have activity against gram-negative bacilli, including *Pseudomonas aeruginosa,* and against *Neisseria meningitidis,* and both would be expected to penetrate neonatal cerebrospinal fluid to treat neonatal meningitis. Cefepime is more active *in vitro* against enteric bacilli (*Escherichia coli*) and *Pseudomonas* than ceftazidime and is stable against ampC β-lactamase often expressed by enteric bacilli, most often *Enterobacter cloacae, Klebsiella aerogenes,* and *Citrobacter freundii.* Cefepime is stable to many, but not all, extended-spectrum β-lactamases (ESBLs), although it is routinely reported as resistant to ESBL-containing gram-negative bacteria. Cefepime also has more *in vitro* activity than ceftazidime against some gram-positive bacteria such as group B streptococci and methicillin-susceptible *Staphylococcus aureus*. There are no meaningful differences in the safety profiles or therapeutic monitoring of cefepime and ceftazidime.[4]

Ceftriaxone is FDA approved for neonates with the following 2 caveats:

1. *Neonates with hyperbilirubinemia should not be treated with ceftriaxone* due to the potential for ceftriaxone to displace albumin-bound bilirubin, creating more free bilirubin that can diffuse into the brain and increase the risk for kernicterus. Our recommendation is to avoid ceftriaxone in any at-risk neonates with hyperbilirubinemia, particularly those who are unstable or acidotic and particularly preterm neonates and infants up to a postmenstrual age of 41 weeks (gestational + chronologic age).[5] Full-term neonates and infants with total bilirubin concentrations less than 10 mg/dL and falling (usually older than 1 week) may be considered for treatment, but no prospective data exist to support this bilirubin cutoff.[6]

2. Ceftriaxone is *contraindicated in neonates younger than 28 days if they require concomitant treatment with calcium-containing IV solutions.* Neonates should not receive IV ceftriaxone while receiving IV calcium-containing products, including parenteral nutrition, by the same or different infusion catheters. Fatal reactions with ceftriaxone-calcium precipitates in lungs and kidneys in neonates have occurred. There are no data on interactions between IV ceftriaxone and PO calcium-containing products or between IM ceftriaxone and IV or PO calcium-containing products.[7]

A. RECOMMENDED THERAPY FOR SELECT NEONATAL CONDITIONS

Condition	Therapy (evidence grade) *See Tables 2B–2D for neonatal dosages.*	Comments
Conjunctivitis		
– Chlamydial[8-11]	Azithromycin 10 mg/kg/day PO for 1 day, then 5 mg/kg/day PO for 4 days (AII), or erythromycin ethylsuccinate PO for 10–14 days (AII)	Macrolides PO preferred to topical eye drops to prevent development of pneumonia; association of macrolides and pyloric stenosis in young neonates.[12] Alternative: 3-day course of higher-dose azithromycin at 10 mg/kg/dose qd, although safety not well-defined in neonates (CIII). PO sulfonamides may be used after the immediate neonatal period for infants who do not tolerate erythromycin.
– Gonococcal[13-17]	Ceftriaxone 25–50 mg/kg (max 250 mg) IV, IM once (AIII)	For adults, ceftriaxone in higher doses is recommended as single-agent therapy. Ceftriaxone should be used for neonates with no risk for hyperbilirubinemia[5] or IV calcium-drug interactions.[7] Cefotaxime or cefepime is preferred for neonates with hyperbilirubinemia[5] and those with risk for calcium-drug interactions (see Notes). Saline irrigation of eyes. Evaluate for chlamydial infection if maternal chlamydial infection not excluded. All neonates born to mothers with untreated gonococcal infection (regardless of symptoms) require therapy. Cefixime and ciprofloxacin not recommended for maternal empiric therapy.
– *Staphylococcus aureus*[18-20]	Topical therapy is sufficient for mild *S aureus* cases (AII), but PO or IV therapy may be considered for moderate to severe conjunctivitis. MSSA: oxacillin/nafcillin IV or cefazolin (for non-CNS infections) IM, IV for 7 days. MRSA: vancomycin IV or ceftaroline IV.	Aminoglycoside ophth drops or oint, polymyxin/TMP drops No prospective data for MRSA conjunctivitis (BIII) Cephalexin PO for mild to moderate disease caused by MSSA Increased *S aureus* resistance with ciprofloxacin/levofloxacin ophth formulations (AII)

A. RECOMMENDED THERAPY FOR SELECT NEONATAL CONDITIONS

Condition	Therapy (evidence grade) See Tables 2B–2D for neonatal dosages.	Comments
– *Pseudomonas aeruginosa*[21–23]	Cefepime/ceftazidime IV or tobramycin/gentamicin IV, IM for 7–10 days (alternatives: meropenem, PIP/TAZO, amikacin) (BIII)	Aminoglycoside or polymyxin B–containing ophth drops or oint as adjunctive therapy
– Other gram-negative	Aminoglycoside or polymyxin B–containing ophth drops or oint if mild (AII) Systemic therapy if moderate to severe or unresponsive to topical therapy (AIII)	Duration of therapy dependent on clinical course and may be as short as 5 days if clinically resolved
Cytomegalovirus[24–28]		
– Congenital[24–28]	For moderately to severely symptomatic neonates with congenital CMV disease: PO valganciclovir at 16 mg/kg/dose bid for 6 mo[27] (AI); IV ganciclovir at 6 mg/kg/dose q12h can be used for some or all of the first 6 wk of PO therapy not advised but provides no added benefit over PO valganciclovir (AII).[29] An "induction period" starting with IV ganciclovir is not recommended if PO valganciclovir can be tolerated. For isolated sensorineural hearing loss secondary to congenital CMV infection: PO valganciclovir at 16 mg/kg/dose bid for 6 wk (AI).[30]	Benefit for hearing loss and neurodevelopmental outcomes (AI). Treatment recommended for neonates with either moderate to severe symptomatic congenital CMV disease (with or without CNS involvement) or isolated sensorineural hearing loss. Note that the durations of therapy differ for these, with 6 mo recommended for the former and 6 wk recommended for the latter. Ideally, treatment should start within 1 mo; treatment after age 1 mo did not improve hearing outcomes in clinical trials (AIII).[28] Treatment is not routinely recommended for "mildly symptomatic" neonates congenitally infected with CMV (eg, only 1 or perhaps 2 manifestations of congenital CMV infection, which are mild in scope [eg, isolated IUGR, mild hepatomegaly] or transient and mild in nature [eg, a single platelet count of 80,000 μL or an ALT of 130 U/L, with these numbers serving only as examples]), as the risks of treatment may not be balanced by benefits in mild disease.[28]

Treatment for asymptomatic neonates congenitally infected with CMV should not be given.

Neutropenia develops in 20% (PO valganciclovir) to 68% (IV ganciclovir) of neonates receiving long-term therapy (responds to G-CSF or temporary discontinuation of therapy).

CMV-IVIG not recommended for infants.

– Perinatally or postnatally acquired[26]	Ganciclovir 12 mg/kg/day IV div q12h for 14–21 days (AIII)

Antiviral treatment has not been studied in this population but can be considered in patients with acute, severe visceral (end-organ) disease, such as pneumonitis, hepatitis, encephalitis, NEC, or persistent thrombocytopenia. If such patients are treated with parenteral ganciclovir, a reasonable approach is to treat for 2 wk and then reassess responsiveness to therapy. If clinical and laboratory data suggest benefit of treatment, an additional 1 wk of parenteral ganciclovir can be considered if symptoms and signs have not fully resolved. PO valganciclovir is not recommended in these more severe disease manifestations. Observe for possible relapse after completion of therapy (AIII).

A. RECOMMENDED THERAPY FOR SELECT NEONATAL CONDITIONS

Condition	Therapy (evidence grade) See Tables 2B–2D for neonatal dosages.	Comments

Fungal infections (See also Ch 5.)

– Candidiasis[31–40]	**Treatment** AmB-D (1 mg/kg/day) is recommended therapy (AII). Fluconazole (25 mg/kg on day 1, then 12 mg/kg q24h) is an alternative if the patient has not been receiving fluconazole prophylaxis (AII).[41] For treatment of neonates and young infants (<120 days) receiving ECMO, fluconazole LD is 35 mg/kg on day 1, then 12 mg/kg q24h (BII).[42] AmB lipid formulation is an alternative but carries a theoretical risk of decreasing urinary tract penetration compared with AmB-D (CIII).[43] Duration of therapy for candidemia without obvious metastatic complications is 2 wk after documented clearance and resolution of symptoms (therefore, generally 3 wk total).	Neonates have high risk for urinary tract and CNS infections, problematic for echinocandins with poor penetration at those sites; therefore, AmB-D is preferred, followed by fluconazole. Echinocandins are discouraged, despite their fungicidal activity. Infants with invasive candidiasis should be evaluated for other sites of infection: CSF analysis, echocardiogram, abdominal ultrasound to include bladder, retinal eye examination (AIII). CT or ultrasound imaging of genitourinary tract, liver, and spleen should be performed if blood culture results are persistently positive (AIII). Meningoencephalitis in the neonate occurs at a higher rate than in older children/adults. Central venous catheter removal strongly recommended. Infected CNS devices, including ventriculostomy drains and shunts, should be removed, if possible. Length of therapy dependent on disease (BIII), usually 2 wk after all clearance. Antifungal susceptibility testing is suggested with persistent disease. *Candida krusei* is inherently resistant to fluconazole; *Candida parapsilosis* may be less susceptible to echinocandins; there is increasing resistance of *Candida glabrata* to fluconazole and echinocandins.

Prophylaxis

In nurseries with high rates of candidiasis (>10%),[44] IV or PO fluconazole prophylaxis (AI) (3–6 mg/kg twice weekly for 6 wk) in high-risk neonates (birth weight <1,000 g) is recommended. PO nystatin, 100,000 U tid for 6 wk, is an alternative to fluconazole in neonates with birth weights <1,500 g if availability or resistance precludes fluconazole use (CII).

Prophylaxis of neonates and children receiving ECMO: fluconazole 12 mg/kg on day 1, then 6 mg/kg/day (BII).

No proven benefit for combination antifungal therapy in candidiasis. Change from AmB or fluconazole to echinocandin if cultures persistently positive (BIII) despite source control.

Although fluconazole prophylaxis has been shown to reduce colonization, it has not reduced mortality.[34]

Echinocandins should be used with caution and generally limited to salvage therapy or situations in which resistance or toxicity precludes use of AmB-D or fluconazole (CIII).

Role of flucytosine in neonates with meningitis is questionable and not routinely recommended due to toxicity concerns. The addition of flucytosine (100 mg/kg/day div q6h) may be considered as salvage therapy in patients who have not had a clinical response to initial AmB therapy, but adverse effects are frequent (CIII).

Serum flucytosine concentrations should be obtained after 3–5 days to achieve a 2-h post-dose peak <100 mcg/mL (ideally 30–80 mcg/mL) to prevent neutropenia.

See Skin and soft tissues later in this table for management of congenital cutaneous candidiasis.

A. RECOMMENDED THERAPY FOR SELECT NEONATAL CONDITIONS

Condition	Therapy (evidence grade) See Tables 2B–2D for neonatal dosages.	Comments
– Aspergillosis (usually cutaneous infection with systemic dissemination)[27,45–47]	Voriconazole dosing never studied in neonates but likely initial dosing same or higher as pediatric ≥2 y: 18 mg/kg/day IV div q12h for an LD on the first day, then 16 mg/kg/day IV div q12h as a maintenance dose. Continued dosing is guided by monitoring of trough serum concentrations (AII). When patient's condition is stable, may switch from voriconazole IV to voriconazole PO 18 mg/kg/day div bid (AII). Unlike in adults, PO bioavailability in children is about only 60%. PO bioavailability in neonates has never been studied. Trough monitoring is crucial after switch.[26] Alternatives for primary therapy when voriconazole cannot be administered: L-AmB 5 mg/kg/day (AII). ABLC is another alternative. Echinocandin primary monotherapy should not be used for treating invasive aspergillosis (CII). AmB-D should be used only in resource-limited settings in which no alternative agent is available (AII).	Aggressive antifungal therapy and early debridement of skin lesions, which are a common manifestation in neonatal aspergillosis (AIII). Voriconazole is preferred antifungal therapy for all clinical forms of aspergillosis (AI). Early initiation of therapy in patients with strong suspicion of disease is important while a diagnostic evaluation is conducted. Therapeutic voriconazole trough serum concentrations of 2–5 mg/L are important for success. It is critical to monitor trough concentrations to guide therapy due to high inter-patient variability.[28] Low voriconazole concentrations are a leading cause of clinical failure. A second agent (eg, AmB) may be added until voriconazole levels are therapeutic. Neonatal and infant voriconazole dosing is not well-defined, but doses required to achieve therapeutic troughs are generally higher than in children >2 y (AIII).[48] Limited experience with posaconazole and no experience with isavuconazole in neonates.[49] Total treatment course is a minimum of 6–12 wk, largely dependent on the degree and duration of immunosuppression and evidence of disease improvement. Salvage antifungal therapy options after failed primary therapy include a change of antifungal class (using L-AmB or an echinocandin), a switch to posaconazole (trough concentrations >1 mcg/mL [see Ch 18 for pediatric dosing]), or use of combination antifungal therapy. Combination therapy with voriconazole + an echinocandin may be considered in select patients. In vitro data suggest some synergy with 2 (but not 3) drug combinations: an azole + an echinocandin is the most well studied. If combination therapy is used, this is likely best done initially when voriconazole trough concentrations may not yet be therapeutic.

Routine susceptibility testing is not recommended but is suggested for patients who are suspected of having an azole-resistant isolate or who are unresponsive to therapy.

Azole-resistant *Aspergillus fumigatus* is increasing. If local epidemiology suggests >10% azole resistance, initial empiric therapy should be voriconazole + echinocandin OR + L-AmB, and subsequent therapy guided based on antifungal susceptibilities.[50]

Micafungin likely has equal efficacy to caspofungin against aspergillosis.[32]

Gastrointestinal infections

– Necrotizing enterocolitis or peritonitis secondary to bowel rupture[51-55]	Ampicillin IV AND gentamicin AND metronidazole IV for ≥10 days (AII). Clindamycin may be used in place of metronidazole (AII). Alternatives: meropenem (AI); PIP/TAZO ± gentamicin (AII). ADD fluconazole if known to have GI colonization with susceptible *Candida* spp (BIII).	Surgical drainage (AII). Possible benefit of laparotomy over peritoneal drain in one randomized controlled trial.[56] Definitive antibiotic therapy based on blood culture results (aerobic, anaerobic, and fungal); meropenem for ESBL-positive GNRs or cefepime for inducible ampC cephalosporinase–producing GNRs; vancomycin rather than ampicillin if MRSA prevalent. *Bacteroides* colonization may occur as early as the first week after birth (AIII). Duration of therapy dependent on clinical response and risk for persisting IAI abscess (AIII). Probiotics may prevent NEC in preterm neonates, but the optimal strain(s), dose, duration, safety, and target subgroups are not fully known.[57,58] Until a product is FDA approved, administration of probiotics to prevent NEC should be limited to participation in a clinical trial.
– *Salmonella* (non-typhoid and *typhi*)[59]	Ampicillin IM, IV (if susceptible) OR ceftriaxone or cefepime IM, IV for 7–10 days (AII)	Observe for focal complications (eg, meningitis, arthritis) (AIII). TMP/SMX for focal GI infection and low risk for unconjugated hyperbilirubinemia due to interaction between sulfa and bilirubin–albumin binding.

A. RECOMMENDED THERAPY FOR SELECT NEONATAL CONDITIONS

Condition	Therapy (evidence grade) *See Tables 2B–2D for neonatal dosages.*	Comments
Herpes simplex infection		
– Central nervous system and disseminated disease[60–62]	Acyclovir 60 mg/kg/day div q8h IV for 21 days (AII). ALT may help identify early disseminated infection.	If CNS involvement, perform CSF HSV PCR near end of 21 days of therapy and continue IV acyclovir until PCR negative. Monitor early in treatment of acute kidney injury, particularly in sicker infants and those receiving additional nephrotoxins.[63]
– Skin, eye, or mouth disease[60–62]	Acyclovir 60 mg/kg/day div q8h IV for 14 days (AII). Obtain CSF PCR for HSV to assess for CNS infection.	Infuse over 1 h and maintain adequate infant hydration to decrease risk for crystal nephropathy. Involve ophthalmologist when acute ocular HSV disease suspected. If present, ADD topical 1% trifluridine or 0.15% ganciclovir ophth gel (AII) (see Ch 18 for pediatric dosing). Acyclovir PO (300 mg/m²/dose tid) suppression for 6 mo recommended following parenteral therapy (AI).[64] Observe for possible cutaneous or CNS relapse after completion of therapy (or, more rarely, during suppression therapy) (BII).[65] Monitor for neutropenia. Different IV acyclovir dosages have been modeled,[66] but no clinical data are available in humans to support their use. Use foscarnet for acyclovir-resistant disease (see Ch 18 for pediatric dosing).

HIV prophylaxis following perinatal exposure[67,68]

– Prophylaxis following low-risk exposure (mother who had HIV infection before pregnancy, received ART during pregnancy, and sustained viral suppression within 4 wk of delivery)	ZDV for the first 4 wk of age (AI). May reduce to 2 wk for some low-risk situations (BII). GA ≥35 wk: ZDV 8 mg/kg/day PO div q12h OR 6 mg/kg/day IV div q8h. GA 30–34 wk: ZDV 4 mg/kg/day PO (OR 3 mg/kg/day IV) div q12h. Increase at 2 wk of age to 6 mg/kg/day PO (OR 4.5 mg/kg/day IV) div q12h. GA ≤29 wk: ZDV 4 mg/kg/day PO (OR 3 mg/kg/day IV) div q12h. Increase at 4 wk of age to 6 mg/kg/day PO (OR 4.5 mg/kg/day IV) div q12h. The preventive ZDV doses listed for neonates are also treatment doses for infants with diagnosed HIV infection. Treatment of HIV-infected neonates should be considered only with expert consultation.	For detailed information: https://clinicalinfo.hiv.gov/en/guidelines/perinatal/whats-new (updated January 31, 2024; accessed August 7, 2024). UCSF Clinician Consultation Center (888-448-8765) provides free clinical consultation. Start prevention therapy as soon after delivery as possible but by 6–8 h of age for best effectiveness (AII). Monitor CBC at birth and 4 wk (AII). Perform HIV-1 DNA PCR or RNA assays at 14–21 days, 1–2 mo, and 4–6 mo (AI). Initiate TMP/SMX prophylaxis for PCP at 6 wk of age if HIV infection not yet excluded (AII). TMP/SMX dosing is 2.5–5 mg/kg/dose of TMP component PO q12h.

A. RECOMMENDED THERAPY FOR SELECT NEONATAL CONDITIONS

Condition	Therapy (evidence grade) See Tables 2B–2D for neonatal dosages.	Comments
– Prophylaxis following higher-risk perinatal exposure (mother who had primary HIV infection during pregnancy OR who was treated before delivery OR who was treated but did not achieve viral suppression within 4 wk of delivery, especially if delivery was vaginal)	Presumptive HIV treatment (BII): ZDV and 3TC for 6 wk AND EITHER NVP or RAL **ZDV dosing** as above; in infants ≥35 wk of gestation, the dosage should be increased to 12 mg/kg/day PO div q12h once the infant is >4 wk of age. **3TC dosing (≥32 wk of gestation at birth):** Birth–4 wk: 4 mg/kg/day PO div q12h >4 wk: 8 mg/kg/day PO div q12h **NVP dosing:** **≥37 wk of gestation at birth:** Birth–4 wk: NVP 12 mg/kg/day PO div q12h. >4 wk: NVP 400 mg/m²/day of BSA PO div q12h; make this dose increase only for infants with confirmed HIV infection. **≥34–<37 wk of gestation at birth:** Birth–1 wk: NVP 8 mg/kg/day PO div q12h. 1–4 wk: NVP 12 mg/kg/day PO div q12h. >4 wk: NVP 400 mg/m²/day of BSA PO div q12h; make this dose increase only for infants with confirmed HIV infection. **RAL dosing:** **≥37 wk of gestation at birth and ≥2,000 g in weight:**	Delivery management varies for women with HIV who are receiving ART and have viral loads between 20 and 999 copies/mL. Data do not show a clear benefit to IV ZDV and cesarean delivery for these women. Decisions about the addition of NVP, 3TC, or RAL for infants born to these mothers should be made in consultation with a pediatric ID specialist. NVP dosing and safety not established for infants with birth weight <1,500 g. The HIV Guidelines Committee recommends using "treatment" ARV regimens for high-risk, exposed neonates in an attempt to preclude infection or to increase the chance of HIV remission or cure. This was initially stimulated by the experience of a baby from Mississippi: high-risk neonate treated within first 2 days after birth with subsequent infection documentation; off therapy at 18 mo of age without evidence of circulating virus until 4 y of age, at which point HIV became detectable.[69] Clinical trials are ongoing to study these issues further. When empiric treatment is used for high-risk infants and HIV infection is subsequently excluded, NVP, 3TC, and/or RAL can be discontinued and ZDV can be continued for 6 wk total. If HIV infection is confirmed, see Ch 7 for treatment recommendations. Consider consultation with a pediatric ID specialist, especially when considering use of RAL (CIII). If the mother has taken RAL within 2–24 h before delivery, the neonate's first dose of RAL should be delayed until 24–48 h after birth; other ARV drugs should be started as soon as possible.

Birth–1 wk: qd dosing at about 1.5 mg/kg/dose: 2–<3 kg: 0.4 mL (4 mg) qd; 3–<4 kg: 0.5 mL (5 mg) qd; 4–<5 kg: 0.7 mL (7 mg) qd

1–4 wk: bid dosing at about 3 mg/kg/dose: 2–<3 kg: 0.8 mL (8 mg) bid; 3–<4 kg: 1 mL (10 mg) bid; 4–<5 kg: 1.5 mL (15 mg) bid

4–6 wk: bid dosing at about 6 mg/kg/dose: 3–<4 kg: 2.5 mL (25 mg) bid; 4–<6 kg: 3 mL (30 mg) bid; 6–<8 kg: 4 mL (40 mg) bid

Influenza A and B viruses[70-73]

Treatment	Oseltamivir: Preterm, <38 wk of PMA: 1 mg/kg/dose PO bid Preterm, 38–40 wk of PMA: 1.5 mg/kg/dose PO bid Preterm, >40 wk of PMA: 3 mg/kg/dose PO bid[71] Full-term, birth–8 mo: 3 mg/kg/dose PO bid[71,74] 9–11 mo: 3.5 mg/kg/dose PO bid[72]	Oseltamivir chemoprophylaxis is not recommended for infants <3 mo unless the situation is judged critical because of limited safety and efficacy data in this age-group. Parenteral peramivir is approved in the United States for use in children ≥6 mo; no PK or safety data exist in neonates.[75] PO baloxavir is approved in the United States for use in people ≥5 y; no PK or safety data exist in neonates.[76]

Omphalitis and funisitis

– Empiric therapy for omphalitis and necrotizing funisitis; direct therapy against coliform bacilli, S aureus (consider MRSA), and anaerobes[77-79]	Cefepime OR gentamicin, AND clindamycin OR metronidazole for ≥10 days (AII)	Appropriate wound management for infected cord and necrotic tissue (AIII). Need to culture to direct therapy. Alternatives for coliform coverage if resistance likely: cefepime, meropenem. For suspect MRSA: ADD ceftaroline or vancomycin. Alternative for combined MSSA and anaerobic coverage: PIP/TAZO.

A. RECOMMENDED THERAPY FOR SELECT NEONATAL CONDITIONS

Condition	Therapy (evidence grade) See Tables 2B–2D for neonatal dosages.	Comments
– Group A or B streptococcus[80]	Penicillin G IV for ≥7–14 days (shorter course for superficial funisitis without invasive infection) (AII)	Group A streptococcus usually causes "wet cord" without pus and with minimal erythema; single dose of penicillin benzathine IM adequate. Consultation with pediatric ID specialist recommended for necrotizing fasciitis (AII).
– *Staphylococcus aureus*[79]	MSSA: oxacillin/nafcillin IV, IM for ≥5–7 days (shorter course for superficial funisitis without invasive infection) (AIII) MRSA: vancomycin (AIII) or ceftaroline (BII)	Assess for bacteremia and other focus of infection. Alternatives for MRSA: clindamycin (if susceptible) (BIII) or linezolid (CIII).
– *Clostridium* or *Bacteroides* spp[81]	Metronidazole OR clindamycin OR penicillin G IV for ≥10 days, with additional agents based on culture results (AII)	Crepitation and rapidly spreading cellulitis around umbilicus Foul-smelling umbilical drainage Mixed infection with other gram-positive and gram-negative bacteria common

Osteomyelitis, suppurative arthritis[81–84]

Obtain cultures (aerobic; fungal if NICU) of bone or joint fluid before antibiotic therapy.
Duration of therapy dependent on causative organism and normalization of ESR and CRP levels; minimum for osteomyelitis 3 wk and arthritis therapy 2–3 wk if no organism identified (AIII).
Surgical drainage of pus (AIII); physical therapy may be needed (BII).

Condition	Therapy (evidence grade) See Tables 2B–2D for neonatal dosages.	Comments
– Empiric therapy	Nafcillin/oxacillin IV (or vancomycin or ceftaroline if MRSA is a concern) AND cefepime OR gentamicin IV, IM (AIII)	Alternatives for MRSA: clindamycin (if susceptible) or linezolid
– Coliform bacteria (eg, *E coli*, *Klebsiella* spp, *Enterobacter* spp)	For *E coli* and *Klebsiella*: cefepime OR ceftazidime OR ampicillin (if susceptible) (AIII) For *Enterobacter*, *Serratia*, or *Citrobacter*: cefepime OR ceftazidime IV (AIII)	Meropenem for ESBL-producing coliforms (AIII)

– Gonococcal arthritis and tenosynovitis[14-17]	Ceftriaxone IV, IM ± azithromycin 10 mg/kg PO q24h for 5 days (AIII; see Comments).	Ceftriaxone no longer recommended as empiric single-agent therapy due to increasing cephalosporin resistance; therefore, addition of azithromycin recommended until susceptibilities are known (no data in neonates; azithromycin dose is that recommended for pertussis). Cefotaxime or cefepime is preferred for neonates with hyperbilirubinemia and those with risk for calcium–drug interactions (see Notes).
– Staphylococcus aureus	MSSA: oxacillin/nafcillin IV (AII) MRSA: vancomycin IV (AIII) OR ceftaroline IV (BII)	Alternative for MSSA: cefazolin (AIII). Alternatives for MRSA: clindamycin (if susceptible) (BII) or linezolid (CIII). Addition of rifampin if persistently positive cultures.
– Group B streptococcus	Ampicillin or penicillin G IV (AII)	
– Haemophilus influenzae	Ampicillin IV OR cefepime/ceftazidime IV, IM if ampicillin resistant	Start with IV therapy and switch to PO therapy when clinically stable. Amox/clav PO OR amoxicillin PO if susceptible (AIII).
Otitis media[85] No controlled treatment trials in neonates; if no response, obtain middle ear fluid for culture.		
– Empiric therapy[86]	Cefepime/ceftazidime OR oxacillin/nafcillin AND gentamicin	Start with IV therapy and switch to amox/clav PO when clinically stable (AIII).
– Escherichia coli (therapy for other coliforms based on susceptibility testing)	Cefepime/ceftazidime	Start with IV therapy and switch to PO therapy when clinically stable. In addition to pneumococcus and Haemophilus, coliforms and S aureus may also cause AOM in neonates (AII). For ESBL-producing strains, use meropenem (AII). Amox/clav if susceptible (AII).
– Staphylococcus aureus	MSSA: oxacillin/nafcillin IV (AII) MRSA: vancomycin IV (AIII) OR ceftaroline IV (BII)	Start with IV therapy and switch to PO therapy when clinically stable. MSSA: cephalexin PO for 10 days or cloxacillin PO (AII). Alternatives for MRSA: clindamycin (if susceptible) (BII) or linezolid (CIII).
– Group A or B streptococcus	Penicillin G or ampicillin IV, IM	Start with IV therapy and switch to PO therapy when clinically stable. Amoxicillin 30–40 mg/kg/day PO div q8h for 10 days.

A. RECOMMENDED THERAPY FOR SELECT NEONATAL CONDITIONS

Condition	Therapy (evidence grade) See Tables 2B–2D for neonatal dosages.	Comments
Parotitis, suppurative[87]	Oxacillin/nafcillin IV AND gentamicin IV, IM for 10 days; consider vancomycin if MRSA suspected (AIII).	Usually staph but occasionally coliform. Antimicrobial regimen without I&D is adequate in >75% of cases.[88]
Pulmonary infections		
– Empiric therapy for the neonate with early onset of pulmonary infiltrates (within the first 48–72 h after birth)	Ampicillin IV, IM AND gentamicin or ceftazidime/cefepime for 7–10 days; consider treating low-risk neonates for <7 days (see Comments).	For neonates with no additional risk factors for bacterial infection (eg, maternal chorioamnionitis) who (1) have negative blood cultures, (2) have no need for >8 h of oxygen, and (3) are asymptomatic at 48 h into therapy, 4 days may be sufficient therapy, based on babies with clinical pneumonia, none of whom had positive cultures.[89]
– Aspiration pneumonia[90]	Ampicillin IV, IM AND gentamicin IV, IM for 7–10 days (AIII)	Early-onset neonatal pneumonia may represent aspiration of amniotic fluid, particularly if fluid is not sterile. Mild aspiration episodes may not require antibiotic therapy.
– *Chlamydia trachomatis*[91]	Azithromycin PO, IV q24h for 5 days OR erythromycin ethylsuccinate PO for 14 days (AII)	Association of erythromycin and azithromycin with pyloric stenosis in infants treated <6 wk of age[92]
– *Mycoplasma hominis*[93,94]	Clindamycin PO, IV for 7–10 days (resistant to macrolides)	Pathogenic role in pneumonia not well-defined and clinical efficacy unknown; no association with BPD (BIII)
– Pertussis[95]	Azithromycin 10 mg/kg PO, IV q24h for 5 days OR erythromycin ethylsuccinate PO for 14 days (AII)	Association of erythromycin and azithromycin with pyloric stenosis in infants treated <6 wk of age[92] Alternatives: for >1 mo of age, clarithromycin for 7 days; for >2 mo of age, TMP/SMX for 14 days
– *Pseudomonas aeruginosa*[96]	Cefepime IV, IM for 7–10 days (AIII)	Alternatives: ceftazidime AND tobramycin, meropenem, OR PIP/TAZO AND tobramycin

– Respiratory syncytial virus[97]	Treatment (see Comments).

Prophylaxis: nirsevimab is approved and recommended over palivizumab. Shortages of nirsevimab during the 2023–2024 RSV season have led the manufacturer to use a reservation program for the 2024–2025 season, but we are still giving palivizumab recommendations in this edition.

Nirsevimab, 50 mg/dose (<5 kg at dose) or 100 mg/dose (≥5 kg at dose) IM once per season (a) within the first week after birth for *all* infants born during October–March and (b) when entering first RSV season and <8 mo of age for all infants born during April–September.

Alternative: palivizumab (a monoclonal antibody) 15 mg/kg IM monthly (max 5 doses).

For high-risk infants:

In first year after birth, recommended for infants born before 29 wk 0 days' gestation.

Not recommended for otherwise healthy infants born at ≥29 wk 0 days' gestation.

In first year after birth, recommended for preterm infants with CLD of prematurity, defined as birth at <32 wk 0 days' gestation and a requirement for >21% oxygen for at least 28 days after birth or at 36 wk of PMA.

Clinicians may administer in the first year after birth to certain infants with hemodynamically significant heart disease.

Aerosol ribavirin (6-g vial to make 20-mg/mL soln in sterile water), aerosolized over 18–20 h daily for 3–5 days (BII), provides little benefit and should be considered for use only in life-threatening RSV infection. Difficulties in administration, complications with airway reactivity, concern for potential toxicities to health care professionals, and lack of definitive evidence of benefit preclude routine use.

Neither palivizumab nor nirsevimab provides benefit in the treatment of an active RSV infection.

Nirsevimab is recommended for all infants during their first RSV season, including well infants. Only those at high risk should receive a second dose before their second RSV season.

For situations where nirsevimab is not available, palivizumab should continue to be used as follows:

- Palivizumab prophylaxis may be considered for children <24 mo who will be profoundly immunocompromised during the RSV season.

- Palivizumab prophylaxis is not recommended in the second year after birth except for children who required at least 28 days of supplemental oxygen after birth and who continue to require medical support (supplemental oxygen, chronic corticosteroid therapy, or diuretic therapy) during the 6-mo period before the start of the second RSV season.

- Monthly prophylaxis should be discontinued in any child who experiences a breakthrough RSV hospitalization.

- Children with pulmonary abnormality or neuromuscular disease that impairs the ability to clear secretions from the upper airways may be considered for prophylaxis in the first year after birth.

Insufficient data are available to recommend palivizumab or nirsevimab prophylaxis for children with CF or Down syndrome.

The burden of RSV disease and costs associated with transport from remote locations may result in a broader use of palivizumab or nirsevimab for RSV prevention in Alaska Native populations and possibly in select other American Indian populations.[98,99]

Palivizumab or nirsevimab prophylaxis is not recommended for prevention of health care–associated RSV disease.

RSV antivirals are currently investigational for neonates and young infants.

A. RECOMMENDED THERAPY FOR SELECT NEONATAL CONDITIONS

Condition	Therapy (evidence grade) See Tables 2B–2D for neonatal dosages.	Comments
– SARS-CoV-2 (COVID-19)	Remdesivir (AIII) 5 mg/kg on day 1, then 2.5 mg/kg/day for up to 10 days	Must be ≥28 days of age and ≥3 kg in weight, with a positive result on SARS-CoV-2 viral testing. Consider corticosteroids.
– *Staphylococcus aureus*[20,100–102]	MSSA: oxacillin/nafcillin IV (AIII). MRSA: ceftaroline IV (BIII) OR vancomycin IV (BII). Duration of therapy depends on extent of disease (pneumonia vs pulmonary abscesses vs empyema) and should be individualized with therapy up to ≥21 days.	Alternative for MSSA: cefazolin IV Alternatives for MRSA: clindamycin (if susceptible) (BII) or linezolid (CIII) Addition of rifampin or linezolid if persistently positive cultures (AIII) Thoracostomy drainage of empyema
– Group B streptococcus[103,104]	Penicillin G IV OR ampicillin IV, IM for 10 days (AIII)	For serious infections, ADD gentamicin for synergy until clinically improved. No prospective, randomized data on the efficacy of a 7-day treatment course.
– *Ureaplasma* spp (*urealyticum* or *parvum*)[105]	Azithromycin[106] IV 20 mg/kg qd for 3 days (BII)[107]	Pathogenic role of *Ureaplasma* not well-defined and BPD prophylaxis not currently recommended. Clinical trials have not shown benefit to azithromycin treatment of *Ureaplasma*-colonized preterm infants.[108] If only the nasogastric route is available, 10 mg/kg PO q12h × 6 can be trialed instead of 20 mg/kg to improve GI tolerability, but the absorption has not been evaluated and this approach may not achieve the same concentrations as IV. Many *Ureaplasma* spp resistant to erythromycin. Association of erythromycin and pyloric stenosis in young infants.

Sepsis and meningitis[102,109,110]

Duration of therapy: 10 days for sepsis without a focus (AIII); minimum of 21 days for gram-negative meningitis (or at least 14 days after CSF is sterile) and 14–21 days for GBS meningitis and other gram-positive bacteria (AIII).

There are no prospective, controlled studies on 5- or 7-day courses for mild or presumed sepsis.

– Initial therapy, organism unknown	Ampicillin IV AND a second agent, either cefepime/ceftazidime IV or gentamicin IV, IM (AII)	Gentamicin preferred over cephalosporins for empiric therapy for sepsis when meningitis has been ruled out.
		Cephalosporin preferred if meningitis suspected or cannot be excluded clinically or by LP (AIII). For locations with a high rate (≥10%) of ESBL-producing *E coli*, and in which meningitis is suspected, empiric therapy with meropenem is preferred over cephalosporins.
		Initial empiric therapy for nosocomial infection should be based on each hospital's pathogens and susceptibilities.
		Essential: Always narrow antibiotic coverage once susceptibility data are available.
– *Bacteroides fragilis*	Metronidazole or meropenem IV, IM (AIII)	Alternative: clindamycin, but increasing resistance reported
– Carbapenem-resistant GNR[111]	CAZ/AVI IV 40 mg/kg q8h (see Ch 18) (BIII)	Combination options: amikacin, colistin IV 2.5 mg/kg q12h.[112] ADD aztreonam if MBL producing (such as NDM or VIM, not currently prevalent in NICUs in the United States).
		Alternative: high-dose meropenem if CRO with MIC 4–8 mg/L.
		Consultation with ID specialist strongly recommended to assist with drug selection, monitoring, and acquisition of investigational agents if needed for emergency use (eg, mero/vabor, IMI/REL, fosfomycin, plazomicin).
– *Enterococcus* spp	Ampicillin IV, IM AND gentamicin IV, IM (AIII); for ampicillin-resistant organisms: vancomycin AND gentamicin IV (AIII)	Gentamicin needed with ampicillin or vancomycin for bactericidal activity; continue until clinical and microbiologic response documented (AIII).
		For vancomycin-resistant enterococci that are also ampicillin resistant: linezolid (AIII).

A. RECOMMENDED THERAPY FOR SELECT NEONATAL CONDITIONS

Condition	Therapy (evidence grade) See Tables 2B–2D for neonatal dosages.	Comments
– Enterovirus	Supportive therapy; no antivirals currently FDA approved	Pocapavir PO is currently under investigation for enterovirus (poliovirus) (see Ch 7) and can be used under an expanded access IND. Pleconaril PO is currently under consideration for submission to the FDA for approval to treat neonatal enteroviral sepsis syndrome.[113] As of June 2024, it is not available for compassionate use.
– *Escherichia coli*[109,110]	Cefepime/ceftazidime IV or gentamicin IV, IM (AII)	Cephalosporin preferred if meningitis suspected or cannot be excluded by LP (AIII) For locations with a high rate (≥10%) of ESBL-producing *E coli*, and in which meningitis is suspected, empiric therapy with meropenem preferred over cephalosporins
– Group A streptococcus or viridans streptococci	Penicillin G or ampicillin IV (AII)	Penicillin resistance increasingly reported for *Streptococcus mitis* isolates; alternatives: vancomycin or linezolid if not cephalosporin susceptible
– Group B streptococcus[103]	Penicillin G or ampicillin IV AND gentamicin IV, IM (AI)	Continue gentamicin until clinical and microbiologic response documented (AIII). Duration of therapy: 10 days for bacteremia/sepsis (AII); minimum of 14 days for meningitis (AII).
– *Listeria monocytogenes*[114]	Ampicillin IV, IM AND gentamicin IV, IM (AIII)	Gentamicin is synergistic in vitro with ampicillin. Continue until clinical and microbiologic response documented (AIII).
– *Neisseria gonorrhoeae*[115]	Ceftriaxone OR cefepime OR ceftazidime IV (AI)	Duration of therapy: 7 days for bacteremia/sepsis (AII), 10–14 days if meningitis is suspected or confirmed (BII). See Gonococcal earlier in this table for recommendations.
– *Neisseria meningitidis*	Ceftriaxone OR cefepime OR ceftazidime IV (AI)	Duration of therapy: 7 days for bacteremia/sepsis (AII), 10–14 days if meningitis is suspected or confirmed (BII)
– *Pseudomonas aeruginosa*	Cefepime IV, IM OR ceftazidime IV, IM AND tobramycin IV, IM (AIII)	Meropenem is a suitable alternative (AIII). PIP/TAZO should not be used for CNS infection.

– *Staphylococcus epidermidis* (or any coagulase-negative staphylococci)	Vancomycin IV (AIII)	Add rifampin if cultures persistently positive.[116] Alternatives: linezolid, ceftaroline.
– *Staphylococcus aureus*[20,100–102,117–119]	MSSA: oxacillin/nafcillin IV, IM or cefazolin IV, IM (AII) MRSA: vancomycin IV or ceftaroline IV (AIII)	Alternatives for MRSA: clindamycin (if susceptible), linezolid
Skin and soft tissues		
– Breast abscess[120]	Oxacillin/nafcillin IV, IM (for MSSA) OR vancomycin IV or ceftaroline IV (for MRSA). ADD cefepime/ceftazidime OR gentamicin if GNRs seen on Gram stain (AIII).	Gram stain of expressed pus guides empiric therapy; vancomycin or ceftaroline if MRSA prevalent in community; other alternatives: clindamycin, linezolid; may need surgical drainage to minimize damage to breast tissue. Treatment duration individualized until clinical findings have completely resolved (AIII).
– Congenital cutaneous candidiasis[121]	AmB for 14 days, or 10 days if CSF culture negative (AII) Alternative: fluconazole if *Candida albicans* or other *Candida* spp with known fluconazole susceptibility	Treat promptly with full IV treatment dose, not prophylactic dosing or topical therapy. Diagnostic workup includes aerobic cultures of skin lesions, blood, and CSF. Pathology examination of placenta and umbilical cord if possible.
– Erysipelas (and other group A strep infections)	Penicillin G IV for 5–7 days, followed by PO therapy (if bacteremia not present) to complete a 10-day course (AIII)	Alternative: ampicillin. GBS may produce similar cellulitis or nodular lesions.
– Impetigo neonatorum	MSSA: oxacillin/nafcillin IV, IM OR cephalexin (AIII) MRSA: vancomycin IV or ceftaroline IV for 5 days (AIII)	Systemic antibiotic therapy not usually required for superficial impetigo; local chlorhexidine cleansing may help with or without topical mupirocin (MRSA) or bacitracin (MSSA). Alternatives for MRSA: clindamycin IV, PO or linezolid IV, PO.

A. RECOMMENDED THERAPY FOR SELECT NEONATAL CONDITIONS

Condition	Therapy (evidence grade) See Tables 2B–2D for neonatal dosages.	Comments
– *Staphylococcus aureus*[20,100,102,122]	MSSA: oxacillin/nafcillin IV, IM (AII) MRSA: ceftaroline IV (AIII) or vancomycin IV	Surgical drainage may be required. Alternatives for MRSA: clindamycin (if susceptible) IV, linezolid IV. Convalescent PO therapy if infection responds quickly to IV therapy.
– Group B streptococcus[103]	Penicillin G IV OR ampicillin IV, IM	Usually no pus formed Treatment duration dependent on extent of infection, 7–14 days

Syphilis, congenital (≤1 mo of age)[123]
When availability of penicillin is compromised, contact the CDC.
Evaluation and treatment do not depend on mother's HIV status.
Obtain follow-up serology q2–3mo until nontreponemal test nonreactive or decreased 4-fold.

– Proven or highly probable disease: (1) abnormal physical examination; (2) serum quantitative nontreponemal serologic titer 4-fold higher than mother's titer; or (3) positive dark field or fluorescent antibody test of body fluid(s)	Aqueous penicillin G 50,000 U/kg/dose q12h (day after birth 1–7), q8h (>7 days) IV OR procaine penicillin G 50,000 U/kg IM q24h for 10 days (AII)	Evaluation to determine type and duration of therapy: CSF analysis (VDRL, cell count, protein), CBC, and platelet count. Other tests, as clinically indicated, including long-bone radiography, chest radiography, LFTs, cranial ultrasonography, ophthalmologic examination, and hearing test (ABR). Infants with positive CSF VDRL test(s) do not routinely need repeat LP unless their serum nontreponemal test(s) remain elevated at age 6–12 mo. If CSF parameters remain abnormal without an alternative explanation, re-treat. If >1 day of therapy is missed, entire course is restarted.

– Normal physical examination, serum quantitative nontreponemal serologic titer ≤ maternal titer, and maternal treatment was (1) none, inadequate, or undocumented; (2) erythromycin, azithromycin, or other non-penicillin regimen; or (3) <4 wk before delivery.	Evaluation abnormal or not done completely: aqueous penicillin G 50,000 U/kg/dose q12h (day after birth 1–7), q8h (>7 days) IV OR procaine penicillin G 50,000 U/kg IM q24h for 10 days (AII) Evaluation normal: aqueous penicillin G 50,000 U/kg/dose q12h (day after birth 1–7), q8h (>7 days) IV OR procaine penicillin G 50,000 U/kg IM q24h for 10 days; OR penicillin G benzathine 50,000 U/kg/dose IM in a single dose (AIII)	Evaluation: CSF analysis, CBC with platelet count, long-bone radiographs. If >1 day of therapy is missed, entire course is restarted. Reliable follow-up important if only a single dose of penicillin benzathine given.
– Normal physical examination, serum quantitative nontreponemal serologic titer ≤ maternal titer, mother treated adequately during pregnancy and >4 wk before delivery; no evidence of reinfection or relapse in mother	Penicillin G benzathine 50,000 U/kg/dose IM in a single dose (AIII)	No evaluation required. Some experts would not treat but provide close serologic follow-up.

A. RECOMMENDED THERAPY FOR SELECT NEONATAL CONDITIONS

Condition	Therapy (evidence grade) See Tables 2B–2D for neonatal dosages.	Comments
– Normal physical examination, serum quantitative nontreponemal serologic titer ≤ maternal titer, mother treated adequately before pregnancy	No treatment	No evaluation required. Some experts would treat with penicillin G benzathine 50,000 U/kg as a single IM injection, particularly if follow-up is uncertain.
Syphilis, congenital (>1 mo of age)[123]	Aqueous penicillin G crystalline 200,000–300,000 U/kg/day IV div q4–6h for 10 days (AII)	Evaluation to determine type and duration of therapy: CSF analysis (VDRL, cell count, protein), CBC, and platelet count. Other tests as clinically indicated, including long-bone radiography, chest radiography, LFTs, neuroimaging, ophthalmologic examination, and hearing evaluation. If there are no clinical manifestations of disease, CSF examination is normal, and CSF VDRL test result is nonreactive, some specialists will treat with up to 3 weekly doses of penicillin G benzathine 50,000 U/kg IM. Some experts will provide a single dose of penicillin G benzathine 50,000 U/kg IM after 10 days of parenteral treatment, but value of this additional therapy is not well-documented.
Tetanus neonatorum[124]	Metronidazole IV, PO (alternative: penicillin G IV) for 10–14 days (AIII) Human TIG 500 U IM for 1 dose (AIII)	Wound cleaning and debridement vital; IVIG (200–400 mg/kg) is an alternative if TIG not available; equine tetanus antitoxin not available in the United States but is alternative to TIG.
Toxoplasmosis, congenital[125,126]	Sulfadiazine 100 mg/kg/day PO div q12h AND pyrimethamine 2 mg/kg PO daily for 2 days (LD), then 1 mg/kg PO q24h for 2–6 mo, then 3×/wk (M-W-F) up to 1 y (AII)	Corticosteroids (1 mg/kg/day div q12h) if active chorioretinitis or CSF protein >1 g/dL (AIII). Round sulfadiazine dose to 125 or 250 mg (¼ or ½ of 500-mg tab); round pyrimethamine dose to 6.25 or 12.5 mg (¼ or ½ of 25-mg tab). OK to crush tabs to give with feeding.

	Folinic acid (leucovorin) 10 mg 3×/wk continuing for 1 wk after pyrimethamine (AII)	Start sulfadiazine after neonatal jaundice has resolved. Clindamycin is an alternative to sulfadiazine in patients with G6PD deficiency or intolerance. Therapy is effective against only active trophozoites, not cysts.
Urinary tract infection[127] No prophylaxis for grades 1–3 reflux.[128,129] In neonates with reflux, prophylaxis reduces recurrences but increases likelihood of recurrences being due to resistant organisms. Prophylaxis does not affect renal scarring.[128]		
– Initial therapy, organism unknown	Ampicillin AND gentamicin; OR ampicillin AND cefepime/ceftazidime, pending culture and susceptibility test results, for 7–10 days	Renal ultrasound and VCUG indicated after first UTI to identify abnormalities of urinary tract PO therapy acceptable once neonate asymptomatic and culture sterile
– Coliform bacteria (eg, E coli, Klebsiella, Enterobacter, Serratia)	Cefepime/ceftazidime IV, IM OR, in absence of renal or perinephric abscess, gentamicin IV, IM for 7–10 days (AII)	Ampicillin or cefazolin used for susceptible organisms
– Enterococcus	Ampicillin IV, IM for 7 days for cystitis (may need 10–14 days for pyelonephritis), add gentamicin until cultures are sterile (AIII); for ampicillin resistance, use vancomycin, add gentamicin until cultures are sterile.	Aminoglycoside needed with ampicillin or vancomycin for synergistic bactericidal activity (assuming organisms are susceptible to an aminoglycoside)
– Pseudomonas aeruginosa	Cefepime IV, IM, OR ceftazidime IV, IM OR, in absence of renal or perinephric abscess, tobramycin IV, IM for 7–10 days (AIII)	Meropenem is an alternative.
– Candida spp[36–38]	See Candidiasis earlier in this table under Fungal infections.	

B. ANTIMICROBIAL DOSAGES FOR NEONATES—Lead author Jason Sauberan; assisted by the editors and John Van Den Anker

NOTE: This table contains empiric dosage recommendations for each agent listed. See Table 2A for more details of dosages for specific pathogens in specific tissue sites and for information on anti-influenza and ARV drug dosages.

Antimicrobial	Route	Dosages (mg/kg/day) and Intervals of Administration				Chronologic Age 29–60 days
		Chronologic Age ≤28 days				
		Body Weight ≤2,000 g		Body Weight >2,000 g		
		0–7 days old	8–28 days old	0–7 days old	8–28 days old	
Acyclovir (treatment of acute disease)	IV	60 div q8h	60 div q8h	60 div q8h	60 div q8h	60 div q8h
Acyclovir (suppression following treatment of acute disease)	PO	—	900/m²/day div q8h	—	900/m²/day div q8h	900/m²/day div q8h
Only IV acyclovir should be used for the treatment of acute neonatal HSV disease. PO suppression therapy for a duration of 6 mo after completion of initial IV treatment.						
Amoxicillin[a]	PO	—	75 div q12h	100 div q12h	100 div q12h	100 div q12h
Amoxicillin/clavulanate[b]	PO	—	—	30 div q12h	30 div q12h	30 div q12h
Amphotericin B						
– Deoxycholate	IV	1 q24h	1 q24h	1 q24h	1 q24h	1 q24h
– Lipid complex	IV	5 q24h	5 q24h	5 q24h	5 q24h	5 q24h
– Liposomal	IV	5 q24h	5 q24h	5 q24h	5 q24h	5 q24h
Ampicillin	IV, IM	100 div q12h	150 div q12h	150 div q8h	150 div q8h	200 div q6h
Ampicillin (GBS meningitis)	IV	300 div q8h	300 div q6h	300 div q8h	300 div q6h	300 div q6h
Azithromycin[c]	IV, PO	10 q24h	10 q24h	10 q24h	10 q24h	10 q24h
Aztreonam	IV, IM	60 div q12h	90 div q8h[d]	90 div q8h	120 div q6h	120 div q6h

Drug	Route					
Cefazolin (Enterobacterales)[e]	IV, IM	50 div q12h	75 div q12h	100 div q12h	150 div q8h	100–150 div q6–8h
Cefazolin (MSSA)	IV, IM	50 div q12h	50 div q12h	75 div q8h	75 div q8h	75 div q8h
Cefepime	IV, IM	60 div q12h	60 div q12h	100 div q12h	100 div q12h	150 div q8h[f]
Cefotaxime	IV, IM	100 div q12h	150 div q8h	100 div q12h	150 div q6h	200 div q6h
Ceftaroline	IV, IM	12 div q12h[g]	18 div q8h[g]	18 div q8h	18 div q8h	18 div q8h
Ceftazidime[h]	IV, IM	100 div q12h	150 div q8h[d]	100 div q12h	150 div q8h	150 div q8h
Ceftazidime/avibactam[i]	IV	60 div q8h[j]	60 div q8h[i]	60 div q8h	60 div q8h	90 div q8h
Ceftolozane/tazobactam	IV	—	—	60 div q8h	60 div q8h	60 div q8h
Ceftriaxone[j]	IV, IM	—	—	50 q24h	50 q24h	50 q24h
Ciprofloxacin	IV	15 div q12h	15 div q12h	25 div q12h	25 div q12h	25 div q12h
Clindamycin	IV, IM, PO	15 div q8h	15 div q8h	21 div q8h	27 div q8h	30 div q8h
Dalbavancin	IV	22.5 once	22.5 once	22.5 once	22.5 once	22.5 once
Daptomycin (Potential neurotoxicity; use cautiously if no other options.)	IV	12 div q12h	12 div q12h	12 div q12h	12 div q12h	12 div q12h
Erythromycin	IV, PO	40 div q6h	40 div q6h	40 div q6h	40 div q6h	40 div q6h
Fluconazole — Treatment[k]	IV, PO	12 q24h	12 q24h	12 q24h	12 q24h	12 q24h
Fluconazole — Prophylaxis	IV, PO	6 mg/kg/dose twice weekly	6 mg/kg/dose twice weekly	6 mg/kg/dose twice weekly	6 mg/kg/dose twice weekly	6 mg/kg/dose twice weekly
Flucytosine[l]	PO	75 div q8h	100 div q6h[d]	100 div q6h	100 div q6h	100 div q6h
Ganciclovir	IV	12 div q12h	12 div q12h	12 div q12h	12 div q12h	12 div q12h
Linezolid	IV, PO	20 div q12h	30 div q8h	30 div q8h	30 div q8h	30 div q8h

B. ANTIMICROBIAL DOSAGES FOR NEONATES

Antimicrobial	Route	Chronologic Age ≤28 days				Chronologic Age 29–60 days
		Body Weight ≤2,000 g		Body Weight >2,000 g		
		0–7 days old	8–28 days old	0–7 days old	8–28 days old	
Meropenem						
– Sepsis, IAI[m]	IV	40 div q12h	60 div q8h[m]	60 div q8h	90 div q8h[m]	90 div q8h
– Meningitis – Carbapenem-resistant organism with MIC 4–8 mg/L	IV	80 div q12h	120 div q8h[m]	120 div q8h	120 div q8h	120 div q8h
Metronidazole[n]	IV, PO	15 div q12h	15 div q12h	22.5 div q8h	30 div q8h	30 div q8h
Micafungin	IV	10 q24h	10 q24h	10 q24h	10 q24h	10 q24h
Nafcillin,[o] oxacillin[o]	IV, IM	50 div q12h	75 div q8h[d]	75 div q8h	100 div q6h	150 div q6h
Penicillin G benzathine	IM	50,000 U	50,000 U	50,000 U	50,000 U	50,000 U
Penicillin G crystalline (GBS sepsis, congenital syphilis)	IV	100,000 U div q12h	150,000 U div q8h	100,000 U div q12h	150,000 U div q8h	200,000 U div q6h
Penicillin G crystalline (GBS meningitis)	IV	450,000 U div q8h	500,000 U div q6h	450,000 U div q8h	500,000 U div q6h	500,000 U div q6h
Penicillin G procaine	IM	50,000 U q24h	50,000 U q24h	50,000 U q24h	50,000 U q24h	50,000 U q24h
Piperacillin/tazobactam	IV	300 div q8h	320 div q6h[p]	320 div q6h	320 div q6h	320 div q6h
Rifampin[q]	IV, PO	10 q24h	15 q24h	10 q24h	15 q24h	15 q24h
Valganciclovir	PO	Insufficient data	Insufficient data	32 div q12h	32 div q12h	32 div q12h
Voriconazole[r]	IV	12 div q12h	12 div q12h	12 div q12h	12 div q12h	16 div q12h

Zidovudine	IV	3 div q12h[s]	3 div q12h[s]	6 div q12h	6 div q12h	See HIV prophylaxis in Table 2A.
	PO	4 div q12h[s]	4 div q12h[s]	8 div q12h	8 div q12h	See HIV prophylaxis in Table 2A.

[a] For streptococcal and enterococcal infections.

[b] FDA approved doses for susceptible *H influenzae* non-CNS infections are shown in the table. Higher dosing 75 mg/kg/day div q8h recommended for IV to PO step-down treatment of susceptible *E coli* (MIC ≤8 mg/L). May use 25- or 50-mg/mL formulation.

[c] See Table 2A for pathogen-specific dosing.

[d] Use 0–7 days old dosing until 14 days old if birth weight <1,000 g.

[e] If isolate MIC 4 mg/L and no CNS focus. If MIC ≤2 mg/L, can use MSSA dosing.

[f] Infusion over 3 h, or 200 mg/kg/day div q6h, to treat organisms with MIC 8 mg/L.

[g] Serum concentration (is available commercially). Goal exposure is a concentration > MIC (usually 0.5 or 1 mg/L) at 60% of the dosing interval.

[h] For treating susceptible *Pseudomonas* infection. If treating non–AmpC-producing Enterobacterales with MIC ≤4 mg/L (eg, susceptible *E coli* or *Klebsiella*), can use one-half the dose given in the table.

[i] FDA approved for GA ≥31 wk. Case reports suggest safety of the 60 mg/kg div q8h dosage for <31 wk. Considering the safety record of ceftazidime alone in very preterm neonates, and the high stakes of a CAZ/AVI-worthy infection, it is reasonable to use this dosage in all neonates up to 28 days postnatally.

[j] Usually avoided in neonates. Can be considered for transitioning to outpatient treatment of GBS bacteremia in well-appearing neonates with low risk for hyperbilirubinemia. Contraindicated if concomitant IV calcium (see Notes at beginning of chapter).

[k] LD 25 mg/kg followed 24 h later by maintenance dose listed if GA ≥30 wk or LD 9 mg/kg if <30 wk.

[l] Desired serum concentrations peak 60–80 mg/L, trough 5–10 mg/L to achieve time-above-MIC of >40% for invasive candidiasis, and trough 10–20 mg/L for *Cryptococcus*. Dose range 50–100 mg/kg/day. Always use in combination with other agents; be alert to development of resistance.

[m] Adjust dosage after 14 days of age rather than after 7 days of age.

[n] LD 15 mg/kg.

[o] Double the dose for meningitis.

[p] When PMA reaches >30 wk.

[q] For either *Staphylococcus* bacteremia or primary TB.

[r] Adjust dose to target trough 2–5 mg/L (see Aspergillosis in Table 2A under Fungal infections).

[s] Starting dose if GA <35 wk 0 days and PNA ≤14 days. See HIV prophylaxis in Table 2A for ZDV dosage after 2 wk of age and for NVP and 3TC recommendations.

C. AMINOGLYCOSIDES

Medication	Route	Empiric Dosage (mg/kg/dose) by Gestational and Postnatal Ages							
		<30 wk		30–34 wk[a]		≥35 wk[a]			
		0–14 days	>14 days	0–10 days	>10 days	0–7 days	>7 days		
Amikacin[b]	IV, IM	15 q48h	15 q36h	15 q36h	15 q24h	15 q24h	17.5 q24h		
Gentamicin[c]	IV, IM	5 q48h	5 q36h	5 q36h	5 q24h	4 q24h	5 q24h		
Tobramycin[c]	IV, IM	5 q48h	5 q36h	5 q36h	5 q24h	4 q24h	5 q24h		

[a] If >60 days of age, see Ch 18.
[b] Desired serum or plasma concentrations: 20–35 mg/L or 10 × MIC (peak), <7 mg/L (trough).
[c] Desired serum or plasma concentrations: 6–12 mg/L or 10 × MIC (peak), <2 mg/L (trough). A 7.5 mg/kg dose q48h, or q36h if ≥30 wk of GA and >7 days of PNA, more likely to achieve desired concentrations if pathogen MIC = 1 mg/L.[130]

D. VANCOMYCIN[a]

	≤28 wk of GA			>28 wk of GA	
Empiric Dosage by Gestational Age and SCr *Begin with a 20 mg/kg LD.*					
SCr (mg/dL)	**Dose (mg/kg)**	**Frequency**	**SCr (mg/dL)**	**Dose (mg/kg)**	**Frequency**
<0.5	15	q12h	<0.7	15	q12h
0.5–0.7	20	q24h	0.7–0.9	20	q24h
0.8–1.0	15	q24h	1.0–1.2	15	q24h
1.1–1.4	10	q24h	1.3–1.6	10	q24h
>1.4	15	q48h	>1.6	15	q48h

[a] SCr concentrations normally fluctuate and are partly influenced by transplacental maternal creatinine in the first week after birth. Cautious use of creatinine-based dosing strategy with frequent reassessment of renal function and vancomycin serum concentrations is recommended in neonates ≤7 days old. Desired serum concentrations: a 24-h AUC:MIC of at least 400 mg·h/L can be considered based on adult studies of invasive MRSA infections. The AUC is best calculated from 2 concentrations (ie, peak and trough) rather than 1 trough serum concentration. When AUC calculation is not feasible, a trough concentration ≥10 mg/L is very highly likely (>90%) to achieve the goal AUC target in neonates when the MIC is 1 mg/L. However, troughs as low as 7 mg/L can still achieve an AUC ≥400 in some preterm neonates due to their slower clearance. Thus, AUC is preferred over trough monitoring to prevent unnecessary overexposure. For centers where invasive MRSA infection is relatively common or where MRSA with MIC of 1 mg/L is common, an online dosing tool is available that may improve the likelihood of empirically achieving AUC ≥400, compared with Table 2D (https://neovanco.insight-rx.com); accessed October 18, 2024). If >60 days of age, see Ch 18.

E. Use of Antimicrobials During Pregnancy or Breastfeeding

The use of antimicrobials during pregnancy and lactation should balance benefit to the mother with the risk for fetal and neonatal toxicity (including anatomic anomalies with fetal exposure). A number of factors determine the degree of transfer of antibiotics across the placenta: lipid solubility, degree of ionization, molecular weight, protein binding, placental maturation, and placental and fetal blood flow. The Pregnancy and Lactation Labeling Rule of 2014 began replacing the traditional A to X risk categories with narrative summaries of risks associated with the use of a drug during pregnancy and lactation for the mother, the fetus, and the breastfeeding newborn/infant/child. The risk categories from A to X were felt to be too simplistic. This transition was completed in 2020. Risks are now all clearly noted, and for drugs with high fetal risk, black box warnings are included (eg, ribavirin).[131] Fetal serum antibiotic concentrations (or cord blood concentrations) following maternal administration have not been systematically studied, but new PK models of transplacental drug transfer and fetal metabolism have recently been developed to provide some insight into fetal drug exposure.[132–134] The following commonly used drugs appear to achieve fetal concentrations that are equal to or only slightly less than those in the mother: penicillin G, amoxicillin, ampicillin, sulfonamides, trimethoprim, tetracyclines, and oseltamivir. The aminoglycoside concentrations in fetal serum are 20% to 50% of those in maternal serum. Cephalosporins, carbapenems, nafcillin, oxacillin, clindamycin, and vancomycin penetrate poorly (10%–30%), and fetal concentrations of erythromycin and azithromycin are less than 10% of those in the mother.

The most current updated information on the PK and safety of antimicrobials and other agents in human milk can be found at the National Library of Medicine LactMed website (www.ncbi.nlm.nih.gov/books/NBK501922; accessed August 7, 2024).[135]

In general, neonatal exposure to antimicrobials in human milk is minimal or insignificant. Aminoglycosides, β-lactams, ciprofloxacin, clindamycin, macrolides, fluconazole, and agents for tuberculosis are considered safe for the mother to take during breastfeeding.[136,137] The most commonly reported neonatal side effect of maternal antimicrobial use during breastfeeding is increased stool output.[138] Clinicians should recommend that mothers alert their pediatric health care professional if stool output changes occur. Maternal treatment with sulfa-containing antibiotics should be approached with caution in the breastfed infant who is jaundiced or ill.

3. Preferred Therapy for Specific Bacterial and Mycobacterial Pathogens

NOTES

- A list of table abbreviations and acronyms can be found at the start of this publication

- For fungal, viral, and parasitic infections, see Chapters 5, 7, and 9, respectively.

- Limitations of space do not permit listing of all possible alternative antimicrobials.

- Again this year, cefotaxime, a third-generation cephalosporin approved by the US Food and Drug Administration for children more than 3 decades ago, is not given as an option for therapy for pathogens, as it is not routinely available in the United States and we believe that it may not return. Ceftriaxone has a virtually identical antibacterial spectrum of activity to cefotaxime; cefepime is very similar in gram-positive activity but adds *Pseudomonas aeruginosa* (and some enhanced activity for *Enterobacter, Serratia,* and *Citrobacter*) to the gram-negative activity of cefotaxime; ceftazidime adds *Pseudomonas* activity but loses gram-positive activity, compared with cefotaxime. Cefepime, ceftazidime, and, of course, ceftriaxone have been documented to be effective in pediatric meningitis clinical trials. We are not aware if these alternative antibiotics, compared with cefotaxime, have resulted in an increased failure rate in treating children, although problems with ceftriaxone and the biliary tract with prolonged therapy, known since the original approval of ceftriaxone, continue to be reported.

A. COMMON BACTERIAL PATHOGENS AND USUAL PATTERN OF SUSCEPTIBILITY TO ANTIBIOTICS (GRAM POSITIVE)

	Commonly Used Antibiotics (One Agent per Class Listed) (scale − to ++ defined in footnote)			
	Penicillin	**Ampicillin/ Amoxicillin**	**Amoxicillin/ Clavulanate**	**Methicillin/ Oxacillin**
Enterococcus faecalis[a]	++	++	+	−
Enterococcus faecium[a]	++	++	+	−
Nocardia spp[b]	−	−	±	−
Staphylococcus, coagulase-negative	−	−	−	±
Staphylococcus aureus, methicillin-resistant	−	−	−	−
Staphylococcus aureus, methicillin-susceptible	−	−	−	++
Streptococcus pneumoniae	++	++	++	+
Streptococcus pyogenes	++	++	++	++

NOTE: ++ = preferred; + = acceptable; ± = possibly effective (see text for further discussion); − = unlikely to be effective.

[a] Need to add gentamicin or other aminoglycoside to ampicillin/penicillin or vancomycin for in vitro bactericidal activity.

[b] *Nocardia* is usually susceptible to TMP/SMX, carbapenems (meropenem), and amikacin.

	Commonly Used Antibiotics (One Agent per Class Listed) (scale − to ++ defined in footnote)					
Cefazolin/ Cephalexin	**Vancomycin**	**Clindamycin**	**Linezolid**	**Daptomycin**	**Ceftaroline**
−	+	−	+	+	−
−	+	−	+	+	−
−	−	−	+	−	−
±	++	+	++	++	++
−	++	++	++	++	++
++	++	+	++	++	++
++	+	+	++	+	++
++	+	++	+	++	++

B. COMMON BACTERIAL PATHOGENS AND USUAL PATTERN OF SUSCEPTIBILITY TO ANTIBIOTICS (GRAM NEGATIVE)[a]

	Antibiotics (One Agent per Class Listed) (scale − to ++ defined in footnote)						
	Ampicillin/ Amoxicillin	Amoxicillin/ Clavulanate	Cefazolin/ Cephalexin	Cefuroxime	Ceftriaxone	CAZ/AVI	Cefiderocol
Acinetobacter spp	−	−	−	−	+	+	++
Burkholderia cepacia	−	−	−	−	−	++	++
Citrobacter spp	−	−	−	+	+	++	++
Enterobacter spp[b]	−	−	−	±	+	++	++
Escherichia coli[c]	+	+	+	++[d]	++[d]	++	++
Haemophilus influenzae[f]	+	++	+	++	++	++	++
Klebsiella spp[c]	−	−	+	++	++	++	++
Neisseria meningitidis	++	++		+	++	+	
Pseudomonas aeruginosa[b]	−	−	−	−	−	++	++
Salmonella, non-typhoid spp	+	++			++	++	++
Serratia spp[b]	−	−	−	±	+	++	++
Shigella spp	+	++	+	+	++	++	++
Stenotrophomonas maltophilia	−	−	−	−	−	+	++

NOTE: ++ = preferred; + = acceptable; ± = possibly effective (see text for further discussion); − = unlikely to be effective; [blank cell] = untested.

[a] CDC (NARMS) statistics for each state, by year, are found for many enteric pathogens on the CDC website at https://wwwn.cdc.gov/narmsnow and are also provided by the SENTRY surveillance system (JMI Laboratories); we also use current pediatric hospital antibiograms from the editors' hospitals to assess pediatric trends. When sufficient data are available, pediatric community isolate susceptibility data are used. Nosocomial resistance patterns may be quite different, usually with increased resistance, particularly in adults; please check your local/regional hospital antibiogram for your local susceptibility patterns.

[b] AmpC will be constitutively produced in low frequency in every population of organisms and will be selected out during therapy with 3rd-generation cephalosporins if used as single-agent therapy.

[c] Rare carbapenem-resistant isolates in pediatrics (KPC, NDM strains).

[d] Will be resistant to virtually all current cephalosporins if ESBL producing.

[e] Follow the MIC, not the report for susceptible (S), intermediate (I), or resistant (R), as some ESBL producers will have low MICs and can be effectively treated with higher dosages.

[f] Will be resistant to ampicillin/amoxicillin if BL producing.

		Antibiotics (One Agent per Class Listed) (scale − to ++ defined in footnote)				
Ceftazidime	**Cefepime**	**Meropenem/ Imipenem**	**Piperacillin/ Tazobactam**	**TMP/ SMX**	**Ciprofloxacin**	**Gentamicin**
+	+	+	+	+	+	−
+	+	+	−	+[d]	−	−
+	++	++	+	++	++	+
+	++	++	+	++	++	+
++[d]	++[e]	++	++	+	++	+
++	++	++	++	++	++	±
++	++[e]	++	++	++	++	++
+	++	++	++		+	
+	++	++	++	−	++	+
++	++	++	++	++	++	+
+	++	++	+	++	++	++
++	++	++	++	±	++	
+	±	−	±	++	+	−

C. COMMON BACTERIAL PATHOGENS AND USUAL PATTERN OF SUSCEPTIBILITY TO ANTIBIOTICS (ANAEROBES)

	Commonly Used Antibiotics (One Agent per Class Listed) (scale — to ++ defined in footnote)				
	Penicillin	**Ampicillin/ Amoxicillin**	**Amoxicillin/ Clavulanate**	**Cefazolin**	**Cefoxitin**
Anaerobic streptococci	++	++	++	++	++
Bacteroides fragilis	±	±	++	—	+
Clostridia (eg, *tetani, perfringens*)	++	++	++		+
Clostridioides (formerly *Clostridium*) *difficile*	—	—	—		—

NOTE: **++** = preferred; **+** = acceptable; **±** = possibly effective (see text for further discussion); **—** = unlikely to be effective; [blank cell] = untested.

Commonly Used Antibiotics (One Agent per Class Listed)					
(scale − to ++ defined in footnote)					
Ceftriaxone/ Cefepime	**Meropenem/ Imipenem**	**Piperacillin/ Tazobactam**	**Metronidazole**	**Clindamycin**	**Vancomycin**
++	++	++	++	++	++
−	++	++	++	+	
±	++	++	++	+	++
−	++		++	−	++

D. PREFERRED THERAPY FOR SPECIFIC BACTERIAL AND MYCOBACTERIAL PATHOGENS; PLEASE CHECK CULTURE SUSCEPTIBILITY PANEL RESULTS FOR INDIVIDUAL CHILDREN

Organism	Clinical Illness	Drug of Choice (evidence grade)	Alternatives
Acinetobacter baumannii[1–7]	Sepsis, meningitis, nosocomial pneumonia, wound infection	Cefepime; meropenem (BIII) or other carbapenem. Use culture results to guide therapy. Consult an ID specialist for highly MDR strains.	Multiple mechanisms of resistance exist, with no single antibiotic that will be routinely effective against all strains. Possible options: ceftazidime ± avibactam, amp/sul, PIP/TAZO, TMP/SMX, ciprofloxacin, tigecycline/ eravacycline, colistin/polymyxin B. Cefiderocol[3] and durlobactam/ sulbactam,[1,2] approved for adults, are currently under active pediatric investigation. Watch for emergence of resistance *during* therapy, including to colistin. Consider combination therapy for life-threatening infection.[7] Inhaled colistin for pneumonia caused by MDR strains (BIII).
Actinomyces israelii[8,9]	Actinomycosis (cervicofacial, thoracic, abdominal)	Penicillin G; ampicillin (CIII)	Amoxicillin, doxycycline, clindamycin, ceftriaxone, meropenem, PIP/TAZO, linezolid
Aeromonas hydrophila[10]	Diarrhea	Ciprofloxacin (CIII)	TMP/SMX, ceftriaxone, cefepime
	Sepsis, cellulitis, necrotizing fasciitis	Cefepime (BIII); ciprofloxacin (BIII)	Meropenem, TMP/SMX

Aggregatibacter (formerly *Actinobacillus*) *actinomycetemcomitans*[11]	Periodontitis, abscesses (including brain), endocarditis	Ceftriaxone (CIII)	Ampicillin/amoxicillin for BL-negative strains, or amox/clav, doxycycline, TMP/SMX, ciprofloxacin. One of the HACEK organisms that cause endocarditis
Aggregatibacter (formerly *Haemophilus*) *aphrophilus*[12]	Sepsis, endocarditis, abscesses (including brain)	Ceftriaxone (AII); OR ampicillin (if BL negative) AND gentamicin (BII)	Ciprofloxacin, amox/clav (for strains resistant to ampicillin). One of the HACEK organisms that cause endocarditis
Anaplasma (formerly *Ehrlichia*) *phagocytophilum*[13,14]	Human granulocytic anaplasmosis	Doxycycline (all ages) (AII)	Rifampin, levofloxacin
Arcanobacterium haemolyticum[15]	Pharyngitis, cellulitis, Lemierre syndrome	Azithromycin (BIII)	Erythromycin, ceftriaxone, clindamycin, vancomycin. Cephalosporin with or without gentamicin or macrolide for invasive disease
Bacillus anthracis[16]	Anthrax (cutaneous, GI, inhalational, meningoencephalitis)	Ciprofloxacin (regardless of age) (AIII). For invasive systemic infection, use combination therapy. Wild-type strains are likely to be susceptible to penicillin.	Doxycycline, amoxicillin, levofloxacin, clindamycin, penicillin G, vancomycin, meropenem. Bioterror strains may be antibiotic resistant.
Bacillus cereus or *subtilis*[17,18]	Sepsis; toxin-mediated gastroenteritis	Vancomycin (BIII)	Clindamycin, meropenem, ciprofloxacin, linezolid, daptomycin
Bacteroides fragilis[19,20]	Peritonitis, sepsis, abscesses	Metronidazole (AI)	Meropenem or imipenem (AI); PIP/TAZO (AI); amox/clav (BII). Recent surveillance suggests resistance of up to 25%–50% globally for clindamycin. Rarely reported carbapenem resistance.

D. PREFERRED THERAPY FOR SPECIFIC BACTERIAL AND MYCOBACTERIAL PATHOGENS; PLEASE CHECK CULTURE SUSCEPTIBILITY PANEL RESULTS FOR INDIVIDUAL CHILDREN

Organism	Clinical Illness	Drug of Choice (evidence grade)	Alternatives
Bacteroides, other spp[19,20]	Pneumonia, sepsis, abscesses	Metronidazole (BII)	Meropenem or imipenem; penicillin G or ampicillin if BL negative
Bartonella henselae[21,22]	CSD	Azithromycin for lymph node disease (BII); gentamicin AND TMP/SMX AND rifampin for hepatosplenic disease and osteomyelitis (BIII). For CNS infection, use ceftriaxone AND gentamicin ± TMP/SMX (BIII).	Ciprofloxacin, doxycycline
Bartonella quintana[22,23]	Bacillary angiomatosis, peliosis hepatis, endocarditis	Gentamicin plus rifampin, OR doxycycline plus rifampin (BIII); erythromycin; ciprofloxacin (BIII)	Azithromycin, doxycycline
Bordetella pertussis, parapertussis[24,25]	Pertussis	Azithromycin (AIII); erythromycin (BII)	Clarithromycin, TMP/SMX, ciprofloxacin (in vitro data)
Borrelia burgdorferi, Lyme disease[26,27]	Treatment based on stage of infection (see Lyme disease in Table 1L), and prophylaxis after high-risk exposure	Doxycycline for all ages (AII); amoxicillin or cefuroxime can be used in children ≤7 y (AIII); ceftriaxone IV for CNS/meningitis (AII).	Azithromycin. A single course of doxycycline is not associated with detectable tooth staining in children.
Borrelia hermsii, turicatae, parkeri; tick-borne relapsing fever[28,29]	Relapsing fever	Doxycycline for all ages (AIII)	Penicillin or erythromycin in children intolerant of doxycycline (BIII). A single course of doxycycline is not associated with detectable tooth staining in children.

Borrelia recurrentis, louse-borne relapsing fever[28]	Relapsing fever	Single-dose doxycycline for all ages (AIII)	Penicillin or erythromycin in children intolerant of doxycycline (BIII). Amoxicillin; ceftriaxone. A single course of doxycycline is not associated with detectable tooth staining in children.
Brucella spp[30-32]	Brucellosis See Ch 1.	Doxycycline AND rifampin (BIII); OR, for children ≤7 y: TMP/SMX AND rifampin (BIII)	For serious infection: doxycycline AND gentamicin AND rifampin; or TMP/SMX AND gentamicin AND rifampin (AIII). May require extended therapy (months).
Burkholderia cepacia complex[33-36]	Pneumonia, sepsis in children with immunocompromise; pneumonia in children with CF[36]	Meropenem (BIII) for severe disease, if susceptible. Consider CAZ/AVI or cefiderocol for severe disease if carbapenem resistant (AII).	Cefiderocol, CAZ/AVI, TOL/TAZ, doxycycline, minocycline, ceftazidime, TMP/SMX. Aerosolized antibiotics may provide higher concentrations in lung.
Burkholderia pseudomallei[37-39]	Melioidosis	Meropenem (AIII) or ceftazidime (BIII), followed by prolonged TMP/SMX for 12 wk (AII)	TMP/SMX, doxycycline, or amox/clav for chronic disease
Campylobacter fetus[40-42]	Sepsis, meningitis in the neonate, endovascular infection	Meropenem (BIII)	Ampicillin, gentamicin, erythromycin, ciprofloxacin
Campylobacter jejuni[42,43]	Diarrhea	Azithromycin (BII); erythromycin (BII)	Amox/clav, doxycycline, ciprofloxacin (very high rates of ciprofloxacin-resistant strains in Thailand, Hong Kong, and Spain)
Capnocytophaga canimorsus[44,45]	Sepsis after dog bite (increased risk with asplenia)	Meropenem OR PIP/TAZO; amox/clav (BIII)	Clindamycin, penicillin G, imipenem, linezolid, ceftriaxone, amp/sul
Capnocytophaga ochracea[46,47]	Neonatal sepsis, abscesses	Ampicillin, ceftriaxone (BIII); amox/clav (BIII)	Meropenem, PIP/TAZO

Preferred Therapy for Bacterial & Mycobacterial Pathogens

3

D. PREFERRED THERAPY FOR SPECIFIC BACTERIAL AND MYCOBACTERIAL PATHOGENS; PLEASE CHECK CULTURE SUSCEPTIBILITY PANEL RESULTS FOR INDIVIDUAL CHILDREN

Organism	Clinical Illness	Drug of Choice (evidence grade)	Alternatives
Cellulosimicrobium (formerly Oerskovia) cellulans[48]	Wound infection; catheter infection	Vancomycin ± rifampin (AIII)	Linezolid; resistant to β-lactams, macrolides, clindamycin, aminoglycosides
Chlamydia trachomatis[49-51]	Lymphogranuloma venereum	Doxycycline (AII)	Azithromycin, erythromycin
	Urethritis, cervicitis	Doxycycline (AII)	Azithromycin, erythromycin, ofloxacin
	Inclusion conjunctivitis of newborn	Azithromycin (AIII)	Erythromycin
	Pneumonia of infancy	Azithromycin (AIII)	Erythromycin, ampicillin
	Trachoma	Azithromycin (AI)	Doxycycline, erythromycin
Chlamydophila (formerly Chlamydia) pneumoniae[49,50,52]	Pneumonia	Azithromycin (AII); erythromycin (AII)	Doxycycline, levofloxacin
Chlamydophila (formerly Chlamydia) psittaci[53]	Psittacosis, pneumonia	Doxycycline (AII) for >7 y; azithromycin (AIII) OR erythromycin (AIII) for ≤7 y	Levofloxacin
Chromobacterium violaceum[54-56]	Sepsis, pneumonia, abscesses	Meropenem ± ciprofloxacin depending on severity of the disease (AIII)	Susceptibility is variable. Other options may include TMP/SMX, cefepime, amikacin, imipenem, ceftriaxone, ceftazidime, and PIP/TAZO.
Citrobacter koseri (formerly diversus), freundii[57,58]	Meningitis; sepsis	C freundii may develop ampC-mediated resistance to 3rd-generation cephalosporins after exposure to these antibiotics; cefepime should be active against most ampC BL-expressing strains; meropenem will be active against both ampC and ESBL-expressing strains.	Ciprofloxacin, PIP/TAZO, ceftriaxone AND gentamicin, TMP/SMX, colistin Carbapenem-resistant strains now reported; may be susceptible to CAZ/AVI, mero/vabor, IMI/REL, or cefiderocol[5,57]

Clostridioides (formerly Clostridium) difficile[59-61]	Antibiotic-associated colitis See Clostridioides difficile in Table 1H under Diarrhea/Gastroenteritis.	Treatment stratified by severity and recurrence For the initial episode Mild to moderate illness: metronidazole PO or vancomycin PO Severe illness: vancomycin PO or fidaxomicin PO[62] Severe and complicated/systemic illness: vancomycin PO or fidaxomicin PO AND metronidazole IV ± vancomycin per rectum	Stop the predisposing antimicrobial therapy, if possible. For relapsing C difficile enteritis, consider pulse therapy with vancomycin (1 wk on/1 wk off for 3–4 cycles) or prolonged tapering therapy. No pediatric data on fecal transplant for recurrent disease. Bezlotoxumab can be considered to reduce the chance of recurrence in high-risk patients.
Clostridium botulinum[63-65]	Botulism: foodborne; wound; potentially bioterror related	Botulism antitoxin heptavalent (equine) types A–G FDA approved in 2013 No antibiotic treatment except for wound botulism when debridement and treatment for vegetative organisms should be provided after antitoxin is administered (penicillin G or metronidazole) (no controlled data)	For more information, call your state health department or the CDC clinical emergency botulism service, 770-488-7100 (www.cdc.gov/botulism/treatment/index.html; accessed October 21, 2024). For bioterror public exposure, treatment recommendations will be emergently posted on the CDC website.
	Infant botulism	Human botulism immune globulin for infants (BabyBIG) (AII) No antibiotic treatment	BabyBIG available nationally from the California Department of Public Health at 510-231-7600 (https://infantbotulism.org; accessed November 11, 2024).

D. PREFERRED THERAPY FOR SPECIFIC BACTERIAL AND MYCOBACTERIAL PATHOGENS; PLEASE CHECK CULTURE SUSCEPTIBILITY PANEL RESULTS FOR INDIVIDUAL CHILDREN

Organism	Clinical Illness	Drug of Choice (evidence grade)	Alternatives
Clostridium perfringens[66,67]	Gas gangrene/necrotizing fasciitis/sepsis (also caused by Clostridium sordellii, septicum, novyi) Food poisoning	Penicillin G AND clindamycin for invasive infection (BII); no antimicrobials indicated for foodborne illness. The clindamycin is recommended by some experts to inhibit toxin production.	Meropenem, metronidazole, clindamycin monotherapy No defined benefit of hyperbaric oxygen over aggressive surgery/antibiotic therapy
Clostridium tetani[68–70]	Tetanus	TIG 500 U (previously 3,000–6,000 U) IM, with part injected directly into the wound (IVIG at 200–400 mg/kg if TIG not available) Metronidazole (AIII) OR penicillin G (BIII)	Prophylaxis for contaminated wounds: 250 U IM for those with <3 tetanus immunizations. Start/continue immunization for tetanus. Alternative antibiotics: meropenem, doxycycline, clindamycin.
Corynebacterium diphtheriae[71]	Diphtheria	Diphtheria equine antitoxin (available through the CDC Emergency Operations Center, 770-488-7100, under an investigational protocol [www.cdc.gov/diphtheria/hcp/dat/index.html; accessed October 21, 2024) AND erythromycin or penicillin G (AIII)	Antitoxin protocol: www.cdc.gov/diphtheria/downloads/protocol.pdf (version 12.0; February 9, 2023; accessed October 21, 2024)
Corynebacterium jeikeium[72,73]	Sepsis, endocarditis, nosocomial infections	Vancomycin (AIII)	Daptomycin (emerging resistance reported), tigecycline, linezolid
Corynebacterium minutissimum[74,75]	Erythrasma; bacteremia in compromised hosts	Erythromycin or clindamycin PO for erythrasma (BIII); OR, for bacteremia,[75] vancomycin OR penicillin IV (BIII)	Topical 1% clindamycin for cutaneous infection; meropenem, penicillin/ampicillin, ciprofloxacin

Organism	Infection/Comment	Preferred Therapy	Alternative Therapy
Coxiella burnetii[76,77]	Q fever See Q fever in Table 1L.	Acute infection: doxycycline (all ages) (AII) Chronic infection or endocarditis (course not well-defined): doxycycline for children >7 y AND hydroxychloroquine for 18–36 mo	Alternative for acute infection: TMP/SMX Alternative for chronic infection: TMP/SMX AND doxycycline (BII); OR levofloxacin AND rifampin
Cutibacterium (formerly *Propionibacterium*) *acnes*[78,79]	In addition to acne, invasive infection: sepsis, postoperative wound/shunt infection	Penicillin G (AIII); vancomycin (AIII)	Ceftriaxone, doxycycline, clindamycin, linezolid, daptomycin Resistant to metronidazole
Ehrlichia chaffeensis,[14,80] *muris*[80,81]	Human monocytic ehrlichiosis	Doxycycline (all ages) (AII)	Rifampin
Ehrlichia ewingii[14,80]	*E ewingii* ehrlichiosis	Doxycycline (all ages) (AII)	Rifampin
Eikenella corrodens[82,83]	Human bite wounds; respiratory tract and GI tract abscesses, meningitis, endocarditis	Amox/clav PO; ceftriaxone; meropenem/imipenem For BL-negative strains: ampicillin; penicillin G (BIII)	PIP/TAZO, amp/sul, ciprofloxacin Resistant to clindamycin, cephalexin, erythromycin
Elizabethkingia (formerly *Chryseobacterium*) *meningoseptica*[84,85]	Sepsis, meningitis (particularly in neonates)	Levofloxacin; TMP/SMX (BIII)	PIP/TAZO, minocycline, vancomycin. Rifampin may be added to another active drug.
Enterobacter spp[5,57,58,86-89]	Sepsis, pneumonia, wound infection, UTI	Cefepime; meropenem; PIP/TAZO (BII)	CAZ/AVI, ertapenem, imipenem, ceftriaxone AND gentamicin, TMP/SMX, ciprofloxacin Emerging carbapenem-resistant strains worldwide[89]

Preferred Therapy for Bacterial & Mycobacterial Pathogens

D. PREFERRED THERAPY FOR SPECIFIC BACTERIAL AND MYCOBACTERIAL PATHOGENS; PLEASE CHECK CULTURE SUSCEPTIBILITY PANEL RESULTS FOR INDIVIDUAL CHILDREN

Organism	Clinical Illness	Drug of Choice (evidence grade)	Alternatives
Enterococcus spp[90-92]	Endocarditis, UTI, intra-abdominal abscess	Ampicillin AND gentamicin (AI), OR vancomycin AND gentamicin (for ampicillin-resistant strains); bactericidal activity present only with combination. Ampicillin AND ceftriaxone in combination also effective[92,93]	For strains resistant to gentamicin on synergy testing, use streptomycin or other active aminoglycoside for invasive infections. For vancomycin-resistant strains that are also ampicillin resistant: daptomycin OR linezolid.[91,92]
Erysipelothrix rhusiopathiae[94]	Cellulitis (erysipeloid), sepsis, abscesses, endocarditis	Invasive infection: ampicillin (BIII); penicillin G; ceftriaxone, meropenem (BIII) Cutaneous infection: penicillin V; amoxicillin; cephalexin; clindamycin	Resistance to penicillin reported. Ciprofloxacin, erythromycin. Resistant to vancomycin, daptomycin, TMP/SMX.
Escherichia coli (See Ch 1 for specific infection entities and references.) Increasing resistance to 3rd-generation cephalosporins due to ESBLs and to carbapenems due to carbapenemases (KPC)[4,5,88,89] See Ch 12.	UTI, community acquired, not hospital acquired	A 1st-, 2nd-, or 3rd-generation cephalosporin PO, IM as empiric therapy (BI)	Amoxicillin; TMP/SMX if susceptible. Ciprofloxacin if resistant to other options. For hospital-acquired UTI, review hospital antibiogram for best empiric choices.
	TD	Azithromycin (AII)	Rifaximin (for nonfebrile, non-bloody diarrhea for children >11 y); cefixime, ciprofloxacin

Sepsis, pneumonia, hospital-acquired UTI	A 2nd-, 3rd-, or 4th-generation cephalosporin IV (BI)	For AmpC-producing strains (ceftriaxone-resistant): cefepime; for ESBL-producing strains: meropenem (AIII) or other carbapenem; PIP/TAZO and ciprofloxacin if resistant to other antibiotics For KPC-producing strains (meropenem-resistant): CAZ/AVI
Meningitis	Ceftriaxone or cefepime (AIII)	For ESBL-producing strains: meropenem (AIII)
Francisella tularensis[95,96] Tularemia	Gentamicin (AII) for invasive disease	Convalescent PO therapy, or treatment of mild disease with doxycycline, ciprofloxacin. Resistant to β-lactam antibiotics. Watch for relapse.
Fusobacterium spp[97-99] Sepsis, soft tissue infection, Lemierre syndrome (See Ch 1.)	Metronidazole (AIII) or clindamycin AND ceftriaxone; meropenem monotherapy is a reasonable option (BIII).	Penicillin G, PIP/TAZO. Combinations often used for Lemierre syndrome. Anticoagulation for ongoing thromboembolic complications.
Gardnerella vaginalis[51,100] Bacterial vaginosis	Metronidazole (BII)	Tinidazole, clindamycin, metronidazole gel, clindamycin cream/gel
Haemophilus ducreyi[51] Chancroid	Azithromycin (AIII); ceftriaxone (BIII)	Erythromycin, ciprofloxacin

D. PREFERRED THERAPY FOR SPECIFIC BACTERIAL AND MYCOBACTERIAL PATHOGENS; PLEASE CHECK CULTURE SUSCEPTIBILITY PANEL RESULTS FOR INDIVIDUAL CHILDREN

Organism	Clinical Illness	Drug of Choice (evidence grade)	Alternatives
Haemophilus influenzae[101]	Nonencapsulated strains: URTIs (otitis media, sinusitis)	BL negative: ampicillin IV (AI); amoxicillin PO (AI) BL positive: ceftriaxone IV, IM (AI); amox/clav (AI) OR 2nd- or 3rd-generation cephalosporins PO (AI)	Levofloxacin, azithromycin, TMP/SMX
	Type b strains in unimmunized children: meningitis, arthritis, cellulitis, epiglottitis, pneumonia	BL negative: ampicillin IV (AI); amoxicillin PO (AI) BL positive: ceftriaxone IV, IM (AI) or cefepime IV; amox/clav (AI) OR 2nd- or 3rd-generation cephalosporins PO (AI)	Other regimens: meropenem IV, levofloxacin IV Full IV course (10 days) for meningitis, but PO step-down therapy well-documented after response to treatment of non-CNS infections Levofloxacin PO as step-down therapy for BL-positive strains
Helicobacter pylori[102-104] See Gastritis in Table 1H under Diarrhea/Gastroenteritis.	Gastritis, peptic ulcer	Triple-agent therapy: clarithromycin (susceptible strains) AND amoxicillin AND omeprazole (AII); ADD metronidazole for suspected resistance to clarithromycin.	For clarithromycin/metronidazole resistance, tetracycline for children >7 y. Other regimens include bismuth in addition to other proton pump inhibitors.
Kingella kingae[105,106]	Osteomyelitis, arthritis	Ampicillin; penicillin G (AII)	Cefazolin, ceftriaxone, TMP/SMX, cefuroxime, ceftaroline, ciprofloxacin. Resistant to clindamycin, vancomycin, linezolid.

Klebsiella spp (*Klebsiella pneumoniae, oxytoca*)[88,89,107–110] *Increasing resistance to 3rd-generation cephalosporins (ESBLs) and carbapenems (KPC), as well as to colistin* See Ch 12.	UTI	A 2nd- or 3rd-generation cephalosporin (AII)	Use most narrow-spectrum agent active against pathogen: TMP/SMX, ciprofloxacin, gentamicin. ESBL producers should be treated with a carbapenem (meropenem, ertapenem, imipenem), but KPC (carbapenemase)-containing bacteria may require ciprofloxacin, CAZ/AVI, colistin.[108,109]
	Sepsis, pneumonia, meningitis, hospital-acquired infection	Ceftriaxone; cefepime (AIII) For carbapenem-resistant KPC strains: CAZ/AVI, mero/vabor, or IMI/REL. For carbapenem-resistant NDM strains, use aztreonam AND CAZ/AVI.	Carbapenem or ciprofloxacin if resistant to other routine antibiotics. Meningitis caused by ESBL producer: meropenem if susceptible. KPC (carbapenemase) producers: ciprofloxacin, colistin, cefiderocol, OR CAZ/AVI (approved by the FDA for children in 2019 and active against current strains of KPC[108–110]). NDMs, VIMs, and IMPs are MBLs resistant to CAZ/AVI, requiring both aztreonam (stable to MBL) AND CAZ/AVI (stable to AmpC and ESBL).
Klebsiella granulomatis[51]	Granuloma inguinale	Azithromycin (AII)	Doxycycline, TMP/SMX, ciprofloxacin
Legionella spp[111]	Legionnaires disease	Azithromycin (AI) OR levofloxacin (AII)	Erythromycin, clarithromycin, TMP/SMX, doxycycline
Leptospira spp[112]	Leptospirosis	Penicillin G IV (AII); ceftriaxone IV (AII)	PO therapy: amoxicillin, doxycycline, azithromycin

3

Preferred Therapy for Bacterial & Mycobacterial Pathogens

3

D. PREFERRED THERAPY FOR SPECIFIC BACTERIAL AND MYCOBACTERIAL PATHOGENS; PLEASE CHECK CULTURE SUSCEPTIBILITY PANEL RESULTS FOR INDIVIDUAL CHILDREN

Organism	Clinical Illness	Drug of Choice (evidence grade)	Alternatives
Leuconostoc[113]	Bacteremia	Penicillin G (AIII); ampicillin (BIII)	Clindamycin, erythromycin, doxycycline (uniformly resistant to vancomycin)
Listeria monocytogenes[114]	Sepsis, meningitis in compromised host; neonatal sepsis	Ampicillin (ADD gentamicin for severe infection, compromised hosts including neonates [new retrospective data in hospitalized adults suggest no benefit from added gentamicin].)[115] (AII)	Ampicillin AND TMP/SMX; ampicillin AND linezolid; levofloxacin. Resistant to cephalosporins including ceftriaxone
Moraxella catarrhalis[116]	Otitis, sinusitis, bronchitis	Amox/clav (AI), as most are BL positive	TMP/SMX; a 2nd- or 3rd-generation cephalosporin
Morganella morganii[57,58,87,117,118]	UTI, neonatal sepsis, wound infection	Cefepime (AIII); meropenem (AIII); levofloxacin (BIII)	Intrinsically resistant to penicillin/ ampicillin and colistin. PIP/TAZO, ceftriaxone AND gentamicin, ciprofloxacin, TMP/ SMX. Has intrinsic inducible ampC BL; 3rd-generation cephalosporins may be selected for resistance. MBLs resistant to CAZ/AVI, requiring both aztreonam (stable to MBL) AND CAZ/AVI (stable to AmpC and ESBL), are now emerging.

| _Mycobacterium abscessus_[119-125] 3 subspecies now identified (_abscessus, bolletii, massiliense_) | Skin and soft tissue infections; pneumonia | All clinical illness presentations: initial treatment depends on whether there is macrolide (eg, clarithromycin or azithromycin) resistance. For susceptible isolates, initial therapy should include azithromycin OR clarithromycin plus amikacin OR imipenem OR cefoxitin plus 2 of the following: omadacycline OR tigecycline, tedizolid OR linezolid, clofazimine. For macrolide-resistant isolates, initial therapy should include amikacin plus imipenem OR cefoxitin plus 2 of the following: omadacycline OR tigecycline, tedizolid OR linezolid, clofazimine. For pneumonia: same as above for initial treatment. Continuation phase: may consider nebulized amikacin AND 2–3 of the following antibiotics guided by drug susceptibility results and patient tolerance: clofazimine, linezolid PO OR tedizolid PO, omadacycline OR, possibly, bedaquiline.[120,123,125] Treatment is for at least 12 mo after sputum cultures become negative. All other forms of disease are treated for at least 6–12 mo. | For patients with pulmonary disease, the decision to treat is based on clinical symptoms, comorbidities, and radiographic and microbiologic findings. All patients with non-pulmonary disease should be treated. Consider consulting an ID physician. Should test for susceptibility to all possible antibiotic options listed as well as cefoxitin. May need pulmonary resection. Initial intensive phase of therapy followed by months of "maintenance" therapy. |

3

Preferred Therapy for Bacterial & Mycobacterial Pathogens

3

D. PREFERRED THERAPY FOR SPECIFIC BACTERIAL AND MYCOBACTERIAL PATHOGENS; PLEASE CHECK CULTURE SUSCEPTIBILITY PANEL RESULTS FOR INDIVIDUAL CHILDREN

Organism	Clinical Illness	Drug of Choice (evidence grade)	Alternatives
Mycobacterium avium complex[119,124,126]	Cervical adenitis	Clarithromycin (AII); azithromycin (AII)	Surgical excision is more likely than sole medical therapy to lead to cure. May increase cure rate with addition of rifampin or ethambutol.
	Pneumonia	For pneumonia, ADD rifampin AND ethambutol AND, for severe disease, amikacin (AIII).[123]	Depending on susceptibilities and severity of the illness, ADD amikacin ± ciprofloxacin.
	Disseminated disease in competent host, or disease in immunocompromised host	Clarithromycin or azithromycin AND ethambutol AND rifampin (AIII), AND, for severe disease, amikacin	Depending on susceptibilities and severity of the illness, ADD additional agents.
Mycobacterium bovis[127-129]	TB (historically not microbiologically or clinically differentiated from Mycobacterium tuberculosis infection; causes adenitis, abdominal TB, meningitis)	INH AND rifampin (AII); ADD ethambutol for suspected resistance (AIII).	M bovis is always resistant to PZA. Consider ADDING streptomycin for severe infection.
Mycobacterium chelonae[119,130]	Abscesses; catheter infection	Clarithromycin or azithromycin (AIII); ADD amikacin for invasive disease, ± imipenem if susceptible (AIII).	Also test for susceptibility to tigecycline, TMP/SMX, doxycycline, tobramycin, imipenem (more active than meropenem),[130] moxifloxacin, linezolid.
Mycobacterium fortuitum complex[118,119,124,126,130]	Skin and soft tissue infections; catheter infection	Amikacin AND cefoxitin ± levofloxacin (AIII)	Also test for susceptibility to clarithromycin, imipenem, tigecycline, minocycline, sulfonamides, doxycycline, linezolid.

Mycobacterium leprae[131]	Leprosy	Dapsone AND rifampin for paucibacillary (1–5 patches) (AII). ADD clofazimine for lepromatous, multibacillary (>5 patches) disease (AII).	Consult HRSA (National Hansen's Disease [Leprosy] Program) at www.hrsa.gov/hansens-disease for advice about treatment and free antibiotics: 800-642-2477 (reviewed August 2024; accessed October 21, 2024).
Mycobacterium marinum, balnei[119,132]	Papules, pustules, abscesses (swimming pool granuloma)	Clarithromycin ± ethambutol (AIII)	TMP/SMX AND rifampin; ethambutol AND rifampin, doxycycline ± 1 or 2 additional antibiotics Surgical debridement
Mycobacterium tuberculosis[127,133] See Tuberculosis in Ch 1 for detailed recommendations for active infection, latent infection, and exposures in high-risk children.	TB (pneumonia; meningitis; cervical adenitis; mesenteric adenitis; osteomyelitis)	For active infection in children without risk factors for resistance: INH AND rifampin AND PZA (AI); ADD ethambutol for suspected resistance. For latent infection: INH AND rifapentine once weekly for 12 wk (AII) OR rifampin daily for 4 mo, OR INH/rifampin combination *daily* (all ages) for 3 mo OR INH daily or biweekly for 9 mo (AII).	Add streptomycin for severe infection. For MDR TB, bedaquiline is FDA approved for adults and for children ≥5 y. The 3-drug PO combination of pretomanid, bedaquiline, and linezolid has orphan drug approval for MDR TB in adults, to be taken together for 26 wk. Corticosteroids should be added to regimens for meningitis, mesenteric adenitis, and endobronchial infection (AIII).
Mycoplasma hominis[51,134,135]	Neonatal infection including meningitis/ventriculitis; nongonococcal urethritis	Neonates: doxycycline; moxifloxacin Urethritis: clindamycin (AIII)	Usually erythromycin resistant
Mycoplasma pneumoniae[136,137]	Pneumonia	Azithromycin (AI); erythromycin (BI); macrolide resistance emerging worldwide[138]	Doxycycline and FQs are usually active against macrolide-susceptible and macrolide-resistant strains.

Preferred Therapy for Bacterial & Mycobacterial Pathogens

3

D. PREFERRED THERAPY FOR SPECIFIC BACTERIAL AND MYCOBACTERIAL PATHOGENS; PLEASE CHECK CULTURE SUSCEPTIBILITY PANEL RESULTS FOR INDIVIDUAL CHILDREN

Organism	Clinical Illness	Drug of Choice (evidence grade)	Alternatives
Neisseria gonorrhoeae[51,139] See Gonorrhea in Table 1I.	Gonorrhea; arthritis	Formerly, ceftriaxone AND azithromycin or doxycycline (AIII), but in 2020, due to increasing resistance to azithromycin (4% in adults), only ceftriaxone is now routinely recommended.	PO cefixime as single-drug therapy is no longer routinely recommended due to increasing resistance but can be used when ceftriaxone cannot.[139] Gentamicin IM + azithromycin for type I allergy to cephalosporins.
Neisseria meningitidis[140,141]	Sepsis, meningitis	Ceftriaxone (AI)	Penicillin G or ampicillin if susceptible with amoxicillin step-down therapy for non-CNS infection For prophylaxis following exposure: rifampin or ciprofloxacin (ciprofloxacin-resistant strains are now reported). Azithromycin may be less effective.
Nocardia asteroides, brasiliensis[142,143]	Pneumonia with abscess, cutaneous cellulitis/abscess, brain abscess	TMP/SMX (AII); sulfisoxazole (BII); for severe infection, ADD imipenem or meropenem AND amikacin (AII).	Linezolid, ceftriaxone, clarithromycin, minocycline, levofloxacin, tigecycline, amox/clav
Pasteurella multocida[144,145]	Sepsis, abscesses, animal bite wound	Penicillin G (AIII); ampicillin (AIII); amoxicillin (AIII)	Amox/clav, PIP/TAZO, doxycycline, ceftriaxone, cefpodoxime, cefuroxime, TMP/SMX, levofloxacin. Cephalexin may not demonstrate adequate activity. Not usually susceptible to clindamycin or erythromycin.

Peptostreptococcus[146]	Sepsis, deep head/neck space and IAI	Penicillin G (AII); ampicillin (AII)	Clindamycin, vancomycin, meropenem, imipenem, metronidazole
Plesiomonas shigelloides[147,148]	Diarrhea, neonatal sepsis, meningitis	Antibiotics may not be necessary to treat diarrhea: amox/clav PO or ciprofloxacin PO (BIII); 2nd- and 3rd-generation cephalosporins (AIII); azithromycin (BII). For meningitis/sepsis: ceftriaxone.	Meropenem Increasing resistance to TMP/SMX
Prevotella (formerly *Bacteroides*) spp,[149] *melaninogenica*	Deep head/neck space abscess; dental abscess	Metronidazole or clindamycin (AII)	PIP/TAZO, cefoxitin, meropenem or imipenem (AII)
Propionibacterium (now *Cutibacterium*) *acnes*[78,79]	In addition to acne, invasive infection: sepsis, postoperative wound/shunt infection	Penicillin G (AIII); vancomycin (AIII)	Ceftriaxone, doxycycline, clindamycin, linezolid, daptomycin Resistant to metronidazole
Proteus mirabilis[150]	UTI, sepsis, meningitis	Ceftriaxone (AII) for AmpC-negative, ESBL-negative strains; cefepime for AmpC-positive, ESBL-negative strains; carbapenem for ESBL-positive strains PO therapy: amox/clav; TMP/SMX, ciprofloxacin	PIP/TAZO; cefiderocol; increasing resistance to TMP/SMX and FQs, particularly in nosocomial isolates Rarely contain plasmid-mediated ampC BL Colistin resistant
Proteus vulgaris, other spp (indole-positive strains)[4–6,57,58,88]	UTI, sepsis, meningitis	Cefepime for AmpC-positive, ESBL-negative strains; meropenem for ESBL producers. Ciprofloxacin; gentamicin if susceptible (BIII). Potential ampC hyperproducer (and some strains with ESBLs), so at risk for resistance to 3rd-generation cephalosporins.	Imipenem, ertapenem, TMP/SMX, cefiderocol, CAZ/AVI for carbapenem resistance Colistin resistant

D. PREFERRED THERAPY FOR SPECIFIC BACTERIAL AND MYCOBACTERIAL PATHOGENS; PLEASE CHECK CULTURE SUSCEPTIBILITY PANEL RESULTS FOR INDIVIDUAL CHILDREN

Organism	Clinical Illness	Drug of Choice (evidence grade)	Alternatives
Providencia spp[57,58,151]	Sepsis	Cefepime; ciprofloxacin, PIP/TAZO, gentamicin (BIII)	Meropenem or other carbapenem for ESBL producer; TMP/SMX; CAZ/AVI for carbapenem resistance Colistin and tigecycline resistant
Pseudomonas aeruginosa[152–154]	UTI	Ceftazidime or cefepime (AII); other antipseudomonal β-lactams; tobramycin	Amikacin, ciprofloxacin
	Nosocomial sepsis, pneumonia	Cefepime (AI), OR meropenem (AI), OR PIP/TAZO AND tobramycin (BI), OR ceftazidime AND tobramycin (BII)	Ciprofloxacin AND tobramycin; cefiderocol; colistin.[57] There is controversy regarding additional clinical benefit in outcomes with combination therapy (including β-lactam/aminoglycoside combinations or double β-lactam combinations), but combinations may increase the likelihood of empiric active coverage and decrease the emergence of resistance.[155–157] Prolonged infusion of β-lactam antibiotics will allow greater therapeutic exposure to high-MIC pathogens.

Pneumonia in CF[158-161] See Cystic Fibrosis in Table 1F.	Cefepime (AII) or meropenem (AII); OR ceftazidime AND tobramycin (BII) (AI). Azithromycin provides benefit in prolonging interval between exacerbations.	Inhalational antibiotics for prevention of acute exacerbations (but insufficient evidence to recommend for treatment of exacerbation): tobramycin; aztreonam; colistin. Many organisms are MDR.

Pseudomonas cepacia, mallei, pseudomallei (See *Burkholderia* entries earlier in this table.)

Ralstonia[162]	Bacteremia, pneumonia, meningitis, osteomyelitis	Ciprofloxacin, meropenem, ceftazidime, TMP/SMX	Often resistant to β-lactams, aminoglycosides. Data lacking on preferred therapeutic regimen.
Rhodococcus (formerly *equi*) *hoagii*[163]	Necrotizing pneumonia	Vancomycin AND imipenem for immunocompromised hosts, single-drug therapy for normal hosts (AIII)	Ciprofloxacin or levofloxacin AND azithromycin or rifampin; doxycycline; linezolid
Rickettsia[164,165]	Rocky Mountain spotted fever, Q fever, typhus, rickettsialpox, *Ehrlichia* infection, *Anaplasma* infection	Doxycycline (all ages) (AII)	Chloramphenicol is less effective than doxycycline. A single course of doxycycline is not associated with detectable dental staining.
Salmonella, non-typhoid spp[166-168] See Salmonellosis in Table 1H under Diarrhea/Gastroenteritis.	Gastroenteritis (may not require therapy if clinically improving and not immunocompromised). Consider treatment for those with higher risk for invasion (<1 y [or, with highest risk, those <3 mo], immunocompromised, and with focal infections or bacteremia).	Azithromycin (AII) OR ciprofloxacin OR ceftriaxone (AII)	For susceptible strains when culture results are available: cefixime (AII), TMP/SMX; ampicillin

D. PREFERRED THERAPY FOR SPECIFIC BACTERIAL AND MYCOBACTERIAL PATHOGENS; PLEASE CHECK CULTURE SUSCEPTIBILITY PANEL RESULTS FOR INDIVIDUAL CHILDREN

Organism	Clinical Illness	Drug of Choice (evidence grade)	Alternatives
Salmonella typhi[167,169,170] See Salmonellosis in Table 1H under Diarrhea/Gastroenteritis.	Typhoid fever	Azithromycin (AIII); ceftriaxone (AII); cefixime (AII); TMP/SMX (AIII); ciprofloxacin (AII)	Obtain blood and stool cultures before treatment to allow for selection of most narrow-spectrum antibiotic. Prefer antibiotics with high intracellular concentrations (eg, TMP/SMX, FQs). Amoxicillin acceptable for susceptible strains.
Serratia marcescens[57,58,87-89]	Nosocomial sepsis, pneumonia	Cefepime; meropenem; PIP/TAZO (BII) Potential AmpC constitutive producer (and some strains with ESBLs)	One of the enteric bacilli that have inducible chromosomal AmpC BLs (active against 1st-, 2nd-, and 3rd-generation cephalosporins) that may be constitutively produced by organisms within a population; ertapenem, imipenem; TMP/SMX, ciprofloxacin, ceftriaxone AND gentamicin Resistant to colistin
Shewanella spp[171,172]	Wound infection, nosocomial pneumonia, peritoneal-dialysis peritonitis, ventricular shunt infection, neonatal sepsis	Ceftazidime (AIII)	Cefepime, meropenem, PIP/TAZO, amp/sul, ciprofloxacin, gentamicin Resistant to TMP/SMX and colistin

Organism	Infection	Therapy	Comments
Shigella spp[173-176]	Enteritis, UTI, prepubertal vaginitis	Mild episodes of enteritis do not require treatment. Azithromycin (unless local resistance is high) OR ciprofloxacin OR cefixime OR ceftriaxone.[176]	Substantial (>30%) resistance to azithromycin now reported in the United States, with ciprofloxacin resistance up to 15% but ceftriaxone resistance low at 5%.[176] Use most narrow-spectrum agent active against pathogen: PO ampicillin (not amoxicillin for enteritis); TMP/SMX.
Sphingomonas paucimobilis[177,178]	Bacteremia, wound infection, ocular infection, osteomyelitis	Antipseudomonal penicillins, carbapenems (BIII)	Aminoglycosides, TMP/SMX
Spirillum minus[179]	Rat-bite fever (sodoku)	Penicillin G IV (AII); for endocarditis, ADD gentamicin or streptomycin (AIII).	Ampicillin, doxycycline, ceftriaxone, vancomycin, streptomycin
Staphylococcus aureus (See Ch 1 for specific infections.)[180,181]			
- Mild to moderate infections	Skin infections, mild to moderate	MSSA: a 1st-generation cephalosporin (cefazolin IV, cephalexin PO) (AI); oxacillin/nafcillin IV (AI), dicloxacillin PO (AI) MRSA: clindamycin (if susceptible) IV or PO, ceftaroline IV;[182] vancomycin IV, or TMP/SMX PO (AII)	For MSSA: amox/clav. For CA-MRSA: linezolid IV, PO; daptomycin IV has been studied and FDA approved for use in children >1 y.[183]

3

D. PREFERRED THERAPY FOR SPECIFIC BACTERIAL AND MYCOBACTERIAL PATHOGENS; PLEASE CHECK CULTURE SUSCEPTIBILITY PANEL RESULTS FOR INDIVIDUAL CHILDREN

Organism	Clinical Illness	Drug of Choice (evidence grade)	Alternatives
- Moderate to severe infections, empiric treatment of CA-MRSA	Pneumonia, sepsis, myositis, osteomyelitis, etc	MSSA: oxacillin/nafcillin IV (AI); a 1st-generation cephalosporin (cefazolin IV) ± gentamicin (AII) MRSA: clindamycin (if susceptible) (AII) OR ceftaroline (AII) OR vancomycin if MIC is ≤2 (AII)[184] Combination therapy with gentamicin and/or rifampin not prospectively studied	For CA-MRSA: linezolid (AII); OR daptomycin[185] for non-pulmonary infection (AII) (studies published on use in children); ceftaroline IV (FDA approved for children) Approved for adults (primarily for treatment of MRSA): dalbavancin (once-weekly dosing), oritavancin (once-weekly dosing), tedizolid (See Ch 12.)
Staphylococcus, coagulase-negative[186,187]	Nosocomial bacteremia (neonatal bacteremia), infected intravascular catheters, CNS shunts, UTI	Empiric: vancomycin (AII) OR ceftaroline (AII)	If susceptible: linezolid; ceftaroline IV; daptomycin for age >1 y (but not for pneumonia)
Stenotrophomonas maltophilia[188–190]	Sepsis	TMP/SMX (AII)	Levofloxacin, doxycycline, minocycline, tigecycline, colistin, and cefiderocol.[190] Consider CAZ/AVI plus aztreonam for severe infection.[88]
Streptobacillus moniliformis[179,191]	Rat-bite fever (Haverhill fever)	Penicillin G (AIII); ampicillin (AIII); for endocarditis, ADD gentamicin or streptomycin (AIII).	Doxycycline, ceftriaxone, carbapenems, clindamycin, vancomycin

Streptococcus, group A[192]	Pharyngitis, impetigo, adenitis, cellulitis, necrotizing fasciitis	A 1st-generation cephalosporin (cefazolin or cephalexin) (AI), clindamycin (AI), a macrolide (AI), vancomycin (AIII). For recurrent strep pharyngitis, clindamycin or amox/clav, or the addition of rifampin to the last 4 days of penicillin therapy (AIII). The addition of clindamycin or linezolid may decrease toxin production in overwhelming infection.
Streptococcus, group B[193]	Neonatal sepsis, pneumonia, meningitis	Penicillin (AII) or ampicillin (AII)	Gentamicin can be used until a clinical/microbiologic response has been documented (AIII).
Streptococcus milleri/anginosus group (*intermedius, anginosus*, and *constellatus*; includes some β-hemolytic group C and group G streptococci)[194–196]	Pneumonia, sepsis, skin and soft tissue infection,[194,195] sinusitis,[197] arthritis, brain abscess, epidural abscess, subdural empyema, meningitis	Penicillin G (AIII); ampicillin (AIII); ADD gentamicin for serious infection (AIII); ceftriaxone. Many strains show decreased susceptibility to penicillin, requiring higher dosages to achieve adequate antibiotic exposure, particularly in the CNS.	Clindamycin, vancomycin
Streptococcus, viridans group (α-hemolytic streptococci, most commonly *Streptococcus sanguinis, oralis* [*mitis*], *salivarius, mutans, morbillorum*)	Endocarditis[198], oropharyngeal, deep head/neck space infections	Penicillin G ± gentamicin (AII) OR ceftriaxone ± gentamicin (AII)	Vancomycin

Preferred Therapy for Bacterial & Mycobacterial Pathogens

D. PREFERRED THERAPY FOR SPECIFIC BACTERIAL AND MYCOBACTERIAL PATHOGENS; PLEASE CHECK CULTURE SUSCEPTIBILITY PANEL RESULTS FOR INDIVIDUAL CHILDREN

Organism	Clinical Illness	Drug of Choice (evidence grade)	Alternatives
Streptococcus pneumoniae[199-201] With widespread use of conjugate pneumococcal vaccines, antibiotic resistance in pneumococci has decreased.[201]	Sinusitis, otitis (outpatient)[202]	Amoxicillin, with or without clavulanate, for first-line therapy. (Adult guidelines recommend amox/clav as first-line therapy.)	Consider initial use of amoxicillin at high dosage (90 mg/kg/day div bid), especially for children at risk for pen-R strains or more than "mild" infection. Other options include cefdinir, with or without clindamycin; doxycycline (age >8 y); or levofloxacin.
	Meningitis	Ceftriaxone (AI); consider addition of vancomycin (ie, ceftriaxone-resistant strains are not common in the post-PCV13 era [AIII]). Vancomycin may not be required. If started, discontinue as soon as susceptibilities are available.	Penicillin G alone for pen-S strains; ceftriaxone alone for ceftriaxone-susceptible strains, but can be given qd for outpatient management for pen-S strains. Corticosteroids may be considered if given concurrently with the first dose of antimicrobial agents, although data are lacking to support this approach.
	Pneumonia, osteomyelitis/arthritis,[199,201] sepsis	Ampicillin (AII); ceftriaxone (AI)	Penicillin G alone for pen-S strains; ceftriaxone alone for ceftriaxone-susceptible strains and for outpatient management
Treponema pallidum[51,202]	Syphilis See Chs 1 and 2.	Penicillin G (AII)	Desensitize to penicillin preferred to alternative therapies. Doxycycline, ceftriaxone.

Ureaplasma urealyticum[51,203]	Genitourinary infections	Azithromycin (AII)	Erythromycin; doxycycline, a quinolone (for adolescent genital infections)
	Neonatal pneumonia	Azithromycin (AIII) (effective clearing of *U urealyticum* cultures in preterm neonates demonstrated, but randomized trial to treat pneumonia not yet performed[203])	
Vibrio cholerae[204,205]	Cholera	Doxycycline (AI), single-dose	A single treatment course of doxycycline is not associated with tooth staining. If susceptible, azithromycin (AII): ciprofloxacin (AII).
Vibrio vulnificus[206–208]	Sepsis, necrotizing fasciitis	Doxycycline AND ceftriaxone (AII) or ciprofloxacin AND ceftriaxone.	Doxycycline or ciprofloxacin for severe diarrhea. TMP/SMX AND aminoglycoside as an alternative. Ceftazidime may be used in place of ceftriaxone.
Yersinia enterocolitica[209,210]	Diarrhea, mesenteric enteritis, reactive arthritis, sepsis	TMP/SMX for enteritis (AIII); ceftriaxone or ciprofloxacin for invasive infection (AIII)	Gentamicin, doxycycline
Yersinia pestis[211–213] See Plague in Table 1L.	Plague	Gentamicin (AII) OR ciprofloxacin (AII) for septicemic plague; OR doxycycline for bubonic plague	Levofloxacin, streptomycin Dual therapy for more severe disease or for bioterrorism-related infection
Yersinia pseudotuberculosis[209]	Mesenteric adenitis; Far East scarlet-like fever[214]; reactive arthritis	Ceftriaxone, TMP/SMX, or ciprofloxacin (AIII)	Gentamicin

Preferred Therapy for Bacterial & Mycobacterial Pathogens

4. Choosing Among Antibiotics Within a Class: β-Lactams and β-Lactamase Inhibitors, Macrolides, Aminoglycosides, and Fluoroquinolones

Antibiotics should be compared with others regarding (1) antimicrobial spectrum; (2) degree of antibiotic exposure (a function of the pharmacokinetics [PK] of the nonprotein-bound drug at the site of infection and the pharmacodynamic impact of the drug); (3) demonstrated efficacy in adequate and well-controlled clinical trials; (4) tolerance, toxicity, and side effects; and (5) cost. When a new antibiotic is first approved by regulatory agencies, it is helpful to compare the new agent with other agents based on publicly available data from controlled clinical trials, particularly relevant to antibiotics in the same class if already approved for children. If there is no substantial benefit for efficacy or safety for one antimicrobial over another for the isolated or presumed bacterial pathogen(s), one should opt for using an older, more extensively used agent (with presumably better-defined efficacy and safety) that is usually less expensive and is preferably narrower in its spectrum of activity. If, however, newer agents provide an enhanced spectrum of activity against antibiotic-resistant isolates, they may be necessary for empiric or definitive therapy.

β-Lactams and β-Lactamase Inhibitors

β-Lactam/β-Lactamase Inhibitor (BLI) Combinations. Increasingly studied and approved by the US Food and Drug Administration (FDA) are β-lactam/BLI combinations that target antibiotic resistance for pathogens with resistance to current β-lactams based on the presence of many newly emerging β-lactamases (BLs). The β-lactam antibiotic may have initially demonstrated activity against a pathogen, but if a new BL is present in that pathogen, it will hydrolyze the β-lactam ring structure and inactivate the antibiotic. The BLI is usually a β-lactam structure, which explains why it binds readily to certain BLs and can inhibit their activity; however, the BLI does not usually demonstrate direct antibiotic activity itself (although some BLIs, like sulbactam, which demonstrates antibacterial activity against *Acinetobacter,* have recently been approved in adults and are being studied in children). Just as different β-lactam antibiotics bind bacterial target sites with varying affinity (creating a range of susceptibilities based on their ability to bind and inhibit function), different BLIs will bind the different bacterial BLs with varying affinity. A BLI that binds well to the *Haemophilus influenzae* BL may not bind to and inhibit a *Staphylococcus aureus* BL or may not bind well to one of the many *Pseudomonas* BLs. As amoxicillin and ampicillin were used extensively against *H influenzae* following their approval, resistance increased based on the presence of a BL that hydrolyzes the β-lactam ring of amoxicillin/ampicillin (with up to 40% of isolates currently demonstrating resistance in some regions). Clavulanate, a BLI that binds to and inactivates the *H influenzae* BL, allows amoxicillin/ampicillin to "survive" and inhibit cell wall formation, leading to the death of the organism. The first oral (PO) β-lactam/BLI combination of amoxicillin/clavulanate, originally known as Augmentin, has been very effective. Similar combinations, primarily intravenous (IV), have now been studied, pairing penicillins, cephalosporins, and carbapenems with BLIs such as tazobactam, sulbactam, avibactam, and relebactam as well as with new increasingly broad-spectrum BLIs including vaborbactam, durlobactam, taniborbactam, and many others in development.

β-Lactam Antibiotics

Oral Cephalosporins (cephalexin, cefadroxil, cefaclor, cefprozil, cefuroxime, cefixime, cefdinir, cefpodoxime, cefditoren [tablet only], and ceftibuten). As a class, the PO cephalosporins have the advantage over PO penicillins of somewhat greater spectrum of activity. The serum half-lives of cefpodoxime, ceftibuten, and cefixime are greater than 2 hours. The spectrum of activity for gram-negative organisms increases as one goes from the first-generation cephalosporins (cephalexin and cefadroxil), to the second-generation (cefaclor, cefprozil, and cefuroxime) that demonstrate activity against *H influenzae* (including BL-producing strains), to the third-generation (cefixime, cefdinir, cefpodoxime, cefditoren, and ceftibuten) that have enhanced coverage of many enteric gram-negative bacilli (GNB; eg, *Escherichia coli, Klebsiella* species). However, ceftibuten and cefixime, in particular, have a disadvantage of less activity against *Streptococcus pneumoniae* than the others, particularly against penicillin non-susceptible strains. Currently, no PO cephalosporins exist with activity against the extended-spectrum β-lactamases (ESBLs) of *E coli*/*Klebsiella, Pseudomonas,* or methicillin-resistant *Staphylococcus aureus* (MRSA).

Parenteral Cephalosporins. First-generation cephalosporins, such as cefazolin, are used mainly for treatment of gram-positive infections caused by *S aureus* (excluding MRSA) and group A streptococcus and for surgical prophylaxis; the gram-negative spectrum is limited but more extensive than for ampicillin. Cefazolin is well tolerated by intramuscular or IV injection.

A second-generation cephalosporin (cefuroxime) and the cephamycins (cefoxitin and cefotetan) provide increased activity against many gram-negative organisms, particularly *H influenzae* and *E coli.* Cefoxitin has additional activity against up to 80% of strains of *Bacteroides fragilis.* In empiric therapy for mild to moderate infections at low risk of being caused by *B fragilis,* cefoxitin can be considered for use in place of the more active agents such as metronidazole or carbapenems.

Third-generation cephalosporins (ceftriaxone and ceftazidime) have enhanced potency against many enteric GNB. As with all cephalosporins, though, they are less active against enterococci and *Listeria* at readily achievable serum concentrations. Only ceftazidime has significant activity against *Pseudomonas.* Ceftriaxone has been used very successfully to treat meningitis caused by pneumococcus (mostly penicillin-susceptible strains), *H influenzae* type b, meningococcus, and susceptible strains of *E coli.* Because ceftriaxone is excreted to a large extent by the liver, it can be used with little dosage adjustment in patients with renal failure. With a serum half-life of 4 to 7 hours, it can be given once a day for infections caused by susceptible organisms. Of great importance, ceftazidime has been paired with the broad-spectrum BLI avibactam, which allows activity against both cephalosporin-resistant (ESBL-producing) and carbapenem-resistant (*Klebsiella pneumoniae* carbapenemase [KPC]–producing) gram-negative pathogens.

Cefepime, a fourth-generation cephalosporin approved for use in children in 1999, exhibits (1) enhanced antipseudomonal activity over ceftazidime; (2) the gram-positive activity of second-generation cephalosporins; (3) better activity than earlier generations against enteric GNB; and (4) stability against the inducible ampC BLs of *Enterobacter* (and some strains of *Citrobacter, Proteus,* and *Serratia*) that can hydrolyze third-generation cephalosporins. It can be used as single-drug antibiotic therapy against these pathogens. However, cefepime is hydrolyzed by many of the most widely circulating ESBL enzymes (and carbapenemases) and should not be used if an ESBL *E coli* or *Klebsiella* is suspected.

Ceftaroline and ceftobiprole are fifth-generation cephalosporins, with activity against MRSA. Ceftaroline was approved by the FDA for adults in 2010, approved for children in 2016 for treatment of complicated skin infections (including MRSA) and community-acquired pneumonia (CAP), and approved for neonates in 2019. Ceftobiprole was approved on April 3, 2024, for CAP in children down to 3 months of age, but it is also approved for *S aureus* bacteremia, endocarditis, and skin infections in adults.[1] The PK of ceftaroline have been evaluated in all pediatric age-groups, including neonates, and in children with cystic fibrosis (CF); clinical studies for pediatric CAP and complicated skin infection are published.[2,3] Based on these published data and postmarketing experience for infants and children, we believe that ceftaroline should be as effective as and perhaps safer than vancomycin for treatment of MRSA infections. Just as β-lactams such as cefazolin are preferred treatment over vancomycin for methicillin-susceptible *S aureus* infections, ceftaroline may be preferred over vancomycin for MRSA infection. Neither renal function nor drug levels need to be followed with ceftaroline therapy. Limited PK and clinical data also support the use of ceftaroline in neonates in which coagulase-negative staphylococci are the most common pathogens causing catheter-related bloodstream infections. Experience with ceftobiprole in children is currently limited. Although ceftobiprole is likely to be comparable in efficacy to ceftaroline, it does not provide significant benefits over ceftaroline, so for now, we continue to recommend ceftaroline as the preferred fifth-generation drug.

Cefiderocol[4,5] is an advanced-spectrum cephalosporin, approved for adults with complicated urinary tract infections (cUTIs) and nosocomial pneumonia (including ventilator-associated pneumonia), with a unique mechanism of entry into bacterial cells. It covers some difficult-to-treat multidrug-resistant gram-negative pathogens, including *Acinetobacter, Pseudomonas,* and *Stenotrophomonas,* so we are looking forward to approval for children, hopefully by next year. Neonatal studies have started.

Penicillinase-Resistant Penicillins (dicloxacillin [capsules only]; nafcillin and oxacillin [parenteral only]). "Penicillinase" refers specifically to the BL produced by *S aureus* in this case and not those produced by gram-negative bacteria. These antibiotics are

4

active against penicillin-resistant (pen-R) *S aureus* but not against MRSA. Nafcillin differs pharmacologically from the others because it is excreted primarily by the liver rather than by the kidneys, which may explain the relative lack of nephrotoxicity when this penicillin is compared with methicillin, which is no longer available in the United States. Nafcillin PK are erratic in people with liver disease, and the drug often causes painful phlebitis with IV infusion.

Antipseudomonal and Anti-Enteric Gram-Negative β-Lactams (ceftazidime, cefepime, meropenem, imipenem, ertapenem, aztreonam, piperacillin/tazobactam [PIP/TAZO], ceftazidime/avibactam [CAZ/AVI], and ceftolozane/tazobactam [TOL/TAZ]). Still under investigation in children, but approved for adults, are cefiderocol, imipenem/relebactam (IMI/REL), meropenem/vaborbactam, sulbactam/durlobactam, and cefepime/enmetazobactam. The BLI (tazobactam, avibactam, vaborbactam, durlobactam, or enmetazobactam in these combinations) binds irreversibly to and neutralizes specific BL enzymes produced by the organism. The combination adds to the spectrum of the original antibiotic only when the mechanism of resistance is a BL enzyme and only when the BLI is capable of binding to and inhibiting that particular organism's BL enzyme(s). The combinations extend the spectrum of activity of the primary antibiotic to include many BL-positive bacteria, including some strains of enteric GNB (*E coli, Klebsiella, Enterobacter,* and *Serratia*), *S aureus,* and *B fragilis*. Strains of *Pseudomonas* may still be resistant to PIP/TAZO, TOL/TAZ, CAZ/AVI, and IMI/REL and other β-lactam/BLI combinations because of many other non-BL mechanisms of resistance.

In general, use ceftazidime and cefepime over meropenem and imipenem, given the narrower spectrum of activity. However, *Pseudomonas* has an intrinsic capacity to develop resistance following exposure to any antibiotic, including β-lactam antibiotics, based on multiple mechanisms of resistance: inducible chromosomal BLs, upregulated efflux pumps, changes in the permeability of the cell wall, and mutational changes in the antibacterial target sites. Because development of resistance during therapy can occur (particularly BL-mediated resistance against ceftazidime), close monitoring is recommended. Cefepime, meropenem, and imipenem are relatively more stable to the BLs, but resistance can still develop to these agents based on other mechanisms. For carbapenem resistance, speak with an infectious diseases specialist, but CAZ/AVI is stable to the more common serine carbapenemases and cefiderocol to the increasingly common metallo-carbapenemases (see Carbapenems later in this section of the chapter).

Aminopenicillins (amoxicillin and amoxicillin/clavulanate [PO formulations only, in the United States], ampicillin [PO and parenteral], and ampicillin/sulbactam [parenteral only]). Amoxicillin is very well absorbed, good tasting, and associated with very few side effects. Augmentin is a combination of amoxicillin and clavulanate (as noted previously) that is available in several fixed proportions that permit amoxicillin to remain active against many BL-producing bacteria, including *H influenzae* and *S aureus* (but not MRSA). Amoxicillin/clavulanate has undergone many changes in formulation since its introduction in 1985. The ratio of amoxicillin to clavulanate was originally 4:1, based on susceptibility data of pneumococcus and *Haemophilus* during the 1970s. With the emergence of pen-R pneumococcus, recommendations for increasing the dosage of amoxicillin were made, particularly for upper respiratory tract infections. If, however, one increases the dosage of clavulanate, the incidence of diarrhea increases. By keeping the dosage of clavulanate constant while increasing the dosage of amoxicillin, one can treat the relatively resistant pneumococci while not increasing gastrointestinal side effects of the combination. The original 4:1 ratio is present in suspensions containing 125 and 250 mg of amoxicillin per 5 mL and the 125- and 250-mg chewable tablets. A higher 7:1 ratio is present in the suspensions containing 200 and 400 mg of amoxicillin per 5 mL and in the 200- and 400-mg chewable tablets. A still higher ratio of 14:1 is present in the suspension formulation Augmentin ES-600 that contains 600 mg of amoxicillin per 5 mL; this preparation is designed to deliver 90 mg/kg/day of amoxicillin, divided twice daily, for the treatment of ear (and sinus) infections. The high serum and middle ear fluid concentrations achieved with 45 mg/kg/dose, combined with the long middle ear fluid half-life (4–6 hours) of amoxicillin, allow for a therapeutic antibiotic exposure to pathogens in the middle ear with a twice-daily regimen. However, the prolonged half-life in the middle ear fluid is not necessarily found in other infection sites (eg, skin, lung tissue, joint tissue), for which dosing of amoxicillin and Augmentin should continue to be 3 times daily for most susceptible pathogens.

For older children who can swallow tablets, the amoxicillin to clavulanate ratios are as follows: 500-mg tablet (4:1); 875-mg tablet (7:1); 1,000-mg tablet (16:1).

Sulbactam, another BLI similar to clavulanate, is combined with ampicillin in a parenteral formulation. The relatively narrow spectrum of activity of ampicillin against enteric bacilli limits the activity of this combination, compared with the more broad spectrum of activity of agents such as piperacillin, ceftazidime, ceftolozane, or carbapenems when used in β-lactam/BLI combinations. Sulbactam, as a BLI, does not increase the spectrum of activity beyond what ampicillin can potentially achieve in organisms without BLs.

Carbapenems. Meropenem, imipenem, and ertapenem are currently available carbapenems with a broader spectrum of activity than of any other class of β-lactam currently available. Meropenem, imipenem, and ertapenem are approved by the FDA for use in children. At present, we recommend them for treatment of infections caused by bacteria resistant to standard therapy or for mixed infections involving aerobes and anaerobes. Imipenem has greater central nervous system (CNS) irritability than other carbapenems, leading to an increased risk for seizures in children with meningitis, but this is not clinically significant in children without underlying CNS inflammation or other predisposing factors. Meropenem was not associated with an increased rate of seizures, compared with cefotaxime in children with meningitis. Imipenem and meropenem are active against virtually all coliform bacilli, including ceftriaxone-resistant (ESBL- or ampC-producing) strains; against *Pseudomonas aeruginosa* (including most ceftazidime-resistant strains); and against anaerobes, including *B fragilis*. While ertapenem lacks the excellent activity against *P aeruginosa* of the other carbapenems, it has the advantage of a prolonged serum half-life, which allows for once-daily dosing in adults and children 13 years and older and twice-daily dosing in younger children. Increasingly emerging strains of *K pneumoniae* (and *E coli*) may contain KPCs that degrade and inactivate all the carbapenems. Less common in North America are the New Delhi metallo–β-lactamase (NDM)–carrying enteric bacilli (*E coli* and *Klebsiella*) that are also resistant to carbapenems. Multidrug-resistant strains have spread to many parts of the world, reinforcing the need to keep track of your local antibiotic susceptibility patterns. Carbapenems have been paired with BLIs (eg, vaborbactam, relebactam) that inhibit serine carbapenemases like KPC but that do not inhibit the metallo-BL enzymes like NDM. New BLIs that can inhibit NDM are under investigation, but cefiderocol, currently approved for adults and under investigation in children, is stable to most metallo-BL like NDM.

Macrolides

Erythromycin is the prototype of macrolide antibiotics. Almost 30 macrolides have been produced, but only 3 are FDA approved for children in the United States: erythromycin, azithromycin (also called an "azalide"), and clarithromycin, while a fourth, telithromycin (also called a "ketolide"), is approved for adults and available only in tablet form. As a class, these drugs achieve greater concentrations intracellularly than in serum, particularly with azithromycin and clarithromycin. As a result, measuring serum concentrations is usually not clinically useful. Gastrointestinal intolerance to erythromycin is caused by the breakdown products of the macrolide. This is much less of a problem with azithromycin and clarithromycin. Azithromycin, clarithromycin, and telithromycin extend the clinically relevant activity of erythromycin to include *Haemophilus;* azithromycin and clarithromycin also have substantial activity against certain mycobacteria. Azithromycin is also active in vitro and effective against many enteric gram-negative pathogens, including *Salmonella* and *Shigella,* when given PO. For many infections, the ability of azithromycin to concentrate intracellularly with drug accumulation over multiple doses allows dosing just once daily for 3 to 5 days to create site-of-infection concentrations that are equivalent to 7 to 10 days for more traditional antibiotics.

Aminoglycosides

Although 5 aminoglycoside antibiotics are available in the United States, only 3 are widely used for systemic therapy for aerobic gram-negative infections and for synergy in the treatment of certain infections: gentamicin, tobramycin, and amikacin. Streptomycin and kanamycin have more limited utility than the other agents due to increased toxicity. Resistance in GNB to aminoglycosides is caused by bacterial enzymes that adenylate, acetylate, or phosphorylate the aminoglycoside, resulting in inactivity. The specific activities of each enzyme against each aminoglycoside in each pathogen are highly variable. As a result, antibiotic susceptibility tests must be done for each aminoglycoside drug separately. There are small differences between aminoglycosides in toxicity to the kidneys and eighth cranial nerve hearing/vestibular function, although it is uncertain whether these small differences are clinically significant. For all children receiving a full treatment course of a week or more, it is advisable to monitor peak and trough serum concentrations early in the course of therapy, as the degree of drug exposure correlates with toxicity and the elevated trough concentrations may predict impending drug accumulation. With amikacin, desired peak concentrations are 20 to 35 mcg/mL and trough drug concentrations are less than 10 mcg/mL; for gentamicin and tobramycin, depending on the frequency of dosing (every 8, 12, or 24 hours), peak concentrations should be 5 to 10 mcg/mL and trough concentrations less than 2 mcg/mL. Decades ago, children with CF required much greater dosages to achieve equivalent therapeutic serum concentrations due to enhanced renal clearance, although with improvements in nutrition and pulmonary function, the differences are far less prominent. Inhaled tobramycin has been very successful in children with CF as prophylaxis for GNB infections. The role of inhaled aminoglycosides in treatment or prevention of other gram-negative pneumonias (eg, ventilator-associated pneumonia) has not yet been defined.

Once-Daily Dosing of Aminoglycosides. Once-daily dosing of 5 to 7.5 mg/kg of gentamicin or tobramycin has been studied in adults and in some neonates and children; peak serum concentrations are greater than those achieved with dosing 3 times daily. Aminoglycosides demonstrate concentration-dependent killing of pathogens, suggesting a potential benefit to higher serum concentrations achieved with once-daily dosing. Regimens giving the daily dosage as a single infusion (rather than as traditionally split doses every 8 hours) are effective and safe for normal adults and immunocompromised hosts with fever and neutropenia and may be less toxic than 8-hourly dosing. Experience with once-daily dosing in children is increasing, with similar encouraging results as noted for adults. A recent Cochrane review for children (and adults) with CF comparing once-daily with 3-times-daily administration showed equal efficacy with decreased toxicity in children.[3] Once-daily dosing should be considered as effective as multiple, smaller doses per day and is likely to be safer for children; therefore, it should be the preferred regimen for treatment.

Fluoroquinolones

Fluoroquinolone (FQ) toxicity to cartilage in weight-bearing joints of experimental juvenile animals was first documented to be dose and duration-of-therapy dependent more than 40 years ago. Pediatric studies were therefore not initially undertaken with ciprofloxacin or other FQs. However, with increasing antibiotic resistance in pediatric pathogens and an accumulating database in pediatrics suggesting that joint toxicity may be uncommon, the FDA allowed prospective studies to proceed in 1998. As of July 2024, no cases of FQ-attributable joint toxicity have been documented to occur in children with FQs that are approved for use in the United States. Limited published data are available from prospective, blinded studies to accurately assess this risk. Retrospective published data are always difficult to interpret but continue to suggest caution.[6] A prospective, randomized, double-blind study of moxifloxacin for intra-abdominal infection, with 1-year follow-up specifically designed to assess tendon/joint toxicity, demonstrated no concern for toxicity.[7] Unblinded studies with levofloxacin for respiratory tract infections (RTIs) and unpublished randomized studies comparing ciprofloxacin with other agents for cUTI suggest the possibility of an uncommon, reversible FQ-attributable arthralgia, but these data should be interpreted with caution. The use of FQs for antibiotic-resistant infections where no other active agent is available is reasonable, while weighing the benefits of treatment against the low risk for toxicity from this class of antibiotics. The use of a PO FQ when the only alternative is parenteral therapy is also justified.[8] For clinicians reading this book, a well-documented case of FQ joint toxicity in a child is publishable (and reportable to the FDA), and the editors would be very happy to support such a report. Feel free to contact us if you have a case.

Ciprofloxacin usually has very good gram-negative activity (with great regional variation in susceptibility) against enteric bacilli (*E coli, Klebsiella, Enterobacter, Salmonella,* and *Shigella*) and against *P aeruginosa*. However, it lacks substantial gram-positive coverage and should not be used to treat streptococcal, staphylococcal, or pneumococcal infections. Levofloxacin and moxifloxacin are more active against these pathogens; levofloxacin has documented efficacy and safety in pediatric clinical trials for RTIs, acute otitis media, and CAP. Children with any question of joint/tendon/bone toxicity in the levofloxacin studies were followed up to 5 years after treatment, with no difference in joint/tendon outcomes compared to the outcomes of standard FDA-approved antibiotics used in these studies.[9] None of the newer-generation FQs are significantly more active against gram-negative pathogens than ciprofloxacin. Quinolone antibiotics are bitter tasting. Ciprofloxacin and levofloxacin are currently available in a suspension form; ciprofloxacin is FDA approved in pediatrics for cUTIs and inhalation anthrax, while levofloxacin is approved for plague and inhalation anthrax. Regarding levofloxacin, Johnson & Johnson chose not to apply to the FDA for approval for pediatric RTI indications, despite successful clinical trials in children. For reasons of safety and to prevent the emergence of widespread resistance, FQs should not be used for primary therapy for pediatric infections and should be limited to situations in which safe and effective alternative PO therapy does not exist.

5. Preferred Therapy for Specific Fungal Pathogens

NOTES

- A list of table abbreviations and acronyms can be found at the start of this publication.
- See Chapter 6 for discussion of the differences between polyenes, azoles, and echinocandins.

A. OVERVIEW OF MORE COMMON FUNGAL PATHOGENS AND THEIR USUAL PATTERN OF ANTIFUNGAL SUSCEPTIBILITIES

Fungal Species	Amphotericin B Formulations	Fluconazole	Itraconazole	Voriconazole	Posaconazole	Isavuconazole	Flucytosine	Caspofungin, Micafungin, Anidulafungin, and Rezafungin
Aspergillus calidoustus	++	−	−	−	−	−	−	++
Aspergillus fumigatus	+	−	±	++	+	++	−	+
Aspergillus terreus	−	−	+	++	+	++	−	+
Blastomyces dermatitidis	++	+	++	+	+	+	−	−
Candida albicans	+	++	+	+	+	+	+	++
Candida auris	±	−	±	±	+	+	±	++
Candida parapsilosis	++	++	+	+	+	+	+	+
Candida tropicalis	+	+	+	+	+	+	+	++
Clavispora (Candida) lusitaniae	−	++	+	+	+	+	+	+
Coccidioides immitis	++	++	+	+	++	+	−	−
Cryptococcus spp	++	+	+	+	+	+	++	−
Fusarium spp	±	−	−	++	+	+	−	−
Histoplasma capsulatum	++	+	++	+	+	+	−	−

Organism								
Lomentospora (formerly Scedosporium) prolificans	–	–	±	±	±	±	–	±
Meyerozyma (Candida) guilliermondii	+	±	+	+	+	+	+	±
Mucor spp	++	–	±	–	+	++	–	–
Nakaseomyces (Candida) glabrata	+	–	±	±	±	±	+	±
Paracoccidioides spp	+	+	++	+	+	+	–	–
Penicillium spp	±	–	++	+	+	+	–	–
Pichia kudriavzevii (Candida krusei)	+	–	–	+	+	+	+	++
Rhizopus spp	++	–	–	–	+	+	–	–
Scedosporium apiospermum	–	–	±	+	+	+	–	±
Sporothrix spp	+	+	++	+	+	+	–	–
Trichosporon spp	–	+	+	++	+	+	–	–

NOTE: ++ = preferred; + = acceptable; ± = possibly effective (see text for further discussion); – = unlikely to be effective.

5

Preferred Therapy for Fungal Pathogens

B. SYSTEMIC INFECTIONS

Infection

When treating invasive fungal disease with azoles, it is important to document therapeutic serum concentrations, particularly when using PO therapy. The editors use laboratories that provide high-performance liquid chromatography/mass spectrometry techniques with more rapid results than from the older microbiologic techniques. One laboratory that provides this service is the University of Texas Health Science Center at the San Antonio Fungus Testing Laboratory (https://lsom.uthscsa.edu/pathology/reference-labs/fungus-testing-laboratory/antifungal-drug-levels [accessed September 9, 2024]; 210-567-4029).

	Therapy (evidence grade)	Comments
Prophylaxis		
Prophylaxis of invasive fungal infection in patients with hematologic malignancies[1-11]	Caspofungin was superior to fluconazole in a randomized controlled trial of neutropenic children with acute myeloid leukemia (AII).[12] yet compared to triazoles, caspofungin did not significantly reduce incidence of invasive fungal disease in pediatric recipients of allogeneic hematopoietic cell transplants.[13] Micafungin is safe and effective as prophylaxis in pediatric autologous hematopoietic stem cell transplant (AII).[14] Fluconazole 6 mg/kg/day for prevention of infection (AII). Posaconazole for prevention of infection has been well studied in adults (AI) and offers anti-mold coverage.[4]	Fluconazole is not effective against molds and some strains of *Candida*. Posaconazole PO, voriconazole PO, and micafungin IV are effective in adults in preventing yeast and mold infections but are not all well studied in children for this indication.[15]
Prophylaxis of invasive fungal infection in patients with solid-organ transplants[16-20]	Fluconazole 6 mg/kg/day for prevention of infection (AII)	AmB, caspofungin, micafungin, voriconazole, or posaconazole may be effective in preventing infection.

Treatment

Aspergillosis[1,21–32]

Voriconazole (AI) 18 mg/kg/day IV div q12h as LD on first day, then 16 mg/kg/day IV div q12h as maintenance dose for children aged 2–12 y or 12–14 y and weighing <50 kg. In children aged ≥15 y or 12–14 y and weighing >50 kg, use adult dosing (load 12 mg/kg/day IV div q12h on first day, then 8 mg/kg/day div q12h as maintenance dose) (AII). When patient's condition is stable, may switch from voriconazole IV to voriconazole PO at a dose of 18 mg/kg/day div bid for children 2–12 y and at least 400 mg/day div bid for children >12 y (AII). Dosing in children <2 y is less clear, but doses are generally higher due to more rapid clearance (AIII). These are only initial dosing recommendations; it is critical to understand that continued dosing in all ages is guided by close monitoring of trough serum voriconazole concentrations in individual patients (AII). Unlike in adults, voriconazole PO bioavailability in children is about only 50%–60%, so trough levels are crucial when using PO.[33]

Alternatives for primary therapy when voriconazole cannot be administered: isavuconazole (AI), posaconazole (AI), or L-AmB 5 mg/kg/day (AII). Dosing of isavuconazole in children <13 y is 10 mg/kg (q8h on days 1 and 2 and qd thereafter).[34] ABLC is another alternative. Echinocandin primary monotherapy should not be used for treating invasive aspergillosis (CII). AmB-D should be used only in resource-limited settings in which no alternative agent is available (AII).

Voriconazole is the current guideline-recommended primary antifungal therapy for all clinical forms of aspergillosis. A recent randomized controlled trial showed that posaconazole is non-inferior to voriconazole for invasive aspergillosis (AI).[35] An earlier randomized controlled trial showed that isavuconazole was non-inferior to voriconazole for invasive aspergillosis (AI).[30]

Early initiation of therapy in patients with strongly suspected disease is important while a diagnostic evaluation is conducted.

Optimal voriconazole trough serum concentrations (generally thought to be 2–5 mcg/mL) are essential. Check trough level 2–5 days after initiation of therapy, and repeat the following week to verify and 4 days after a change of dose.[32] It is critical to monitor trough concentrations to guide therapy due to high inter-patient variability.[36] Low voriconazole concentrations are a consistent leading cause of clinical failure. Younger children (especially <3 y) often have lower trough voriconazole levels and need much higher dosing. Dosing for younger children should begin as listed but will invariably need to be increased.

Total treatment course is a minimum of 6 wk, largely dependent on the degree and duration of immunosuppression and evidence of disease improvement.

A recent expert panel agreed that primary therapy, with confirmed appropriate therapeutic drug levels, should be given for at least 8 days to show an effect.[37]

(Continued on next page)

B. SYSTEMIC INFECTIONS

Therapy (evidence grade)	Comments
SYSTEMIC INFECTIONS	
Aspergillosis[1,21–32] *(continued)*	Current guidelines recommend that salvage antifungal therapy options after failed primary therapy include a change of antifungal class (by using L-AmB or an echinocandin), a switch to isavuconazole, a switch to posaconazole (serum trough concentrations ≥1 mcg/mL), or use of combination antifungal therapy. Most experts would recommend a switch to L-AmB.
	Azole monotherapy is not usually recommended after azole prophylaxis has failed.
	Combination antifungal therapy with voriconazole plus an echinocandin may be considered in select patients. The addition of anidulafungin to voriconazole as combination therapy showed some statistical benefit to the combination over voriconazole monotherapy in only certain patients.[38] In vitro data suggest some synergy with 2 (but not 3) drug combinations: an azole plus an echinocandin is the most well studied. If combination therapy is used, this is likely best done initially, when voriconazole trough concentrations may not yet be appropriate.
	Routine antifungal susceptibility testing is not recommended but is suggested for patients who are suspected of having an azole-resistant isolate or who are unresponsive to therapy.
	Azole-resistant *A fumigatus* is increasing. If local epidemiology suggests >10% azole resistance, initial empiric therapy should be voriconazole + echinocandin OR + L-AmB, and subsequent therapy should be guided by antifungal susceptibilities.[39]
	Micafungin likely has equal efficacy to caspofungin against aspergillosis.[40]

		Return of immune function is paramount to treatment success; for children receiving corticosteroids, decreasing the corticosteroid dosage or changing to steroid-sparing protocols is important.
Bipolaris, Cladophialophora, Curvularia, Exophiala, Alternaria, and other agents of **phaeohyphomycosis** (dematiaceous, pigmented molds)[41–48]	Voriconazole (AI) 18 mg/kg/day IV div q12h as LD on first day, then 16 mg/kg/day IV div q12h as maintenance dose for children aged 2–12 y or 12–14 y and weighing <50 kg. In children aged ≥15 y or 12–14 y and weighing >50 kg, use adult dosing (load 12 mg/kg/day IV q12h on first day, then 8 mg/kg/day div q12h as maintenance dose) (AII). When patient's condition is stable, may switch from voriconazole IV to voriconazole PO at a dose of 18 mg/kg/day div bid for children 2–12 y and at least 400 mg/day div bid for children >12 y (AII). Dosing in children <2 y is less clear, but doses are generally higher due to more rapid clearance (AIII). These are only initial dosing recommendations; continued dosing in all ages is guided by close monitoring of trough serum voriconazole concentrations in individual patients (AII). Unlike in adults, voriconazole PO bioavailability in children is about only 50%–60%, so trough levels are crucial.[33] Alternatives could include posaconazole (trough concentrations >1 mcg/mL) or combination therapy with an echinocandin + azole or an echinocandin + L-AmB (BIII).	Aggressive surgical debulking/excision is essential for CNS lesions. These can be highly resistant infections, so strongly recommend antifungal susceptibility testing to guide therapy and consultation with a pediatric ID expert. Antifungal susceptibilities are often variable, but empiric therapy with voriconazole is the best start. Optimal voriconazole trough serum concentrations (generally thought to be 2–5 mcg/mL) are important for success. Check trough level 2–5 days after initiation of therapy and repeat the following week to verify and 4 days after a change of dose. It is critical to monitor trough concentrations to guide therapy due to high inter-patient variability.[36] Low voriconazole concentrations are a leading cause of clinical failure. Younger children (especially <3 y) often have lower voriconazole levels and need much higher dosing. Some experts will recommend higher trough levels for difficult CNS lesions.

B. SYSTEMIC INFECTIONS

	Therapy (evidence grade)	Comments
Blastomycosis (North American)[49-55]	For moderate to severe pulmonary disease: L-AmB 5 mg/kg IV daily for 1–2 wk or until improvement noted, then step-down therapy with itraconazole PO soln 10 mg/kg/day div bid (max 400 mg/day) for a total of 6–12 mo (AIII). ABLC is an alternative formulation if L-AmB is not available. Itraconazole LD (double dose for first 2 days) is recommended in adults but has not been studied in children (but is likely helpful). For mild to moderate pulmonary disease: itraconazole PO soln 10 mg/kg/day div bid (max 400 mg/day) for a total of 6–12 mo (AIII). Itraconazole LD (double dose for first 2 days) is recommended in adults but has not been studied in children (but is likely helpful). For CNS blastomycosis: L-AmB or ABLC (preferred over AmB-D) for 4–6 wk, followed by an azole (fluconazole is preferred, at 12 mg/kg/day after an LD of 25 mg/kg; alternatives for CNS disease are voriconazole or itraconazole), for a total of at least 12 mo and until resolution of CSF abnormalities (AII). Some experts suggest combination therapy with L-AmB/ABLC plus high-dose fluconazole as induction therapy in CNS blastomycosis until clinical improvement (BIII).	New international guidelines exist.[56] All forms of blastomycosis should be treated. Itraconazole PO soln provides greater and more reliable absorption than caps, and only the PO soln should be used (on an empty stomach); serum concentrations of itraconazole should be determined 5 days after start of therapy to ensure adequate drug exposure. For blastomycosis, maintain trough itraconazole concentrations 1–2 mcg/mL (values for both itraconazole and hydroxyl-itraconazole are added together). If only itraconazole caps are available, use 20 mg/kg/day div q12h taken with cola drink to increase gastric acidity and bioavailability. Alternative to itraconazole: 12 mg/kg/day fluconazole (BIII) after an LD of 25 mg/kg/day. A case series has shown that outcomes of voriconazole are similar to those of itraconazole, and there is little experience with posaconazole or isavuconazole. Patients with extrapulmonary blastomycosis should receive at least 12 mo of total therapy; long courses are recommended for CNS or bone involvement. If induction with L-AmB alone is failing, add itraconazole or high-dose fluconazole until clinical improvement. Lifelong itraconazole if immunosuppression cannot be reversed.
Candidiasis[57-61] (See Ch 6.)		
– Cutaneous	Topical therapy (alphabetic order): ciclopirox, clotrimazole, econazole, haloprogin, ketoconazole, miconazole, oxiconazole, sertaconazole, sulconazole	Fluconazole 6 mg/kg/day PO qd for 5–7 days Relapse common with chronic mucocutaneous disease, and antifungal susceptibilities critical to drive appropriate therapy

– Disseminated infection, acute (including catheter fungemia)	An echinocandin is recommended as initial therapy. Caspofungin 70 mg/m² IV LD on day 1 (max dose 70 mg), followed by 50 mg/m² IV (max dose 70 mg) on subsequent days (AII); OR micafungin 2 mg/kg/day q24h (children weighing <40 kg), with max dose 100 mg/day (AII).[62] ABLC or L-AmB 5 mg/kg/day IV q24h (BII) is an effective but less attractive alternative due to potential toxicity (AII).
	Fluconazole (12 mg/kg/day q24h, after an LD of 25 mg/kg/day) is an alternative for patients who are not critically ill and have had no prior azole exposure (CIII). A fluconazole LD is standard of care in adult patients but has been studied only in infants (not yet in children)[63]; however, it is very likely that the beneficial effect of an LD extends to children. Fluconazole can be used as step-down therapy in stable neutropenic patients with susceptible isolates and documented bloodstream clearance (CIII). For children of all ages receiving ECMO, fluconazole is dosed as a 35 mg/kg LD on day 1, followed by 12 mg/kg/day (BII).[64]
	Transition from an echinocandin to fluconazole (usually within 5–7 days) is recommended for non-neutropenic patients who are clinically stable, have isolates that are susceptible to fluconazole (eg, C albicans), and have negative repeat blood cultures following initiation of antifungal therapy (AII).
	Prompt removal of an infected IV catheter or any infected devices is absolutely critical to success (AII). Biofilms form early, so prompt removal is preferred.
	For infections with C krusei or C glabrata, an echinocandin is preferred; however, there are increasing reports of some C glabrata resistance to echinocandins (treatment would, therefore, be L-AmB or ABLC) (BIII). There are increasing reports of some C tropicalis resistance to fluconazole.
	L-AmB (5 mg/kg daily) is a reasonable alternative if there is intolerance, limited availability, or resistance to other antifungal agents (AI). Transition from a lipid AmB to fluconazole is recommended after 5–7 days among patients who have isolates that are susceptible to fluconazole, who are clinically stable, and in whom repeat cultures during antifungal therapy are negative (AI).
	Voriconazole (18 mg/kg/day div q12h LD, followed by 16 mg/kg/day div q12h) is effective for candidemia but offers little advantage over fluconazole as initial therapy. Voriconazole is recommended as PO step-down therapy for select cases of candidemia due to C krusei or if mold coverage is needed.
	Follow-up blood cultures should be performed qd or qod to establish the time point at which candidemia has been cleared (AIII).
	Duration of therapy is for 2 wk AFTER negative cultures in pediatric patients without obvious metastatic complications and after symptom resolution (AII).
	In neutropenic patients, ophthalmologic findings of choroidal and vitreous infection are minimal until recovery from neutropenia; therefore, dilated funduscopic examinations should be performed within the first week after recovery from neutropenia (AIII).

(Continued on next page)

5

B. SYSTEMIC INFECTIONS

	Therapy (evidence grade)	Comments
- Disseminated infection, acute (including catheter fungemia) (continued)	For CNS infections: L-AmB/ABLC (5 mg/kg/day), and AmB-D (1 mg/kg/day) as an alternative, combined with or without flucytosine 100 mg/kg/day PO div q6h (AII) until initial clinical response, then step-down therapy with fluconazole (12 mg/kg/day q24h, after an LD of 25 mg/kg/day); echinocandins do not achieve therapeutic concentrations in CSF.	All non-neutropenic patients with candidemia should ideally have a dilated ophthalmologic examination, preferably performed by an ophthalmologist, within the first week after diagnosis (AIII).
- Disseminated infection, chronic (hepatosplenic)	Initial therapy with lipid formulation AmB (L-AmB or ABLC, 5 mg/kg daily) OR an echinocandin (caspofungin 70 mg/m² IV LD on day 1 [max dose 70 mg], followed by 50 mg/m² IV [max dose 70 mg] on subsequent days OR micafungin 2 mg/kg/day q24h in children weighing <40 kg [max dose 100 mg]) for several weeks, followed by PO fluconazole in patients unlikely to have a fluconazole-resistant isolate (12 mg/kg/day q24h, after an LD of 25 mg/kg/day) (AIII). Therapy should continue until lesions resolve on repeat imaging; they usually resolve after several months. Premature discontinuation of antifungal therapy can lead to relapse (AIII).	If chemotherapy or hematopoietic cell transplant is required, it should not be delayed because of the presence of chronic disseminated candidiasis, and antifungal therapy should be continued throughout the period of high risk to prevent relapse (AIII).
- Neonatal[60] See Ch 2.	AmB-D (1 mg/kg/day) is recommended therapy (AII).[65] Fluconazole (12 mg/kg/day q24h, after an LD of 25 mg/kg/day) is an alternative if patient has not been receiving fluconazole prophylaxis (AII).[66] For treatment of neonates and young infants (<120 days) receiving ECMO, fluconazole is loaded with 35 mg/kg on day 1, followed by 12 mg/kg/day q24h (BII).	In nurseries with high rates of candidiasis (>10%), IV or PO fluconazole prophylaxis (AI) (3–6 mg/kg twice weekly for 6 wk) in high-risk neonates (birth weight <1,000 g) is recommended. PO nystatin, 100,000 U tid for 6 wk, is an alternative to fluconazole in neonates with birth weights <1,500 g when availability or resistance precludes the use of fluconazole (CII).

L-AmB is an alternative but carries a theoretical risk of penetrating the urinary tract less than AmB-D (CIII) would.

Duration of therapy for candidemia without obvious metastatic complications is for 2 wk AFTER documented clearance and resolution of symptoms (therefore, generally 3 wk total).

Echinocandins should be used with caution and generally limited to salvage therapy or to situations in which resistance or toxicity precludes the use of AmB-D or fluconazole (CIII). A recent randomized trial of caspofungin vs AmB-D showed similar fungal-free survival.[67]

Role of flucytosine in neonates with meningitis is questionable and not routinely recommended due to toxicity concerns. The addition of flucytosine (100 mg/kg/day div q6h) may be considered as salvage therapy in patients who have not had a clinical response to initial AmB therapy, but adverse effects are frequent (CIII).

LP and dilated retinal examination recommended for neonates with cultures positive for *Candida* spp from blood and/or urine (AIII). Same recommended for all neonates with birth weight <1,500 g with candiduria with or without candidemia (AIII).

CT or ultrasound imaging of genitourinary tract, liver, and spleen should be performed if blood cultures are persistently positive (AIII).

Meningoencephalitis in the neonate occurs at a higher rate than in older children/adults.

Central venous catheter removal is strongly recommended.

Infected CNS devices, including ventriculostomy drains and shunts, should be removed if possible.

Condition	Therapy
– Oropharyngeal, esophageal[57]	Mild oropharyngeal disease: clotrimazole 10-mg troches PO 5 times daily OR nystatin 100,000 U/mL, 4–6 mL qid for 7–14 days. Alternatives also include miconazole mucoadhesive buccal 50-mg tab to the mucosal surface over the canine fossa qd for 7–14 days OR 1–2 nystatin pastilles (200,000 U each) qid for 7–14 days (AII). Moderate to severe oropharyngeal disease: fluconazole 6 mg/kg PO qd for 7–14 days (AII). Esophageal candidiasis: PO fluconazole (6–12 mg/kg/day, after an LD of 25 mg/kg/day) for 14–21 days (AI). If cannot tolerate PO therapy, use fluconazole IV OR ABLC/L-AmB/AmB-D OR an echinocandin (AI).	A meta-analysis showed that clotrimazole is less effective than fluconazole but as effective as other topical therapies.[68] For fluconazole-refractory oropharyngeal or esophageal disease: itraconazole PO soln OR posaconazole OR AmB IV OR an echinocandin for up to 28 days (AII). Esophageal disease always requires systemic antifungal therapy. A diagnostic trial of antifungal therapy for esophageal candidiasis is appropriate before performing an endoscopic examination (AI). Chronic suppressive therapy (3×/wk) with fluconazole is recommended for recurrent infections (AI).

B. SYSTEMIC INFECTIONS

	Therapy (evidence grade)	Comments
– Urinary tract infection	Cystitis: fluconazole 6 mg/kg qd IV or PO for 2 wk (AII). For fluconazole-resistant C glabrata or C krusei, AmB-D for 1–7 days (AIII). Pyelonephritis: fluconazole 12 mg/kg qd IV or PO for 2 wk (AIII) after an LD of 25 mg/kg/day. For fluconazole-resistant C glabrata or C krusei, AmB-D with or without flucytosine for 1–7 days (AIII).	Treatment is NOT recommended in asymptomatic candiduria unless high risk for dissemination; neutropenic low birth weight neonate (<1,500 g); or patient to undergo urologic manipulation (AIII). Neutropenic patients and low birth weight neonates should be treated as recommended for candidemia (AIII). Removing Foley catheter, if present, may lead to a spontaneous cure in the normal host; check for additional upper urinary tract disease. AmB-D bladder irrigation is not generally recommended due to high relapse rate (an exception may be in fluconazole-resistant Candida) (CIII). For renal collecting-system fungus balls, surgical debridement may be required in non-neonates (BIII). Echinocandins have poor urinary concentrations. AmB-D has greater urinary penetration than L-AmB/ABLC.
– Vulvovaginal[66]	Topical vaginal cream/tabs/suppositories (alphabetic order): butoconazole, clotrimazole, econazole, fenticonazole, miconazole, sertaconazole, terconazole, or tioconazole for 3–7 days (AI) OR fluconazole 10 mg/kg (max 150 mg) as a single dose (AII)	For uncomplicated vulvovaginal candidiasis, no topical agent is clearly superior. Avoid azoles during pregnancy. For severe disease, fluconazole 150 mg given q72h for 2–3 doses (AI). For recurring disease, consider 10–14 days of induction with topical agent or fluconazole, followed by fluconazole once weekly for 6 mo (AI). In a phase 2 study, ibrexafungerp was effective and well tolerated (AII).[69]

| **Chromoblastomycosis** (SUBQ infection by dematiaceous fungi)[70–74] | Itraconazole PO soln 10 mg/kg/day div bid for 12–18 mo, in combination with surgical excision or repeat cryotherapy (AII). Itraconazole PO soln provides greater and more reliable absorption than caps, and only the PO soln should be used (on an empty stomach); serum concentrations of itraconazole should be determined 5 days after start of therapy to ensure adequate drug exposure. Maintain trough itraconazole concentrations 1–2 mcg/mL (values for both itraconazole and hydroxyl-itraconazole are added together). | Alternative: terbinafine plus surgery; heat and potassium iodide; posaconazole. Lesions are recalcitrant and difficult to treat. |

B. SYSTEMIC INFECTIONS

	Therapy (evidence grade)	Comments
Coccidioidomycosis[75–83]	For moderate infections: fluconazole 12 mg/kg IV/PO q24h (AII) after an LD of 25 mg/kg/day. For severe pulmonary disease: AmB-D 1 mg/kg/day IV q24h OR ABLC/L-AmB 5 mg/kg/day IV q24h (AIII) as initial therapy for several weeks until clear improvement, followed by a PO azole for total therapy of at least 12 mo, depending on genetic or immunocompromised risk factors. For meningitis: fluconazole 12 mg/kg/day IV q24h (AII) after an LD of 25 mg/kg/day (AII). Itraconazole has also been effective (BII). If no response to azole, use intrathecal AmB-D (0.1–1.5 mg/dose) with or without fluconazole (AIII). Lifelong azole suppressive therapy required due to high relapse rate. Adjunctive corticosteroids in meningitis have resulted in less secondary cerebrovascular events.[84] For extrapulmonary (non-meningeal), particularly for osteomyelitis, a PO azole such as fluconazole or itraconazole soln 10 mg/kg/day bid for at least 12 mo (AIII), and L-AmB/ABLC as an alternative (less toxic than AmB-D) for severe disease or if worsening. Itraconazole PO soln provides greater and more reliable absorption than caps, and only the PO soln should be used (on an empty stomach); serum concentrations of itraconazole should be determined 5 days after start of therapy to ensure adequate drug exposure. Maintain trough itraconazole concentrations 1–2 mcg/mL (values for both itraconazole and hydroxyl-itraconazole are added together).	New international guidelines exist.[56] Mild pulmonary disease does not require routine therapy in the normal host and only requires periodic reassessment. Treatment with fluconazole or itraconazole should be given to all patients with underlying immunosuppression, prolonged infection, underlying cardiopulmonary comorbidities, or complement fixation titers of ≥1:32. There is experience with posaconazole for disease in adults but little experience in children. Isavuconazole experience in adults is increasing. Treat until titers of serum cocci complement fixation drop to 1:8 or 1:4, at about 3–6 mo. Disease in immunocompromised hosts may need to be treated longer, including potentially lifelong azole secondary prophylaxis. Watch for relapse up to 1–2 y after therapy.

Cryptococcosis[85-89]

For mild to moderate pulmonary disease: fluconazole 12 mg/kg/day (max 400 mg) IV/PO q24h after an LD of 25 mg/kg/day for 6–12 mo (AII). Itraconazole is an alternative if cannot tolerate fluconazole.

For meningitis or severe pulmonary disease: induction therapy with L-AmB 3–4 mg/kg/day q24h; AND flucytosine 100 mg/kg/day PO div q6h for a minimum of 2 wk and a repeat CSF culture is negative. In low-resource settings, use L-AmB 10 mg/kg as a single dose and flucytosine. This is followed by consolidation therapy with fluconazole (12 mg/kg/day with max dose 400–800 mg after an LD of 25 mg/kg/day) for a minimum of 8 more wk (AI). Then use maintenance therapy with fluconazole (6 mg/kg/day) or 200 mg daily for 12 mo (AI).

Alternative induction therapies for meningitis or severe pulmonary disease (order of preference): AmB product plus flucytosine for 4–6 wk (AII); AmB product plus fluconazole for 2 wk, followed by fluconazole for 8 wk (BII); fluconazole plus flucytosine for 6 wk (BII).

New international guidelines exist.[90]

Serum flucytosine concentrations should be obtained after 3–5 days to achieve a 2-h post-dose peak <100 mcg/mL (ideally 30–80 mcg/mL) to prevent neutropenia.

For HIV-positive patients, continue maintenance therapy with fluconazole (6 mg/kg/day) indefinitely. Initiate HAART 2–10 wk after commencement of antifungal therapy to avoid immune reconstitution inflammatory syndrome.

In organ transplant recipients, continue maintenance fluconazole (6 mg/kg/day) for 6–12 mo after consolidation therapy with higher-dose fluconazole.

For cryptococcal relapse, restart induction therapy (this time for 4–10 wk), repeat CSF analysis q2wk until sterile, and determine antifungal susceptibility of relapse isolate.

Successful use of voriconazole, posaconazole, and isavuconazole for cryptococcosis has been reported in adult patients.

In resource-limited settings, a recent clinical trial of a single 10 mg/kg dose of L-AmB plus 14 days of flucytosine + fluconazole was non-inferior to standard therapy.[91]

B. SYSTEMIC INFECTIONS

	Therapy (evidence grade)	Comments
Fusarium, Lomentospora (formerly **Scedosporium prolificans,** **Pseudallescheria boydii** (and its asexual form, **Scedosporium apiospermum**)[,41,92–96] and other agents of **hyalohyphomycosis**	Voriconazole (AII) 18 mg/kg/day IV div q12h as LD on first day, then 16 mg/kg/day IV div q12h as maintenance dose for children aged 2–12 y or 12–14 y and weighing <50 kg. In children aged ≥15 y or 12–14 y and weighing >50 kg, use adult dosing (load 12 mg/kg/day IV div q12h on first day, then 8 mg/kg/day div q12h as maintenance dose) (AII). When patient's condition is stable, may switch from voriconazole IV to voriconazole PO at a dose of 18 mg/kg/day div bid for children 2–12 y and at least 400 mg/day div bid for children >12 y (AII). Dosing in children <2 y is less clear, but doses are generally higher due to more rapid clearance (AIII). These are only initial dosing recommendations; continued dosing in all ages is guided by close monitoring of trough serum voriconazole concentrations in individual patients (AII). Unlike in adults, voriconazole PO bioavailability in children is about only 50%–60%, so trough levels are crucial at this stage.[33]	These can be highly resistant infections, so strongly recommend antifungal susceptibility testing against a wide range of agents to guide specific therapy and consultation with a pediatric ID expert. Optimal voriconazole trough serum concentrations (generally thought to be 2–5 mcg/mL) are important for success. Check trough level 2–5 days after initiation of therapy and repeat the following week to verify and 4 days after a change of dose. It is critical to monitor trough concentrations to guide therapy due to high inter-patient variability.[36] Low voriconazole concentrations are a leading cause of clinical failure. Younger children (especially <3 y) often have lower voriconazole levels and need much higher dosing. Often resistant to AmB in vitro. Alternatives: posaconazole (trough concentrations >1 mcg/mL) can be active; echinocandins have been reportedly successful as salvage therapy in combination with azoles; while there are reports of promising in vitro combinations with terbinafine, terbinafine does not obtain therapeutic tissue concentrations required for these disseminated infections; miltefosine (for leishmaniasis) use has been reported. Olorofim is an investigational agent with excellent activity against these recalcitrant pathogens.

Histoplasmosis[97–99]

For severe acute pulmonary disease: ABLC/L-AmB 5 mg/kg/day q24h for 1–2 wk, followed by itraconazole 10 mg/kg/day div bid (max 400 mg daily) to complete a total of 12 wk (AIII). Add methylprednisolone (0.5–1.0 mg/kg/day) for first 1–2 wk in patients with hypoxia or significant respiratory distress.

For mild to moderate acute pulmonary disease: if symptoms persist for >1 mo, itraconazole PO soln 10 mg/kg/day div bid for 6–12 wk (AIII).

For progressive disseminated histoplasmosis: ABLC/L-AmB 5 mg/kg/day q24h for 4–6 wk; alternative treatment is L-AmB for 1–2 wk followed by itraconazole 10 mg/kg/day div bid (max 400 mg daily) to complete a total of at least 12 mo (AIII).

New international guidelines exist.[56] Mild pulmonary disease may not require therapy and, in most cases, resolves in 1 mo.

CNS histoplasmosis requires initial L-AmB/ABLC (less toxic than AmB-D) therapy for 4–6 wk, followed by itraconazole for at least 12 mo and until CSF antigen resolution.

Itraconazole PO soln provides greater and more reliable absorption than caps, and only the PO soln should be used (on an empty stomach); serum concentrations of itraconazole should be determined 5 days after start of therapy to ensure adequate drug exposure. Maintain trough itraconazole concentrations at >1–2 mcg/mL (values for both itraconazole and hydroxyl-itraconazole are added together). If only itraconazole caps are available, use 20 mg/kg/day div q12h taken with cola drink to increase gastric acidity and bioavailability.

Potential lifelong suppressive itraconazole if cannot reverse immunosuppression.

Corticosteroids recommended for 2 wk for pericarditis with hemodynamic compromise.

Voriconazole and posaconazole use has been reported. Fluconazole is inferior to itraconazole.

B. SYSTEMIC INFECTIONS

	Therapy (evidence grade)	Comments
Mucormycosis (previously known as zygomycosis)[31,100–106]	Aggressive surgical debridement combined with induction antifungal therapy: L-AmB at 5–10 mg/kg/day q24h (AII) for 3 wk. Lipid formulations of AmB are preferred to AmB-D due to increased penetration and decreased toxicity. Some experts advocate induction or salvage combination therapy with combination of L-AmB plus posaconazole[107] or L-AmB plus an echinocandin (although data are largely in diabetic patients with rhinocerebral disease) (CIII).[108] For salvage therapy, isavuconazole (AII)[109] or posaconazole (AII). Following successful induction antifungal therapy (for at least 3 wk), can continue consolidation therapy with posaconazole (or use intermittent L-AmB) (BI).	Latest international mucormycosis guidelines recommend L-AmB as primary therapy.[110] Following clinical response with AmB, long-term PO step-down therapy with posaconazole (trough concentrations ideally for mucormycosis at >2 mcg/mL) can be attempted for 2–6 mo. Dosing of isavuconazole in children <13 y is 10 mg/kg (q8h on days 1 and 2 and qd thereafter).[34] Voriconazole has NO activity against mucormycosis or other zygomycetes. Return of immune function is paramount to treatment success; for children receiving corticosteroids, decreasing the corticosteroid dosage or changing to steroid-sparing protocols is also important. Antifungal susceptibility is key if it can be obtained. CNS disease likely benefits from higher doses such as L-AmB at 10 mg/kg/day q24h. Likely no benefit at >10 mg/kg/day and only increased toxicity.
Paracoccidioido-mycosis[111–114]	Itraconazole PO soln 10 mg/kg/day (max 400 mg daily) div bid for 6 mo (AIII) OR voriconazole (for dosing, see Aspergillosis earlier in this table under Treatment) (BI). Itraconazole is superior to TMP/SMX.	New international guidelines exist.[56] Alternatives: fluconazole; isavuconazole; sulfadiazine or TMP/SMX for 3–5 y. Voriconazole is similarly efficacious and useful in cases with CNS involvement. AmB is recommended for immunocompromised patients.

Pneumocystis jirovecii (formerly ***carinii***) pneumonia[115–117]	Severe disease: preferred regimen is TMP/SMX 15–20 mg TMP component/kg/day IV div q8h (AI) OR, for TMP/SMX intolerance or TMP/SMX treatment failure, pentamidine isethionate 4-mg base/kg/day IV qd (BII), for 3 wk.	Alternatives: TMP AND dapsone; OR primaquine AND clindamycin; OR atovaquone.
	Mild to moderate disease: start with IV therapy, then, after acute pneumonitis is resolved, TMP/SMX 20 mg TMP component/kg/day PO div qid for 3-wk total treatment course (AII).	Prophylaxis: preferred regimen is TMP/SMX (5 mg TMP component/kg/day) PO bid 3×/wk on consecutive days; OR same dose, given qd; OR atovaquone: 30 mg/kg/day for infants 1–3 mo; 45 mg/kg/day for infants/children 4–24 mo; and 30 mg/kg/day for children >24 mo; OR dapsone 2 mg/kg (max 100 mg) PO qd, OR dapsone 4 mg/kg (max 200 mg) PO once weekly.
		Use steroid therapy for more severe disease.
Sporotrichosis[118,119]	For cutaneous/lymphocutaneous: itraconazole PO soln 10 mg/kg/day div bid for 2–4 wk after all lesions gone (generally total of 3–6 mo) (AII)	New international guidelines exist.[56] If no response for cutaneous disease, treat with higher itraconazole dose, terbinafine, or saturated soln of potassium iodide.
	For serious pulmonary or disseminated infection or disseminated sporotrichosis: ABLC/L-AmB at 5 mg/kg/day q24h until favorable response, then step-down therapy with itraconazole PO for at least a total of 12 mo (AIII)	Fluconazole is less effective.
		Obtain serum concentrations of itraconazole after 2 wk of therapy; want serum trough concentration >1 mcg/mL.
	For less severe disease, itraconazole for 12 mo	For meningeal disease, initial L-AmB/ABLC (less toxic than AmB-D) should be 4–6 wk before change to itraconazole for at least 12 mo of therapy.
		Surgery may be necessary in osteoarticular or pulmonary disease.

C. LOCALIZED MUCOCUTANEOUS INFECTIONS

Infection	Therapy (evidence grade)	Comments
Dermatophytoses		
– Scalp (tinea capitis, including kerion)[120-125]	Griseofulvin ultramicrosize 10–15 mg/kg/day or microsize 20–25 mg/kg/day PO qd for 6–12 wk (AII) (taken with milk or fatty foods to augment absorption) generally for 8 wk. For kerion, treat concurrently with prednisone (1–2 mg/kg/day for 1–2 wk) (AIII). Terbinafine can be used for only 2–4 wk. 125 mg/day (20–40 kg), or 250 mg/day (>40 kg) (AII).	Griseofulvin is superior for *Microsporum* infections, but terbinafine is superior for *Trichophyton* infections.[126] *Trichophyton tonsurans* predominates in the United States. No need to routinely follow LFTs in healthy children taking griseofulvin. Alternatives: itraconazole PO soln 5 mg/kg qd or fluconazole. 2.5% selenium sulfide shampoo, or 2% ketoconazole shampoo, 2–3×/wk should be used concurrently to prevent recurrences.
– Tinea corporis (infection of the trunk/limbs/face) – Tinea cruris (infection of the groin) – Tinea pedis (infection of the toes/feet)	Topical agents (alphabetic order): butenafine, ciclopirox, clotrimazole, econazole, haloprogin, ketoconazole, miconazole, naftifine, oxiconazole, sertaconazole, sulconazole, terbinafine, and tolnaftate (AII); apply daily for 4 wk.	For unresponsive tinea lesions, use griseofulvin PO in dosages provided for scalp (tinea capitis, including kerion); fluconazole PO; itraconazole PO; OR terbinafine PO. For tinea pedis: terbinafine PO or itraconazole PO is preferred over other PO agents. Keep skin as clean and dry as possible, particularly for tinea cruris and tinea pedis.
– Tinea unguium (onychomycosis)[122,127,128]	Terbinafine 62.5 mg/day (<20 kg), 125 mg/day (20–40 kg), or 250 mg/day (>40 kg). Use for at least 6 wk (fingernails) or 12–16 wk (toenails) (AII).	Recurrence or partial response common. Pulse terbinafine (1 wk per mo or 1 wk q3mo) or itraconazole has similar efficacy to that of continuous treatment.[129,130] Alternative: itraconazole pulse therapy with 10 mg/kg/day div q12h for 1 wk per mo. Two pulses for fingernails and 3 pulses for toenails. Alternatives: fluconazole, griseofulvin.

– Tinea versicolor (also called "pityriasis versicolor")[122,131,132]	Apply topically: selenium sulfide 2.5% lotion or 1% shampoo daily, leave on 30 min, then rinse; for 7 days, then monthly for 6 mo (AIII); OR ciclopirox 1% cream for 4 wk (BII); OR terbinafine 1% soln (BII); OR ketoconazole 2% shampoo daily for 5 days (BII). For small lesions, topical clotrimazole, econazole, haloprogin, ketoconazole, miconazole, or naftifine.	For lesions that fail to clear with topical therapy or for extensive lesions: fluconazole PO or itraconazole PO is equally effective. Recurrence common.

6. Choosing Among Antifungal Agents: Polyenes, Azoles, and Echinocandins

Separating antifungal agents by class, much like navigating the myriad of antibacterial agents, allows one to best understand the underlying mechanisms of action and then appropriately choose which agent is optimal for empiric therapy or a targeted approach. There are certain helpful generalizations that should be considered; for example, echinocandins are fungicidal against yeasts and fungistatic against molds, while azoles are the opposite. Coupled with these concepts is the need for continued surveillance for fungal epidemiology and resistance patterns. While some fungal species are inherently or very often resistant to specific agents or even classes, there are an increasing number of fungal isolates that are developing resistance due to environmental pressure or chronic use in individual patients. Additionally, new (often resistant) fungal species emerge that deserve special attention, such as *Candida auris,* which can be multidrug resistant. In 2024, there are now 17 individual antifungal agents approved by the US Food and Drug Administration (FDA) for systemic use, including entirely new classes. That includes several recently approved agents, such as rezafungin and oteseconazole. In addition, many new antifungals are currently in development, likely to be approved and available soon (fosmanogepix, olorofim, encochleated amphotericin B [AmB], opelconazole, and others). This chapter focuses on only the most commonly used systemic agents and will not highlight the many anticipated new agents until they are approved for use in patients. For each agent, there are sometimes several formulations, each with unique pharmacokinetics (PK) that one must understand to optimize the agent, particularly in patients who are critically ill. Therefore, it is more important than ever to establish a firm conceptual foundation in understanding both how these antifungal agents work to optimize PK and pharmacodynamics (PD) and where they work best to target fungal pathogens most appropriately.

Polyenes

Amphotericin B is a polyene antifungal antibiotic that has been available since 1958. A *Streptomyces* species, isolated from the soil in Venezuela, produced 2 antifungals whose names originated from the drug's amphoteric property of reacting as an acid as well as a base. Amphotericin A was not as active as AmB, so only AmB is used clinically. Nystatin is another polyene antifungal, but, due to systemic toxicity, it is used only in topical preparations. Nystatin was named after the New York State Department of Health, where the discoverers were working at the time. AmB remains the most broad-spectrum antifungal available for clinical use. This lipophilic drug binds to ergosterol, the major sterol in the fungal cell membrane, and for years it was thought to create transmembrane pores that compromise the integrity of the cell membrane and create a rapid fungicidal effect through osmotic lysis. However, new biochemical studies suggest a mechanism of action more related to inhibiting ergosterol synthesis. Toxicity is likely due to cross-reactivity with the human cholesterol bi-lipid membrane, which resembles fungal ergosterol. The toxicity of the conventional formulation, amphotericin B deoxycholate (AmB-D)—the parent molecule coupled with an ionic detergent for clinical use—can be substantial from the standpoints of systemic reactions (eg, fever, rigors) and acute and chronic renal toxicity. Premedication with acetaminophen, diphenhydramine, and meperidine has historically been used to prevent systemic reactions during infusion. Renal dysfunction develops primarily as decreased glomerular filtration with a rising serum creatinine concentration, but substantial tubular nephropathy is associated with potassium and magnesium wasting, requiring supplemental potassium for many neonates and children, regardless of clinical symptoms associated with infusion. Fluid loading with saline pre– and post–AmB-D infusion seems to somewhat mitigate renal toxicity. A recent age analysis suggests that there is a greater chance of adverse events in patients older than 13 months, suggesting that this potentially toxic agent is somewhat comparatively less toxic in the smallest children.[1]

Three lipid preparations approved in the mid-1990s decrease toxicity with no apparent decrease in clinical efficacy. Decisions on which lipid AmB preparation to use should, therefore, largely focus on side effects and costs. Two clinically useful lipid formulations exist: one in which ribbonlike lipid complexes of AmB are created (amphotericin B lipid complex [ABLC]), Abelcet, and one in which AmB is incorporated into true liposomes (liposomal amphotericin B [L-AmB], AmBisome). The classic clinical dosage used of these preparations is 5 mg/kg/day, in contrast to the 1 mg/kg/day of AmB-D. In most studies, the side effects of L-AmB were somewhat less than for ABLC, but both have significantly fewer side effects than AmB-D. The advantage of the lipid preparations is the ability to safely deliver a greater overall dose of the parent AmB drug. The cost of conventional AmB-D is substantially less than for either lipid formulation. A colloidal dispersion of AmB in cholesteryl sulfate, Amphotec, which is no longer available in the United States, with decreased nephrotoxicity but infusion-related side effects, is closer to AmB-D than to the lipid formulations and precludes recommendation for its use. The decreased nephrotoxicity of the 3 lipid preparations is thought to be due to the preferential binding of its AmB to high-density lipoproteins, compared to AmB-D binding to low-density lipoproteins. Despite in vitro concentration-dependent killing, a clinical trial comparing L-AmB at doses of 3 mg/kg/day with 10 mg/kg/day showed no efficacy benefit for the higher dose and only greater toxicity.[2] Recent PK analyses of L-AmB showed that while children receiving L-AmB at lower doses exhibit linear PK, a significant proportion of children receiving L-AmB at daily doses greater than 5 mg/kg/day exhibit nonlinear PK with significantly higher peak concentrations and some toxicity.[3,4] Therefore, it is generally not recommended to use any lipid AmB preparations at very high dosages (>5 mg/kg/day), as it will likely incur only greater toxicity with no real therapeutic advantage. There are reports of using higher dosing in very difficult infections where a lipid AmB formulation is the first-line therapy (eg, mucormycosis), and while experts remain divided on this practice, it is clear that at least 5 mg/kg/day of a lipid AmB formulation should be used in such a setting. AmB has a long terminal half-life, and, coupled with the concentration-dependent killing, the agent is best used as single daily doses. These PK/PD explain the use in some studies of once-weekly, or even once-every-2-weeks,[5] AmB for antifungal prophylaxis or preemptive therapy, albeit with mixed clinical results. If the overall AmB exposure needs to be decreased due to toxicity, it is best to increase the dosing interval (eg, move from daily to only 3 times weekly) but retain the full milligram per kilogram dose for optimal PK for concentration-dependent killing. There are ongoing efforts to develop novel delivery mechanisms for AmB, such as nanoparticles with encochleated AmB as an oral (PO) formulation, which are not ready for clinical use yet.

AmB-D has been used for nonsystemic purposes, such as bladder washes, intraventricular instillation, intrapleural instillation, and other modalities, but there are no firm data supporting those clinical indications, and it is likely that the local toxicities outweigh the theoretic benefits. One exception is aerosolized AmB for antifungal prophylaxis (not treatment) in lung transplant recipients due to the different pathophysiology of invasive aspergillosis (often originating at the bronchial anastomotic site, more so than parenchymal disease) in that specific patient population. This aerosolized prophylaxis approach, while indicated for lung transplant recipients, has not been shown to be effective in other patient populations. Due to the lipid chemistry, the L-AmB does not interact well with renal tubules and L-AmB is recovered from the urine at lower levels than AmB-D, so there is a theoretic concern for decreased microbiologic efficacy when using a lipid formulation, as opposed to AmB-D, in the treatment of isolated urinary fungal disease. This theoretic concern is likely outweighed by the real concern of toxicity with AmB-D. Most experts believe AmB-D should be reserved for use in resource-limited settings in which no alternative agents (eg, lipid formulations) are available. An exception is in neonates, for whom limited retrospective data suggest that the AmB-D formulation has better efficacy for invasive candidiasis.[6] Importantly, there are several pathogens that are inherently or functionally resistant to AmB, including *Candida lusitaniae*, *Trichosporon* species, *Aspergillus terreus*, *Fusarium* species, and *Pseudallescheria boydii* (*Scedosporium apiospermum*) or *Lomentospora prolificans*.

Azoles

This class of systemic agents was first approved in 1981 and is divided into imidazoles (ketoconazole), triazoles (fluconazole and itraconazole), and second-generation triazoles (voriconazole, posaconazole, and isavuconazole) based on the number of nitrogen atoms in the azole ring. All the azoles work by inhibition of ergosterol synthesis (fungal cytochrome P450 [CYP] sterol 14-demethylation) that is required for fungal cell membrane integrity. While the polyenes are rapidly fungicidal, the azoles are fungistatic against yeasts and fungicidal against molds. However, it is important to note that ketoconazole and fluconazole have no mold activity. The only systemic imidazole is ketoconazole, which is primarily active against *Candida* species and is available in a PO formulation. Three azoles (itraconazole, voriconazole, and posaconazole) need therapeutic drug monitoring (TDM) with trough levels within the first 4 to 7 days (when the patient is at a PK steady state); at present, it is unclear if isavuconazole will require drug-level monitoring, but an increasing number of reports suggest it might be needed. It is less clear if TDM is required during primary azole prophylaxis, although low levels have been associated with a higher probability of breakthrough infection.

Fluconazole is active against a broader range of fungi than ketoconazole and includes clinically relevant activity against *Cryptococcus, Coccidioides,* and *Histoplasma.* The pediatric treatment dose is 12 mg/kg/day, which targets exposures that are observed in critically ill adults who receive 800 mg of fluconazole per day. Like most other azoles, fluconazole requires a loading dose (LD) on the first day, and this approach is routinely used in adult patients. An LD of 25 mg/kg on the first day has been nicely studied in infants[7,8] but has not been definitively studied in all children; yet it is likely also beneficial and the patient will reach steady-state concentrations more quickly based on adult and neonatal studies. The exception where it has been formally studied is children of all ages receiving extracorporeal membrane oxygenation, for whom, because of the higher volume of distribution, a higher LD (35 mg/kg) is required to achieve comparable exposure.[9,10] Compared with AmB, fluconazole achieves relatively high concentrations in urine and cerebrospinal fluid (CSF) due to its low lipophilicity, with urinary concentrations often so high that treatment against even "resistant" pathogens that are isolated only in the urine is possible. Fluconazole remains one of the most active and, so far, one of the safest systemic antifungal agents for the treatment of most *Candida* infections. *Candida albicans* remains generally susceptible to fluconazole, although resistance is increasingly present in many non-*albicans Candida* species as well as in *C albicans* in children repeatedly exposed to fluconazole. *Candida krusei* is considered inherently resistant to fluconazole, *Candida glabrata* demonstrates dose-dependent resistance to fluconazole (and, usually, voriconazole), *Candida tropicalis* is developing more resistant strains, and the newly identified *C auris* is generally fluconazole resistant. Fluconazole is available in parenteral and PO (with >90% bioavailability) formulations, and toxicity is unusual and primarily hepatic.

Itraconazole is active against an even broader range of fungi and, unlike fluconazole, includes molds such as *Aspergillus.* It is currently available as a capsule or a PO solution (the intravenous [IV] form was discontinued); the PO solution provides about 30% higher and more consistent serum concentrations than capsules and should be used preferentially. Absorption using itraconazole PO solution is improved on an empty stomach and not influenced by gastric pH (unlike with the capsule form, which is best administered under fed conditions or with a more acidic cola beverage to increase absorption). Monitoring itraconazole serum concentrations, as with most azole antifungals, is a key principle in management. Generally, itraconazole serum trough levels should be 1 to 2 mcg/mL, greater than 1 mcg/mL for treatment, and greater than 0.5 mcg/mL for prophylaxis; trough levels greater than 5 mcg/mL may be associated with increased toxicity. Concentrations should be checked after 5 days of therapy to ensure adequate drug exposure. When measured by high-pressure liquid chromatography, itraconazole and its bioactive hydroxy-itraconazole metabolite are reported, the sum of which should be considered in assessing drug levels. In adult patients, itraconazole is loaded at 200 mg twice daily for 2 days, followed by 200 mg daily starting on the third day. Loading dose studies have not been performed in children. Itraconazole in children requires twice-daily dosing throughout treatment, compared with once-daily maintenance dosing in adults, and the key to treatment success is following drug levels. Limited PK data are available in children; itraconazole has not been approved by the FDA for pediatric indications. Itraconazole is indicated in adults for therapy for mild to moderate disease with blastomycosis, histoplasmosis, and others. Although it possesses some mold antifungal activity, itraconazole is not indicated as primary therapy against invasive aspergillosis, as voriconazole is a far superior option. Itraconazole is not active against mucormycosis. A recent guideline on allergic bronchopulmonary aspergillosis (ABPA) in children and adolescents with asthma suggests that itraconazole is preferred over voriconazole due to the increased toxicity seen with voriconazole.[11] Revised worldwide clinical practice guidelines for ABPA reaffirm itraconazole preference. Toxicity in adults is primarily hepatic.[12]

Voriconazole was approved in 2002 and is FDA approved for children 2 years and older.[13] Voriconazole is a fluconazole derivative, so think of it as having the greater tissue and CSF penetration of fluconazole but the added antifungal spectrum of itraconazole to include molds. While the bioavailability of voriconazole in adults is about 96%, multiple studies have shown that it is about only 50% to 60% in children, requiring clinicians to carefully monitor voriconazole trough concentrations in patients taking the PO formulation, further complicated by great inter-patient variability in clearance. Voriconazole serum concentrations are tricky to interpret, but monitoring these concentrations is essential to using this drug, as with all azole antifungals, and is especially important in circumstances of suspected treatment failure or possible toxicity. Most experts suggest voriconazole trough concentrations of 2 mcg/mL (at a minimum, 1 mcg/mL) or greater, which would generally exceed the pathogen's minimum inhibitory concentration. Generally, toxicity will not be seen until concentrations of about 6 mcg/mL or greater. Trough levels should be monitored 2 to 5 days after initiation of therapy and monitored again the following week to confirm that the patient remains in the therapeutic range or again 4 days after a change of dose. One important point is the acquisition of an accurate trough concentration, one obtained just before the next dose is due (not hours before solely for phlebotomy convenience) and not obtained through a catheter infusing the drug. These simple trough parameters will make interpretation possible. The fundamental voriconazole PK are different in adults versus children; in adults, voriconazole is metabolized in a nonlinear fashion, whereas in children, the drug is metabolized in a linear fashion. This explains the increased pediatric loading dosing for voriconazole at 9 mg/kg/dose versus loading with 6 mg/kg/dose in adult patients. Younger children, especially those younger than 2 years, require even higher dosages of voriconazole and have a larger therapeutic window for dosing. The youngest patients (aged <2 years) likely also require higher initial starting doses.[14] However, many studies have shown an inconsistent relationship, on a population level, between dosing and levels, highlighting the need for close monitoring after the initial dosing scheme and then dose adjustment as needed in the individual patient. A recent study highlighted the need for not only larger doses but often multiple dose adjustments in children to obtain therapeutic trough concentrations.[15] For children younger than 2 years, some studies have even proposed 3-times-daily dosing to achieve sufficient serum levels.[16] Given the poor clinical and microbiologic response of *Aspergillus* infections to AmB, voriconazole is clearly the treatment of choice for invasive aspergillosis and many other invasive mold infections (eg, pseudallescheriasis, fusariosis). Importantly, infections with mucormycosis are resistant to voriconazole. Voriconazole retains activity against most *Candida* species, including some that are fluconazole resistant, but it is unlikely to replace fluconazole for treatment of fluconazole-susceptible *Candida* infections. Importantly, there are increasing reports of *C glabrata* resistance to voriconazole. Voriconazole produces some unique transient visual field abnormalities in about 10% of adults and children. There are an increasing number of reports, seen in as high as 20% of patients, of a photosensitive sunburn-like erythema that is not prevented by sunscreen (only sun avoidance). In some rare long-term use (mean of 3 years of therapy) cases, voriconazole phototoxicity has developed into cutaneous squamous cell carcinoma. Discontinuing voriconazole is recommended in patients experiencing chronic phototoxicity. Rash is the most common indication for switching from voriconazole to posaconazole/isavuconazole if a triazole antifungal is required. Other voriconazole chronic toxicities reported include fluorosis and periostitis. Hepatotoxicity is uncommon, occurring in only 2% to 5% of patients. Voriconazole is CYP metabolized (CYP2C19), and allelic polymorphisms in the population could lead to personalized dosing.[17] Results have shown that some patients of certain ethnicities will face higher toxic serum concentrations than other patients, again reiterating the need for close trough level monitoring. Voriconazole also interacts with many similarly P450-metabolized drugs to produce some profound changes in serum concentrations of many concurrently administered drugs.

Posaconazole, an itraconazole derivative, was FDA approved in 2006 as a PO suspension for adolescents 13 years and older. A delayed-release (DR) tablet formulation was approved in November 2013, also for adolescents 13 years and older, and an IV formulation was approved in March 2014 for patients 18 years and older. Effective absorption of the PO suspension strongly requires taking the medication with food, ideally a high-fat meal; taking posaconazole on an empty stomach will result in about one-fourth of the absorption as in the fed state. In one study, the PO suspension had only 16% bioavailability.[18] The tablet formulation has significantly better absorption (66% in one study)[19] due to its delayed release in the small intestine, but absorption will still be slightly increased with food. If the patient can take the (relatively large) tablets, the DR tablet is the much-preferred form due to the ability to easily obtain higher and more consistent drug levels. Due to the low pH (<5) of IV posaconazole, a central venous catheter is required for administration. The IV formulation contains only slightly lower amounts of the cyclodextrin vehicle than voriconazole, so similar theoretic renal accumulation concerns exist. The pediatric PO suspension dose recommended by some experts for treating invasive disease is estimated to be at least 18 mg/kg/day divided 3 times daily, but even that dose has not achieved target levels.[20] A study with a new pediatric formulation for suspension, essentially the tablet form that is able to be suspended, has recently been completed and showed good tolerability. In that study, a dose of 6 mg/kg (given twice daily as an LD on the first day and then once daily) as an IV or formulation for PO suspension achieved target exposures that were necessary for antifungal prophylaxis, with a safety profile similar to that for adult patients.[21] In that study, the IV formulation led to greater levels than the formulation for suspension, but both achieved target levels. Pharmacokinetic modeling also revealed that 6-mg/kg dosing was appropriate, and for those patients weighing more than 40 kg, the 300-mg/day tablet was predicted to be effective.[22] A subsequent study suggests that posaconazole dosing for the DR tablets and IV formulation requires likely greater daily doses for children younger than 13 years.[23] However, the exact pediatric dosing for posaconazole requires consultation with a pediatric infectious disease expert. Importantly, the DR tablet cannot be broken for use due to its chemical coating. Pediatric dosing with the current IV or extended-release (ER) tablet dosing is not yet fully defined, but adolescents can likely follow the adult dosing schemes. In adult patients, IV posaconazole is loaded at 300 mg twice daily on the first day and then 300 mg once daily starting on the second day. Similarly, in adult patients, the ER tablet is dosed as 300 mg twice daily on the first day and then 300 mg once daily starting on the second day. In adult patients, the maximum amount of posaconazole PO suspension given is 800 mg/day due to its excretion, and that has been given as 400 mg twice daily or 200 mg 4 times daily in severely ill patients due to saturable absorption and findings of a marginal increase in exposure with more frequent dosing. Greater than 800 mg/day is not indicated in any patient. As with voriconazole and itraconazole, trough levels should be monitored, and most experts feel that posaconazole levels for treatment should be greater than or equal to 1 mcg/mL (and >0.7 mcg/mL for prophylaxis). Monitor posaconazole trough levels on day 5 of therapy or soon after. For in vitro activity against *Candida* species, posaconazole is better than fluconazole and equivalent to voriconazole. For overall in vitro antifungal activity against *Aspergillus,* posaconazole is also equivalent to voriconazole, but, notably, it is the first triazole with substantial activity against some mucormycosis pathogens, including *Rhizopus* species and *Mucor* species, as well as activity against *Coccidioides, Histoplasma,* and *Blastomyces* and the pathogens of phaeohyphomycosis. Posaconazole treatment of invasive aspergillosis in patients with chronic granulomatous disease appears to be superior to voriconazole in this specific patient population for an unknown reason. Posaconazole is eliminated by hepatic glucuronidation but does demonstrate inhibition of the CYP3A4 enzyme system, leading to many drug interactions with other P450-metabolized drugs. It is currently approved for prophylaxis of *Candida* and *Aspergillus* infections in high-risk adults and for treatment of *Candida* oropharyngeal disease or esophagitis in adults. Posaconazole, like itraconazole, has generally poor CSF penetration.

Isavuconazole is a new triazole that was FDA approved in March 2015 for treatment of invasive aspergillosis and invasive mucormycosis with PO (capsules only) and IV formulations. Isavuconazole has not only a similar antifungal spectrum as voriconazole but also, very importantly, activity against mucormycosis. A phase 3 clinical trial in adult patients demonstrated non-inferiority versus voriconazole against invasive aspergillosis and other mold infections,[24] and an open-label study showed activity against mucormycosis.[25] New international mucormycosis guidelines recommend isavuconazole in the setting of preexisting renal compromise (when L-AmB, the recommended primary therapy, is, therefore, not recommended).[26] Isavuconazole is actually dispensed as the prodrug isavuconazonium sulfate. Dosing in adult patients is loading with isavuconazole at 200 mg (equivalent to 372-mg isavuconazonium sulfate) every 8 hours for 2 days (6 doses), followed by 200 mg once daily for maintenance dosing. A recently completed pediatric PK study reports that a dose of 10 mg/kg (every 8 hours on days 1 and 2 and once daily thereafter) resulted in similar exposures and safety as seen in adults.[27] The half-life is long (>5 days), there is 98% bioavailability in adults, and there is no reported food effect with PO isavuconazole. The manufacturer suggests no need for TDM, but some experts suggest trough levels may be needed in difficult-to-treat infections, and, absent well-defined therapeutic targets, the mean concentrations from phase II/III studies suggest that a range of 2 to 3 mcg/mL after day 5 is adequate exposure. Another study suggests a range of 2 to 5 mcg/mL.[28] To date, it seems that isavuconazole requires less dose modifications than voriconazole. Unlike voriconazole, the IV formulation does not contain the vehicle cyclodextrin, a difference that could make it more attractive in patients with renal failure. Early experience suggests a much lower rate of photosensitivity and skin disorders as well as visual disturbances, compared with voriconazole. Pediatric studies for treatment of invasive aspergillosis and mucormycosis are currently ongoing.

Oteseconazole is a PO azole approved in 2022 to reduce the incidence of recurrent vulvovaginal candidiasis. However, this agent is contraindicated in females of reproductive potential based on animal studies in that it may cause fetal harm when administered to a pregnant woman or potential harm to the breastfed infant.

Echinocandins

This class of systemic antifungal agents was first approved in 2001. The echinocandins inhibit cell wall formation (in contrast to acting on the cell membrane by the polyenes and azoles) by noncompetitively inhibiting beta-1,3-glucan synthase, an enzyme present in fungi but absent in mammalian cells. These agents are generally very safe, as there is no beta-1,3-glucan in humans. The echinocandins are not metabolized through the CYP system, so fewer drug interactions occur, compared with the azoles. There is no need to adjust dose in renal failure, but one needs a lower dosage in the setting of very severe hepatic dysfunction. As a class, these antifungals generally have poor CSF penetration, although animal studies have shown adequate brain parenchyma levels, and do not concentrate well in the urine. While the 3 clinically available echinocandins each individually have some unique and important dosing and PK parameters, especially in children, efficacy is generally equivalent. Opposite the azole class, the echinocandins are fungicidal against yeasts but fungistatic against molds. The fungicidal activity against yeasts has elevated the echinocandins to the preferred therapy against invasive candidiasis. Echinocandins are best used against invasive aspergillosis only as salvage therapy if a triazole fails or in a patient with suspected triazole resistance, never as primary monotherapy against invasive aspergillosis or any other invasive mold infection. Improved efficacy with combination therapy with the echinocandins and triazoles against *Aspergillus* infections is unclear, with disparate results in multiple smaller studies and a definitive clinical trial demonstrating minimal benefit over voriconazole monotherapy in only certain patient populations. Some experts have used combination therapy in invasive aspergillosis with a triazole plus echinocandin only during the initial phase of waiting for triazole drug levels to be appropriately high. There are reports of echinocandin resistance in *Candida* species, as high as 12% in *C glabrata* in some studies, and the echinocandins as a class have previously been shown to be somewhat less active against *Candida parapsilosis* isolates (about 10%–15% respond poorly, but most are still susceptible, and guidelines still recommend echinocandin empiric therapy for invasive candidiasis). There is no TDM required for the echinocandins.

Caspofungin received FDA approval for children and teens aged 3 months to 17 years in 2008 for empiric therapy for presumed fungal infections in febrile, neutropenic patients; treatment of candidemia as well as *Candida* esophagitis, peritonitis, and empyema; and salvage therapy for invasive aspergillosis. A study in children with acute myeloid leukemia demonstrated that caspofungin prophylaxis resulted in significantly lower incidence of invasive fungal disease, compared with fluconazole prophylaxis.[29] A study comparing caspofungin with triazole prophylaxis in pediatric allogeneic hematopoietic cell transplant recipients showed no difference in the agents.[30] Due to its earlier approval, there are generally more reports with caspofungin than with the other echinocandins. Caspofungin dosing in children is calculated according to body surface area (BSA), with an LD on the first day of 70 mg/m², followed by daily maintenance dosing of 50 mg/m², and not to exceed 70 mg regardless of the calculated dose. Dose adjustment is unnecessary in children with mild liver dysfunction.[31] Significantly higher doses of caspofungin have been studied in adult patients without any clear added benefit in efficacy, but if the 50 mg/m² dose is tolerated and does not provide adequate clinical response, the daily dose can be increased to 70 mg/m². One study suggested a cutoff of a BSA of 1.3 m², whereby below that size, a BSA-based LD is indicated, and above that size, a fixed LD is indicated.[32] Dosing for caspofungin in neonates is 25 mg/m²/day.

Micafungin was approved in 2005 for adults for treatment of candidemia, *Candida* esophagitis and peritonitis, and prophylaxis of *Candida* infections in stem cell transplant recipients and in 2013 for pediatric patients 4 months and older. Micafungin has the most pediatric and neonatal data available of all 3 echinocandins, including more extensive PK studies surrounding dosing and several efficacy studies.[33-35] Micafungin dosing in children is age dependent, as clearance increases dramatically in the younger age-groups (especially neonates), necessitating higher doses for younger children. Dosages for children are generally thought to be 2 mg/kg/day, with higher dosages likely needed for neonates, infants,[36] and younger patients and 10 mg/kg/day given to preterm neonates. Adult micafungin dosing (100 or 150 mg once daily) is used in patients who weigh more than 40 kg. Unlike with the other echinocandins, an LD is not required for micafungin. Micafungin twice-weekly dosing for prophylaxis has been initially shown to be effective in children,[37] and a prospective pediatric study showed that micafungin prophylaxis was safe and effective in children with autologous hematopoietic stem cell transplant.[38]

Anidulafungin was approved for adults for candidemia and *Candida* esophagitis in 2006 and is not officially approved for pediatric patients. Like the other echinocandins, anidulafungin is not P450 metabolized and has not demonstrated significant drug interactions. Limited pediatric PK data suggest weight-based dosing (3 mg/kg/day LD, followed by 1.5 mg/kg/day maintenance dosing).[39] This dosing achieves similar exposure levels in neonates and infants.[39] The adult dose for invasive candidiasis is an LD of 200 mg on the first day, followed by 100 mg daily. An open-label study of pediatric invasive candidiasis in children showed similar efficacy and minimal toxicity, comparable to those of the other echinocandins.[40] An additional study showed similar and acceptable PK in patients 1 month to 2 years of age.[41]

Rezafungin was approved in 2023 for adults with limited or no alternative options for treatment of candidemia or candidiasis. Administration is unique in that it consists of an LD of 400 mg followed by a once-***weekly*** 200-mg dose. The ReSTORE randomized, double-blind clinical trial investigators studied a total of 199 patients and compared rezafungin administered once weekly to caspofungin administered daily in the treatment of candidemia and candidiasis and found rezafungin to be non-inferior, with rezafungin (59%) and caspofungin (61%) showing similar global cure rates at 14 days.[42] There are no completed trials in pediatrics, but a phase 1 pediatric PK study is in development.

Triterpenoid

Ibrexafungerp was approved in June 2021 for adults with vulvovaginal candidiasis following 2 phase III studies (VANISH 203 and VANISH 306). This is the first new class of antifungals (also called "fungerps") approved since 2001. Enfumafungin, structurally distinct from the echinocandins, was discovered through screening of natural products and modified to develop this semisynthetic derivative for clinical use. Like the echinocandins, ibrexafungerp not only noncompetitively inhibits beta-1,3-glucan synthase but also destroys the fungi *Candida* and inhibits the fungi *Aspergillus*. The binding site on the glucan-synthase enzyme is not the same as on the echinocandins. Resistance or reduced susceptibility to the echinocandins is largely through 2 hot spot alterations in the *FKS1* gene, while many resistance alterations to ibrexafungerp are due to the *FKS2* gene, and ibrexafungerp has activity against some echinocandin-resistant isolates. Ibrexafungerp is the first PO available glucan-synthase inhibitor and has a long half-life, suggesting once-daily dosing for clinical use. A liposomal IV formulation is in clinical development. As with the echinocandins, initial studies show limited to no distribution to the central nervous system and variable distribution to the eye. In a phase II study, ibrexafungerp as step-down therapy following initial echinocandin therapy for invasive candidiasis was well tolerated and achieved a favorable global response, like the standard of care.[43] There is an ongoing coadministration study with voriconazole in pulmonary invasive aspergillosis (SCYNERGIA), as well as an ongoing recurrent vulvovaginal candidiasis study (CANDLE), yet no completed or ongoing pediatric studies.

7. Preferred Therapy for Specific Viral Pathogens

NOTE

- A list of table abbreviations and acronyms can be found at the start of this publication.

Preferred Therapy for Viral Pathogens

7

A. OVERVIEW OF NON-HIV, NON-HEPATITIS B OR C VIRAL PATHOGENS AND USUAL PATTERN OF SUSCEPTIBILITY TO ANTIVIRALS

Virus	Acyclovir	Baloxavir	Cidofovir	Famciclovir	Foscarnet	Ganciclovir
Cytomegalovirus			+		+	+
Herpes simplex virus	++			+	+	+
Influenza A and B viruses		+				
SARS-CoV-2						
Varicella-zoster virus	++			+	+	+

Virus	Letermovir	Maribavir	Nirmatrelvir Plus Ritonavir	Oseltamivir	Peramivir	Remdesivir	Valacyclovir	Valganciclovir	Zanamivir
Cytomegalovirus	+	+						++	
Herpes simplex virus							++	+	
Influenza A and B viruses				++	+				+
SARS-CoV-2			++			++			
Varicella-zoster virus							++		

NOTE: ++ = preferred; + = acceptable; [blank cell] = untested.

B. OVERVIEW OF HEPATITIS B OR C VIRAL PATHOGENS AND USUAL PATTERN OF SUSCEPTIBILITY TO ANTIVIRALS

Virus	Elbasvir/Grazoprevir (Zepatier)	Entecavir	Glecaprevir/Pibrentasvir (Mavyret)	Interferon Alfa-2b
Hepatitis B virus		++		+
Hepatitis C virus[a]	+[b,c]		++[d,e]	

Virus	Lamivudine	Pegylated Interferon Alfa-2a	Sofosbuvir/Ledipasvir (Harvoni)	Sofosbuvir (Sovaldi) Plus Ribavirin
Hepatitis B virus	+	+		
Hepatitis C virus[a]			++[d,f]	++[d,g]

Virus	Sofosbuvir/Velpatasvir (Epclusa)	Sofosbuvir/Velpatasvir/Voxilaprevir (Vosevi)	Tenofovir
Hepatitis B virus			++
Hepatitis C virus[a]	++[d,e]	+[e,h]	

NOTE: ++ = preferred; + = acceptable; [blank cell] = untested.

[a] HCV treatment guidelines from the IDSA and the AASLD available at www.hcvguidelines.org (accessed August 15, 2024).

[b] Approved ≥12 y of age.

[c] Treats genotypes 1 and 4.

[d] Approved ≥3 y of age.

[e] Treats genotypes 1 through 6.

[f] Treats genotypes 1, 4, 5, and 6.

[g] In children, treats genotypes 2 and 3; in adults, 1 through 4.

[h] Not approved for children.

7

C. PREFERRED THERAPY FOR SPECIFIC VIRAL PATHOGENS

Infection	Therapy (evidence grade)	Comments
Adenovirus (pneumonia or disseminated infection in immunocompromised hosts)[1]	Cidofovir and ribavirin are active in vitro, but no prospective clinical data exist and both have significant toxicity. Two cidofovir dosing schedules have been used in clinical settings: (1) 5 mg/kg/dose IV once weekly or (2) 1–1.5 mg/kg/dose IV 3×/wk. If parenteral cidofovir is used, IV hydration and PO probenecid should be used to reduce renal toxicity.	Brincidofovir, the PO bioavailable lipophilic derivative of cidofovir, has been evaluated for the treatment of adenovirus in immunocompromised hosts. It has been approved for use in smallpox and is available only in the US stockpile for use in the event of a bioterrorism attack.
Coronavirus (SARS-CoV-2)	Remdesivir is approved for use in patients aged ≥28 days and weighing at least 3 kg with positive results of direct SARS-CoV-2 viral testing, who are hospitalized or who are not hospitalized and have mild to moderate COVID-19 and risk factors for progression to severe COVID-19: Adults and pediatric patients weighing ≥40 kg: single IV LD of 200 mg on day 1, followed by maintenance IV doses of 100 mg qd on and after day 2 Pediatric patients aged ≥28 days and weighing 3–<40 kg: single IV LD of 5.0 mg/kg on day 1, followed by maintenance IV doses of 2.5 mg/kg qd on and after day 2 Nirmatrelvir/ritonavir (Paxlovid) is approved for use in adults to treat mild to moderate COVID-19; in people aged 12–17 y weighing ≥40 kg, it is available by EUA from the FDA: 300 mg nirmatrelvir with 100 mg ritonavir PO bid for 5 days	Treatment duration for remdesivir is 10 days for hospitalized patients requiring invasive mechanical ventilation and/or ECMO. Treatment duration for remdesivir is 5 days for hospitalized patients not requiring invasive mechanical ventilation and/or ECMO (can be extended for up to 5 additional days based on initial clinical response). Treatment duration for remdesivir is 3 days for nonhospitalized patients diagnosed with mild to moderate COVID-19 and having risk factors for progression to severe COVID-19. Nirmatrelvir/ritonavir (Paxlovid) has numerous drug-drug interactions. Consult the listing on the FDA or Pfizer website before prescribing.

Cytomegalovirus	
– Congenital and postnatal[2]	See Ch 2.
– Immunocompromised (HIV, chemotherapy, transplant-related)[3-15]	For induction: ganciclovir 10 mg/kg/day IV div q12h for 14–21 days (AII) (may be increased to 15 mg/kg/day IV div q12h). For maintenance: 5 mg/kg IV q24h for 5–7 days per week. Duration dependent on degree of immunosuppression (AII). CMV hyperimmune globulin may decrease morbidity in bone marrow transplant patients with CMV pneumonia (AII).	Use foscarnet or cidofovir for ganciclovir-resistant strains; for HIV-positive children undergoing HAART, CMV may resolve without anti-CMV therapy. Also used for prevention of CMV disease posttransplant for 100–120 days. Data on valganciclovir dosing in young children for treatment of retinitis are unavailable, but consideration can be given to transitioning from IV ganciclovir to PO valganciclovir after improvement of retinitis is noted. Limited data on PO valganciclovir in infants[16,17] (32 mg/kg/day PO div bid) and children (dosing by BSA [dose (milligrams) = 7 × BSA × CrCl]).[5] Maribavir (400 mg PO bid) is approved for the treatment of adult and pediatric patients (aged ≥12 y and weighing at least 35 kg) with posttransplant CMV infection/disease that is refractory to treatment (with or without genotypic resistance) with ganciclovir, valganciclovir, cidofovir, or foscarnet.

7

C. PREFERRED THERAPY FOR SPECIFIC VIRAL PATHOGENS

Infection	Therapy (evidence grade)	Comments
– Prophylaxis of infection in immunocompromised hosts[4,18]	Ganciclovir 5 mg/kg IV daily (or 3×/wk) (started at engraftment for stem cell transplant patients) (BII) Valganciclovir at total dose in milligrams = 7 × BSA × CrCl (use max CrCl 150 mL/min/1.73 m²) PO qd with food for children and teens 4 mo–16 y (max dose 900 mg/day) for primary prophylaxis in HIV patients[19] who are CMV antibody positive and have severe immunosuppression (CD4 count <50/mm³ in children ≥6 y; CD4 percentage <5% in children <6 y) (CIII) Letermovir (adults ≥18 y, CMV-seropositive recipients [R+] of an allogeneic hematopoietic stem cell transplant) 480 mg administered PO qd or as IV infusion over 1 h through 100 days posttransplant (BI)[20]	Neutropenia is a complication with ganciclovir and valganciclovir prophylaxis and may be addressed with G-CSF. Prophylaxis and preemptive treatment strategies are effective, but preemptive treatment in high-risk adult liver transplant recipients is superior to prophylaxis.[9] Letermovir being studied in children, but no dosing information available at this time.
Ebola	Atoltivimab/maftivimab/odesivimab-ebgn (brand name: Inmazeb) Ansuvimab-zykl (brand name: Ebanga)	For treatment of *Zaire ebolavirus* infections
Enterovirus	Supportive therapy; no antivirals currently FDA approved	Pocapavir PO is currently under investigation for enterovirus (poliovirus) and can be used under an expanded access IND. Pleconaril PO is currently under consideration for submission to the FDA for approval to treat neonatal enteroviral sepsis syndrome.[21] As of August 2024, it is not available for compassionate use.

Epstein-Barr virus

– Mononucleosis, encephalitis[22-24]

Limited data suggest small clinical benefit of valacyclovir in adolescents for mononucleosis (3 g/day div tid for 14 days) (CIII).

For EBV encephalitis: ganciclovir IV OR acyclovir IV (AIII).

No prospective data on benefits of acyclovir IV or ganciclovir IV in EBV clinical infections of normal hosts.

Patients suspected to have infectious mononucleosis should not be given ampicillin or amoxicillin, which causes nonallergic morbilliform rashes in a high proportion of patients with active EBV infection (AII).

Therapy with short-course corticosteroids (prednisone 1 mg/kg/day PO [max 20 mg/day] for 7 days with subsequent tapering) may have a beneficial effect on acute symptoms in patients with marked tonsillar inflammation with impending airway obstruction, massive splenomegaly, myocarditis, hemolytic anemia, or hemophagocytic lymphohistiocytosis (BIII).

– Posttransplant lymphoproliferative disorder[25,26]

Ganciclovir (AIII)

Decrease immunosuppression if possible, as this approach has the most effect on control of EBV; rituximab, methotrexate have been used but without controlled data. Preemptive treatment with ganciclovir may decrease PTLD in solid-organ transplants.

7

C. PREFERRED THERAPY FOR SPECIFIC VIRAL PATHOGENS

Infection	Therapy (evidence grade)	Comments
Hepatitis B virus (chronic)[27-45]	AASLD-preferred treatments of children and adolescents[46]: Interferon alfa-2b for children and adolescents 1–18 y: 3 million U/m² BSA SUBQ 3x/wk for 1 wk, followed by dose escalation to 6 million U/m² BSA (max 10 million U/dose); OR entecavir for children ≥2 y (optimum duration of therapy unknown) [BII] Entecavir dosing IF no prior nucleoside therapy: ≥16 y: 0.5 mg qd 2–15 y: 10–11 kg: 0.15 mg PO soln qd >11–14 kg: 0.2 mg PO soln qd >14–17 kg: 0.25 mg PO soln qd >17–20 kg: 0.3 mg PO soln qd >20–23 kg: 0.35 mg PO soln qd >23–26 kg: 0.4 mg PO soln qd >26–30 kg: 0.45 mg PO soln qd >30 kg: 0.5 mg PO soln or tab qd If prior nucleoside therapy: Double the dosage in each weight bracket for entecavir listed previously; OR tenofovir dipivoxil fumarate for adolescents ≥12 y and adults: 300 mg qd. **NOTE:** TAF is also a preferred treatment of adults (25 mg daily) but has not been studied in children.	AASLD-nonpreferred treatments of children and adults: Lamivudine (3TC) 3 mg/kg/day (max 100 mg) PO q24h for 52 wk for children ≥2 y (children coinfected with HIV and HBV should use the approved dose for HIV) (AII). 3TC approved for children ≥2 y, but antiviral resistance develops during therapy in 30%; OR adefovir for children ≥12 y (10 mg PO q24h for a minimum of 12 mo; optimum duration of therapy unknown) (BII). There are not sufficient clinical data to identify the appropriate dose for use in children. Indications for treatment of chronic HBV infection, with or without HIV coinfection, are (1) evidence of ongoing HBV viral replication, as indicated by serum HBV DNA (>20,000 IU/mL without HBeAg positivity or >2,000 IU/mL with HBeAg positivity) for >6 mo and persistent elevation of serum transaminase levels for >6 mo, or (2) evidence of chronic hepatitis on liver biopsy (BII). Antiviral therapy is not warranted in children without necroinflammatory liver disease (BIII). Treatment is not recommended for children with immunotolerant chronic HBV infection (ie, normal serum transaminase levels despite detectable HBV DNA) (BII). All patients with HBV and HIV coinfection should initiate ART, regardless of CD4 count. This should include 2 drugs that have HBV activity as well, specifically tenofovir (dipivoxil fumarate or alafenamide) plus 3TC or emtricitabine.[46] Patients who are already receiving effective ART that does not include a drug with HBV activity should have treatment changed to include tenofovir (dipivoxil fumarate or alafenamide) plus 3TC or emtricitabine; alternatively, entecavir is reasonable if patients are receiving a fully suppressive ART regimen.

Hepatitis C virus (chronic)[47-54]	Genotypes 1–6: daily fixed-dose combination of sofosbuvir/velpatasvir (Epclusa) (<17 kg: 37.5 mg velpatasvir with 150 mg sofosbuvir qd; 17–<30 kg: 50 mg velpatasvir with 200 mg sofosbuvir; ≥30 kg: 100 mg velpatasvir with 400 mg sofosbuvir) for patients ≥3 y with genotype 1–6 who are treatment naive or interferon experienced without cirrhosis or with compensated cirrhosis OR Daily fixed-dose combination of glecaprevir/pibrentasvir (Mavyret) for patients ≥3 y with genotype 1–6 who are treatment naive or treatment experienced without cirrhosis or with compensated cirrhosis: ≥12 y or ≥45 kg: glecaprevir 300 mg with pibrentasvir 120 mg qd 3–11 y: <20 kg: glecaprevir 150 mg with pibrentasvir 60 mg qd 20–<30 kg: glecaprevir 200 mg with pibrentasvir 80 mg qd 30–<45 kg: glecaprevir 250 mg with pibrentasvir 100 mg qd Genotype 1: daily fixed-dose combination of ledipasvir (90 mg)/sofosbuvir (400 mg) (Harvoni) for patients with genotype 1 who are treatment naive without cirrhosis or with compensated cirrhosis or are treatment experienced with or without cirrhosis OR, for patients ≥12 y, elbasvir (50 mg)/grazoprevir (100 mg) (Zepatier) qd	Treatment of HCV infections in adults has been revolutionized in recent years with the licensure of numerous highly effective DAAs for use in adults, adolescents, and children as young as 3 y. Given the efficacy of these new treatment regimens in adults (AI),[55-70] treatment of children should consist only of interferon-free regimens, and an age-appropriate antiviral should be given to all HCV-infected children ≥3 y. The following treatment is recommended, based on viral genotype[71]: Sofosbuvir (Sovaldi) and sofosbuvir in a fixed-dose combination tab with ledipasvir (Harvoni) are now approved for patients ≥3 y; sofosbuvir/velpatasvir (Epclusa) is now approved for patients ≥3 y; and glecaprevir/pibrentasvir (Mavyret) is now approved for patients ≥3 y. See www.hcvguidelines.org/unique-populations/children (accessed August 15, 2024) for additional information (BI).

(Continued on next page)

7

C. PREFERRED THERAPY FOR SPECIFIC VIRAL PATHOGENS

Infection	Therapy (evidence grade)	Comments
Hepatitis C virus (chronic)[47-54] (*continued*)	Genotype 2: daily sofosbuvir (400 mg) plus weight-based ribavirin (as below) for patients with genotype 2 who are treatment naive or treatment experienced without cirrhosis or with compensated cirrhosis Genotype 3: daily sofosbuvir (400 mg) plus weight-based ribavirin (as below) for patients with genotype 3 who are treatment naive or treatment experienced without cirrhosis or with compensated cirrhosis Genotype 4 in patients ≥12 y: elbasvir (50 mg)/grazoprevir (100 mg) (Zepatier) qd Genotype 4, 5, or 6: daily fixed-dose combination of ledipasvir (90 mg)/sofosbuvir (400 mg) (Harvoni) for patients with genotype 4, 5, or 6 who are treatment naive or treatment experienced without cirrhosis or with compensated cirrhosis Dosing for ribavirin in combination therapy with sofosbuvir for adolescents ≥12 y or ≥35 kg: <47 kg: 15 mg/kg/day in 2 div doses 47–59 kg: 800 mg/day in 2 div doses 60–73 kg: 400 mg in morning and 600 mg in evening >73 kg: 1,200 mg/day in 2 div doses	

Herpes simplex virus

– Third trimester maternal suppressive therapy[72-74]	Acyclovir or valacyclovir maternal suppressive therapy in pregnant women reduces HSV recurrences and viral shedding at the time of delivery but does not fully prevent neonatal HSV[73] (BIII).
– Neonatal	See Ch 2.
– Mucocutaneous (normal host)	Acyclovir 80 mg/kg/day PO div qid (max dose 800 mg) for 5–7 days, or 15 mg/kg/day IV as 1- to 2-h infusion div q8h (AII). Valacyclovir 20 mg/kg/dose (max dose 1 g) PO bid[75] for 5–7 days (BII). Suppressive therapy for frequent recurrence (no pediatric data): acyclovir 20 mg/kg/dose bid or tid (max dose 400 mg) for 6–12 mo, then reevaluate need (AIII).	Foscarnet for acyclovir-resistant strains. Immunocompromised hosts may require 10–14 days of therapy. Topical acyclovir not efficacious and, therefore, not recommended.
– Genital	Adult doses: acyclovir 400 mg PO tid for 7–10 days; OR valacyclovir 1 g PO bid for 10 days; OR famciclovir 250 mg PO tid for 7–10 days (AI)	All 3 drugs have been used as prophylaxis to prevent recurrence. Topical acyclovir not efficacious and, therefore, not recommended.
– Encephalitis	Acyclovir 60 mg/kg/day IV as 1- to 2-h infusion div q8h; for 21 days for infants ≤4 mo. For older infants and children, 45 mg/kg/day IV as 1- to 2-h infusion div q8h (AIII).	Safety of high-dosage acyclovir (60 mg/kg/day) not well-defined beyond the neonatal period; can be used, but monitor for neurotoxicity and nephrotoxicity.
– Keratoconjunctivitis	1% trifluridine OR 0.15% ganciclovir ophthalmic gel (AII)	Consultation with ophthalmologist required for assessment and management (eg, concomitant use of topical steroids in certain situations)

7

C. PREFERRED THERAPY FOR SPECIFIC VIRAL PATHOGENS

Infection	Therapy (evidence grade)	Comments
HIV		
Current information on HIV treatment and opportunistic infections in children[76] is posted at https://clinicalinfo.hiv.gov/en/guidelines (accessed August 15, 2024); other information on HIV programs is available at www.cdc.gov/hiv/policies/index.html (accessed August 15, 2024). Consult with an HIV expert, if possible, for current recommendations, as treatment options are complicated and constantly evolving.		
– Therapy for HIV infection		
State-of-the-art therapy is rapidly evolving with introduction of new agents and combinations; currently there are many individual and fixed-dose combination ARV agents approved for use by the FDA that have pediatric indications and that continue to be actively used; guidelines for children and adolescents are continually updated on the ClinicalInfo.HIV.gov and CDC websites given previously.	Effective therapy (HAART) consists of ≥3 agents, including 2 NRTIs, plus a protease inhibitor, a non-NRTI, or an integrase inhibitor; many different combination regimens give similar treatment outcomes; choice of agents depends on the age of the child, viral load, consideration of potential viral resistance, and extent of immune depletion, in addition to judging the child's ability to adhere to the regimen. "Rapid initiation" of ART is recommended for all children, meaning initiation within days of HIV diagnosis.	Assess drug toxicity (based on the agents used) and virologic/immunologic response to therapy (quantitative plasma HIV and CD4 count) initially monthly and then q3–6mo during the maintenance phase.
– Children of any age	Any child with AIDS or significant HIV-related symptoms (clinical category C and most B conditions) should be treated (AI). Guidance from the WHO and HHS guidelines committees now recommends treatment of **all children** regardless of age, CD4 count, or clinical status.	Adherence counseling and appropriate ARV formulations are critical for successful implementation. Recently, the combination of an integrase inhibitor with 2 NRTIs has become the preferred treatment regimen for children (as well as adults). Alternative regimens may use either an NNRTI or a protease inhibitor.

– First 4 wk after birth	HAART with ≥3 drugs is recommended for **all infants and children** regardless of clinical status or laboratory values (AI).
	Preferred therapy in the first 2 wk after birth is ZDV or abacavir PLUS 3TC or emtricitabine PLUS either NVP or RAL.
	Preferred therapy from 2–4 wk: ZDV or abacavir PLUS 3TC or emtricitabine PLUS either lopinavir/ritonavir (toxicity concerns preclude its use until a PMA of 42 wk and a PNA of at least 14 days are reached) or RAL.
– HIV-infected children 1 mo–12 y	**Treat all** with any CD4 count (AI).
	Preferred regimens:
	4 wk–2 y: 2 NRTIs PLUS dolutegravir (Alternatives to dolutegravir include RAL or elvitegravir [>25 kg].)
	>2 y: 2 NRTIs PLUS dolutegravir OR bictegravir (Alternatives to dolutegravir or bictegravir include RAL OR elvitegravir OR atazanavir/ritonavir OR darunavir/ritonavir.)
– HIV-infected youth ≥12 y	**Treat all** regardless of CD4 count (AI).
	Preferred regimens comprise TAF plus emtricitabine OR abacavir plus 3TC PLUS dolutegravir, RAL, or bictegravir.
	NOTE: Cabenuva (injectable, long-acting cabotegravir plus rilpivirine) has recently been approved to treat HIV infection in 12- to 18-year-olds, which has some appeal for youth with PO adherence challenges. It requires a PO lead-in dosing period followed by injections q2mo (one each for cabotegravir and rilpivirine). For this treatment regimen, initiation by a pediatric/adult HIV specialist team is strongly recommended.
– Antiretroviral-experienced child	Consult with HIV specialist.
	Consider treatment history and drug resistance testing and assess adherence.

7

C. PREFERRED THERAPY FOR SPECIFIC VIRAL PATHOGENS

Infection	Therapy (evidence grade)	Comments
– HIV exposures, nonoccupational	Therapy recommendations for exposures available on the CDC website at www.cdc.gov/hiv/guidelines/preventing.html (accessed August 15, 2024)	PEP remains unproven, but substantial evidence supports its use; consider individually regarding risk, time from exposure, and likelihood of adherence; prophylactic regimens administered for 4 wk.
– Negligible exposure risk (urine, nasal secretions, saliva, sweat, or tears—no visible blood in secretions) OR >72 h since exposure	Prophylaxis not recommended (BIII)	
– Significant exposure risk (blood, semen, vaginal, or rectal secretions from a known HIV-infected individual) AND <72 h since exposure	Prophylaxis recommended (BIII) Preferred regimens: 4 wk–<2 y: ZDV PLUS 3TC PLUS either RAL or lopinavir/ritonavir 2–12 y: tenofovir PLUS emtricitabine PLUS RAL ≥13 y: tenofovir PLUS emtricitabine PLUS either RAL or dolutegravir	Consultation with a pediatric HIV specialist is advised.
– Significant exposure risk PrEP	Truvada (tenofovir [300 mg]/emtricitabine [200 mg]): 1 tab daily	Daily PrEP has proven efficacy for prevention of HIV infection in individuals at high risk. It is FDA approved for adolescents/youth (13–24 y; ≥35 kg). Strategies for use include both episodic and continuous administration. Baseline HIV and renal function testing is indicated, and it is recommended to evaluate HIV infection status and renal function about q3mo while receiving PrEP.
– HIV exposure, occupational[77]	See guidelines on the CDC website at www.cdc.gov/hiv/guidelines/preventing.html (accessed August 15, 2024).	
Human herpesvirus 6		
– Immunocompromised children[78]	No prospective comparative data; ganciclovir 10 mg/kg/day IV div q12h used in case report (AIII)	May require high dose to control infection; safety and efficacy not defined at high doses

Influenza virus

Recommendations for the treatment of influenza can vary from season to season; access the AAP website (www.aap.org) and the CDC website (www.cdc.gov/flu/hcp/antivirals/summary-clinicians.html; accessed November 26, 2024) for the most current, accurate information.

Influenza A and B

– Treatment[79–81]	Oseltamivir	Oseltamivir is currently drug of choice for treatment of influenza.
	Preterm, <38 wk of PMA: 1 mg/kg/dose PO bid[79]	For patients 12–23 mo, the original FDA-approved unit dose
	Preterm, 38–40 wk of PMA: 1.5 mg/kg/dose PO bid[79]	of 30 mg/dose may provide inadequate drug exposure; 3.5 mg/kg/dose PO bid has been studied,[80] but study
	Preterm, >40 wk of PMA: 3 mg/kg/dose PO bid	population sizes were small.
	Full-term, birth–8 mo: 3 mg/kg/dose PO bid	Studies of parenteral zanamivir have been completed in
	9–11 mo: 3.5 mg/kg/dose PO bid[80]	children.[82] However, this formulation of the drug is not
	12–23 mo: 30 mg/dose PO bid	approved in the United States and is not available for
	2–12 y:	compassionate use.
	≤15 kg: 30 mg bid	The adamantanes, amantadine and rimantadine, are
	16–23 kg: 45 mg bid	currently not effective for treatment due to near-universal
	24–40 kg: 60 mg bid	resistance of influenza A virus.
	>40 kg: 75 mg bid	Resistance to baloxavir is being monitored carefully across
	≥13 y: 75 mg bid	the world. Problems with resistance have limited use of
	OR	baloxavir in Japan.
	Zanamivir	
	≥7 y: 10 mg by inhalation bid for 5 days	
	OR	
	Peramivir (BII)	
	6 mo–<13 y: single IV dose 12 mg/kg, up to 600 mg	
	≥13 y: single IV dose 600 mg	
	OR	
	Baloxavir (BII)	
	≥5 y:	
	<20 kg: single dose 2 mg/kg PO	
	20–79 kg: single dose 40 mg PO	
	≥80 kg: single dose 80 mg PO	

7

C. PREFERRED THERAPY FOR SPECIFIC VIRAL PATHOGENS

Infection	Therapy (evidence grade)	Comments
– Chemoprophylaxis	Oseltamivir 3 mo–12 y: the milligram dose given for prophylaxis is the same as for the treatment dose for all ages, but it is given qd for prophylaxis rather than bid for treatment. Zanamivir ≥5 y: 10 mg by inhalation qd for as long as 28 days (community outbreaks) or 10 days (household setting) Baloxavir ≥5 y: <20 kg: single dose 2 mg/kg PO 20–79 kg: single dose 40 mg PO ≥80 kg: single dose 80 mg PO	Oseltamivir is currently drug of choice for chemoprophylaxis of influenza. Unless the situation is judged critical, oseltamivir chemoprophylaxis is not routinely recommended for patients <3 mo because of limited safety and efficacy data in this age-group. The adamantanes, amantadine and rimantadine, are currently not effective for chemoprophylaxis due to near-universal resistance of influenza A virus.
Measles[83]	No prospective data on antiviral therapy. Ribavirin is active against measles virus in vitro. Vitamin A is beneficial in children with measles and is recommended by the WHO for all children with measles regardless of their country of residence (qd dosing for 2 days); for children ≥1 y: 200,000 IU (60,000 mcg RAE); for infants 6–12 mo: 100,000 IU (30,000 mcg RAE); for infants <6 mo: 50,000 IU (15,000 mcg RAE) (BII). An additional (ie, a third) age-specific dose of vitamin A should be given 2–6 wk later to children with clinical signs and symptoms of vitamin A deficiency. Even in countries where measles is not usually severe, vitamin A should be given to all children with severe measles (eg, requiring hospitalization). Parenteral and PO formulations are available in the United States.	Immune globulin prophylaxis for exposed, unimmunized children: 0.5 mL/kg/kg (max 15 mL) IM

Mpox (monkeypox)	There are no FDA-approved treatments for mpox. Tecovirimat and brincidofovir are approved to treat smallpox based on the FDA Animal Rule regulations, which provide a pathway for approval of certain drugs and biologic products when it is not ethical or feasible to conduct efficacy studies in humans. For use in mpox, they are available only through clinical trial(s) or under the FDA expanded access program (www.fda.gov/emergency-preparedness-and-response/mcm-issues/mpox; accessed August 15, 2024). Following consultation with the CDC, treatment may be considered in patients experiencing severe disease that prompts hospitalization or in patients likely to experience severe disease (ie, immunocompromised patients, children <8 y, pregnant/breastfeeding women); CDC-held expanded access IND protocol allows use of VIGIV for non–variola *Orthopoxvirus* infection (eg, mpox).	PrEP vaccination may be available for health care professionals, and PEP vaccination (within 4 days from date of exposure) may be available with the 2 attenuated virus vaccines that are FDA approved, through the CDC (800-CDC-INFO [800-232-4636]).
Respiratory syncytial virus[84,85]		
– Therapy (severe disease in compromised host)	Ribavirin (6-g vial to make 20-mg/mL soln in sterile water), aerosolized over 18–20 h daily for 3–5 days (BII)	Aerosol ribavirin provides only a small benefit and should be considered only for use for life-threatening infection with RSV. Airway reactivity with inhalation precludes routine use.

C. PREFERRED THERAPY FOR SPECIFIC VIRAL PATHOGENS

Infection	Therapy (evidence grade)	Comments
– Prophylaxis (nirsevimab or palivizumab) (BI)[84,85]	Prophylaxis: Nirsevimab is approved and recommended over palivizumab. For infants aged <8 mo: Nirsevimab, 50 mg/dose (<5 kg at dose) or 100 mg/dose (≥5 kg at dose) IM once per season (a) at birth for *all* infants born during October–March and (b) when entering first RSV season and <8 mo of age for all infants born during April–September. For infants aged 8–19 mo, a second dose of nirsevimab is given October–March for children with • Chronic lung disease who required medical support (chronic corticosteroid therapy, diuretic therapy, or supplemental oxygen) anytime during the 6-mo period before the start of the second RSV season • Severe immunocompromise • CF who have either manifestations of severe lung disease (previous hospitalization for pulmonary exacerbation in the first year after birth or abnormalities on chest imaging that persist when stable) or weight-for-length <10th percentile • American Indian or Alaska Native heritage	Neither palivizumab nor nirsevimab provides benefit in the treatment of an active RSV infection. Nirsevimab is recommended for all infants during their first RSV season, including well infants. Only those at high risk should receive a second dose before their second RSV season.

Varicella-zoster virus[86]		
– Infection in a normal host	For prophylaxis/preemptive therapy following exposure in an asymptomatic child, see Ch 15.	The sooner antiviral therapy can be started, the greater the clinical benefit.
	Acyclovir 80 mg/kg/day (max single dose 800 mg) PO div qid for 5 days (AI)	
– Severe primary chickenpox, disseminated infection (cutaneous, pneumonia, encephalitis, hepatitis); immunocompromised host with primary chickenpox or disseminated zoster	Acyclovir 30 mg/kg/day IV as 1- to 2-h infusion div q8h for 10 days (acyclovir doses of 45–60 mg/kg/day in 3 div doses IV should be used for disseminated or CNS infection). Dosing can also be provided as 1,500 mg/m²/day IV div q8h. Duration in immunocompromised children: 7–14 days, based on clinical response (AI).	PO valacyclovir, famciclovir, foscarnet also active

8. Choosing Among Antiviral Agents

As a general rule, antiviral agents are specific to certain families of viruses. That is, the anti-herpesvirus drugs do not work against influenza, the anti–hepatitis C drugs do not work against hepatitis B, and so on. While some antiviral agents (eg, ribavirin, remdesivir, molnupiravir) may have cross-family coverage, an antiviral drug that is broad enough in spectrum to cover multiple types of viruses and thus be used empirically in many situations simply does not exist at this point. It is therefore imperative that clinicians think through what viruses need to be covered when they are selecting which specific antiviral agent to use. For this reason, this chapter is structured by virus family.

Anti-Herpesvirus Drugs

Broadly speaking, anti-herpesvirus drugs should be considered by subfamily within the broader Herpesviridae family. Herpes simplex virus (HSV) and varicella-zoster virus (VZV) are in the alpha subfamily, cytomegalovirus (CMV) and human herpesvirus 6 (HHV-6) are in the beta subfamily, and Epstein-Barr virus (EBV) is in the gamma subfamily.

The antiviral drug of choice for the alpha herpesviruses (ie, HSV, gingivostomatitis/fever blisters, genital infection, neonatal infection; VZV, chickenpox, shingles) is acyclovir, a nucleoside analogue that is available intravenously (IV) or orally (PO). Orally administered acyclovir (given in divided doses 4 or 5 times daily as tablets, capsules, or suspension) is poorly absorbed. However, the valine ester prodrug of acyclovir, valacyclovir, has enhanced bioavailability and twice-daily dosing that makes it an attractive option if the patient is old enough to be able to take it. Valacyclovir does not come in a liquid formulation, but there is a recipe for creation of a suspension in the package insert that allows for the compounding of a product that has a 28-day shelf life. There are data for dosing of valacyclovir in pediatric patients, although not in very young infants. Famciclovir (the prodrug of penciclovir), also a nucleoside analogue like acyclovir, is approved in adults for genital HSV and shingles, but there are far less pediatric data on efficacy. Although pediatric dosing recommendations are provided in the package label for infants and children, no suspension formulation has been approved; we prefer acyclovir to famciclovir based on much more extensive published pediatric data. Resistance to this class of antiviral may occur with repeat treatment courses. Alternatives include cidofovir and foscarnet, but each of these has significant toxicity issues that limit their use more widely.

For the beta herpesviruses, ganciclovir (another nucleoside analogue) is the antiviral agent of choice for parenteral use. When PO dosing is an option, the valine ester prodrug of ganciclovir, valganciclovir, is used. Valganciclovir has improved bioavailability relative to PO ganciclovir. Cidofovir and foscarnet also have activity against the beta herpesviruses but, as mentioned previously, have toxicity issues that limit the use. Recently, letermovir, a DNA terminase complex inhibitor, and maribavir, a pUL97 kinase inhibitor, have been approved for use in children 12 years and older (maribavir) and adults (both drugs) in specific situations. Studies of letermovir in the pediatric population are underway.

There are no antiviral agents with excellent activity against the gamma herpesviruses. In general, ganciclovir or its prodrug, valganciclovir, is used when activity is desired against EBV. The degree of benefit that either of these drugs provides, though, is unproven.

Anti-Influenza Drugs

The drug of choice for influenza treatment in children is oseltamivir, a neuraminidase inhibitor, which is available only as a PO formulation. Zanamivir, also a neuraminidase inhibitor, is an active antiviral agent against most current strains of influenza but is available only in the United States as an inhalation formulation. Zanamivir is about as effective as oseltamivir, but its inhaled delivery mechanism has limited its use. Peramivir is another neuraminidase inhibitor given only IV as a single dose for uncomplicated outpatient influenza for patients down to 6 months of age; starting an IV catheter and infusing peramivir over 15 to 30 minutes may be difficult in many clinic settings. All the neuraminidase inhibitors should be given as early as possible in the influenza illness, preferably within 48 hours of onset of illness. Influenza may mutate to develop resistance to the neuraminidase inhibitors at any time, but the Centers for Disease Control and Prevention keeps track of global resistance patterns and shares current information on its website.

Baloxavir is the first approved endonuclease inhibitor drug in this class for influenza, for use in children 5 years and older and in adults; it prevents replication of virus at a very early stage in cell infection. It requires only a single dose for treatment of uncomplicated outpatient influenza infection in adults, with published data in children down to 1 year of age documenting similar efficacy. Experience with this drug is limited in the United States at this time.

In addition to treating active infection, oseltamivir, zanamivir, and baloxavir are also approved for prophylaxis following influenza exposure.

Anti-Hepatitis Drugs

The development of drugs that are active against hepatitis C virus (HCV) has been one of the most remarkable aspects of antiviral drug development over the past 10 years. There are currently 4 antiviral drugs with activity against HCV that are approved for use in children 3 years and older: sofosbuvir/ledipasvir (Harvoni), sofosbuvir plus ribavirin, sofosbuvir/velpatasvir (Epclusa), and glecaprevir/pibrentasvir (Mavyret). Mavyret and Epclusa demonstrate transgenotype activity and, therefore, can be used with any genotype of HCV. There is also 1 HCV antiviral drug approved for use in children 12 years and older: elbasvir/grazoprevir (Zepatier). Given the pace of development, it is reasonable to anticipate that additional antiviral drugs with HCV activity are likely to be approved in children over the upcoming years. The American Academy of Pediatrics recommends that all HCV-infected children 3 years and older be treated with an age-approved antiviral regimen.

Anti-Coronavirus Drugs

As of August 2024, remdesivir is the only antiviral drug with activity against coronaviruses approved for use in children. In addition, nirmatrelvir/ritonavir (Paxlovid) has been approved for use in adults and is available by Emergency Use Authorization from the US Food and Drug Administration for adolescents 12 through 17 years of age. Paxlovid is indicated for the treatment of mild to moderate COVID-19 disease in people 12 years and older weighing 40 kg or more.

9. Preferred Therapy for Specific Parasitic Pathogens

NOTES

- A list of table abbreviations and acronyms can be found at the start of this publication.

- Many of the parasitic infections listed in this chapter are not common, and current advice from your local infectious disease/tropical medicine/global health specialist may be invaluable. For some parasitic diseases, therapy may be available only from the Centers for Disease Control and Prevention (CDC), as noted. The CDC also provides up-to-date information about parasitic diseases and current treatment recommendations at www.cdc.gov/parasites. Consultation is available from the CDC for parasitic disease diagnostic services (www.cdc.gov/dpdx), for parasitic disease diagnosis and management (404-718-4745 or parasites@cdc.gov), and for malaria (770-488-7788 or 855-856-4713 toll-free, Monday through Friday, 9:00 am to 5:00 pm [ET]; after-hours emergency number 770-488-7100 for after hours, weekends, and holidays; or malaria@cdc.gov). Antiparasitic drugs available from the CDC Drug Service can be reviewed and requested at www.cdc.gov/laboratory/drugservice/formulary.html.

- Some of the drugs listed can be obtained only from the US Food and Drug Administration or specialized pharmacies; contact information has been provided when available.

- Albendazole is taken with food, preferably fatty food, to enhance bioavailability but is taken on an empty stomach when used as a luminal agent. We have noted when it should be taken on an empty stomach; if not noted, it should be taken with food.

- Additional information about many of the organisms and diseases mentioned here, along with treatment recommendations, can be found in the appropriate sections in the American Academy of Pediatrics *Red Book*.

9

Preferred Therapy for Parasitic Pathogens

A. SELECT COMMON PATHOGENIC PARASITES AND SUGGESTED AGENTS FOR TREATMENT

	Albendazole/ Mebendazole	Triclabendazole	Metronidazole/ Tinidazole	Praziquantel	Ivermectin	Nitazoxanide	DEC	Pyrantel Pamoate	Paromomycin	TMP/SMX
Ascariasis	++				+	+		+		
Blastocystis spp			+			+			+	+
Cryptosporidiosis						+			+	
Cutaneous larva migrans	++				++					
Cyclosporiasis			−			+				++
Cystoisospora spp						+				++
Dientamoebiasis	−		++			+			+	
Liver fluke *Clonorchis/ Opisthorchis*	+			++						
Fasciola hepatica, gigantica		++				+				
Lung fluke	−			++						
Giardia spp	+		++			++			+	
Hookworm	++				−			+		
Loiasis	+						++			
Mansonella ozzardi	−				+		−			
Mansonella perstans	±				−		±			

Pathogen					
Onchocerciasis				++	
Pinworm	++				++
Schistosomiasis			++		
Strongyloides spp	+			++	
Tapeworm			++	+	
Toxocariasis	++ (Albendazole preferred)			−	+
Trichinellosis	++				
Trichomoniasis		++			
Trichuriasis	++				
Wuchereria bancrofti	+				++

NOTE: ++ = preferred; **+** = acceptable; **±** = possibly effective (see text for further discussion); **−** = unlikely to be effective; [blank cell] = untested.

B. PREFERRED THERAPY FOR SPECIFIC PARASITIC PATHOGENS

Disease/Organism	Treatment (evidence grade)	Comments
Acanthamoeba	See Amebic meningoencephalitis later in this table.	
Amebiasis[1–5]		
Entamoeba histolytica		
– Asymptomatic intestinal colonization	Paromomycin 25–35 mg/kg/day PO tid for 7 days; OR iodoquinol 30–40 mg/kg/day (max 650 mg/dose) PO div tid for 20 days; OR diloxanide furoate (not commercially available in the United States) 20 mg/kg/day PO div tid (max 500 mg/dose) for 10 days (CII)	Follow-up stool examination to ensure eradication of carriage; screen/treat positive close contacts. *Entamoeba dispar* and *Entamoeba polecki* do not require treatment; need for treatment of *Entamoeba moshkovskii* and *Entamoeba bangladeshi* is uncertain. Nitazoxanide may be an option as an alternative luminal agent.
– Mild to moderate intestinal disease	Metronidazole 35–50 mg/kg/day (max 500–750 mg/dose) PO div tid for 7–10 days; OR tinidazole (age >3 y) 50 mg/kg/day PO (max 2 g) qd for 3 days; OR nitazoxanide (age ≥12 y, 500 mg bid for 3 days; 4–11 y, 200 mg bid for 3 days; 1–3 y, 100 mg bid for 3 days) FOLLOWED BY paromomycin or iodoquinol, as above, to eliminate cysts (BII). For mild to moderate intestinal disease, secnidazole (FDA approved but not for this indication) 2 g once PO in adults and 30 mg/kg once PO in children or ornidazole (not approved in the United States) 500 mg PO qd in adults and 40 mg/kg/day PO qd in children for 3 days are alternatives.	Treatment options for severe and extraintestinal disease are similar to those for mild to moderate disease except that the need for broad-spectrum antibiotics should be considered in the event of superimposed bacterial infection, and the need for site-specific treatment should be considered in extraintestinal infection such as liver abscess. Use of paromomycin for clearance of intestinal infection should be delayed if there is concern for intestinal perforation. Avoid antimotility drugs, steroids. Tinidazole (evaluated by the FDA for children ≥3 y), when available, may be more effective with fewer adverse events than metronidazole. Take tinidazole with food to decrease GI side effects; pharmacists can crush tabs and mix with syrup for those unable to take tabs. Avoid alcohol ingestion with nitroimidazole drugs.

– Liver abscess, extraintestinal disease	Metronidazole 35–50 mg/kg/day IV q8h, with a switch to PO when tolerated, for 7–10 days; OR tinidazole (age >3 y) 50 mg/kg/day PO (max 2 g) qd for 5 days; OR nitazoxanide (age ≥12 y, 500 mg bid for 3 days; 4–11 y, 200 mg bid for 3 days; 1–3 y, 100 mg bid for 3 days) FOLLOWED BY paromomycin or iodoquinol, as above, to eliminate cysts (BII)	Serologic assays >95% positive in extraintestinal amebiasis. Percutaneous or surgical drainage may be indicated for large liver abscesses or inadequate response to medical therapy. Avoid alcohol ingestion with nitroimidazole drugs. Take tinidazole with food to decrease GI side effects; pharmacists can crush tabs and mix with syrup for those unable to take tabs.
Amebic meningoencephalitis[6–10]		
Naegleria fowleri	AmB 1.5 mg/kg/day IV div q12h for 3 days, then 1 mg/kg/day qd for 11 days; PLUS AmB intrathecally 1.5 mg qd for 2 days, then 1 mg/day qod for 8 days; PLUS azithromycin 10 mg/kg/day IV or PO (max 500 mg/day) for 28 days; PLUS fluconazole 10 mg/kg/day IV or PO qd (max 600 mg/day) for 28 days; PLUS rifampin 10 mg/kg/day qd IV or PO (max 600 mg/day) for 28 days; PLUS miltefosine <45 kg 50 mg PO bid; ≥45 kg 50 mg PO tid (max 2.5 mg/kg/day) for 28 days PLUS dexamethasone 0.6 mg/kg/day div qid for 4 days	Treatment recommendations based on regimens used for 5 known survivors; available at www.cdc.gov/naegleria/hcp/clinical-care (accessed August 9, 2024). Conventional amphotericin preferred; L-AmB is less effective in animal models. Treatment outcomes usually unsuccessful; early therapy (even before diagnostic confirmation if indicated) may improve survival. Miltefosine is available commercially (www.impavido.com); the CDC provides expertise in treatment of patients with *N fowleri* infection (770-488-7100).

B. PREFERRED THERAPY FOR SPECIFIC PARASITIC PATHOGENS

Disease/Organism	Treatment (evidence grade)	Comments
Acanthamoeba	Combination regimens including miltefosine, fluconazole, and pentamidine favored by some experts; TMP/SMX, metronidazole, and a macrolide may be added. Other drugs that have been used alone or in combination include rifampin, other azoles, sulfadiazine, flucytosine, and caspofungin. Keratitis: topical therapies include PHMB (0.02%) or chlorhexidine, combined with propamidine isethionate (0.1%) or hexamidine (0.1%) (topical therapies not approved in the United States but available at compounding pharmacies).	Optimal treatment regimens uncertain; combination therapy favored. Miltefosine is available commercially (www.impavido.com). The CDC is available for consultation about management of these infections (770-488-7100). Keratitis should be evaluated by an ophthalmologist. Prolonged treatment often needed.
Balamuthia mandrillaris	Combination regimens preferred. Drugs that have been used alone or in combination include pentamidine, 5-flucytosine, fluconazole, macrolides, sulfadiazine, miltefosine, and itraconazole.	Optimal treatment regimen uncertain; regimens based on case reports; prolonged treatment often needed. Surgical resection of skin or CNS lesions may be beneficial. The CDC is available for consultation about management of these infections (770-488-7100).
Ancylostoma braziliense	See Cutaneous larva migrans later in this table.	
Ancylostoma caninum	See Cutaneous larva migrans later in this table.	
Ancylostoma duodenale	See Hookworm later in this table.	

Angiostrongyliasis[11–14]

	Preferred Therapy	Comments
Angiostrongylus cantonensis (cerebral disease)	Supportive care. Most patients recover without antiparasitic therapy; anthelmintic treatment alone may provoke worsening of neurologic symptoms.	Corticosteroids, analgesics, and repeat LP may be of benefit. Prednisolone (1–2 mg/kg/day, up to 60 mg qd, in 2 div doses, for 2 wk) may shorten duration of headache and reduce need for repeat LP. Ocular disease may require surgery or laser treatment.
Angiostrongylus costaricensis (eosinophilic enterocolitis)	Supportive care	Surgery may be pursued to exclude another diagnosis, such as appendicitis, or to remove inflamed intestine.
Ascariasis (*Ascaris lumbricoides*)[15]	First line: albendazole 400 mg PO once OR mebendazole 500 mg once or 100 mg bid for 3 days (BII) Pregnant women: pyrantel pamoate 11 mg/kg, max 1 g once Alternatives: ivermectin 150–200 mcg/kg PO once (CII); nitazoxanide Ages 1–3 y: 100 mg PO bid for 3 days Ages 4–11 y: 200 mg PO bid for 3 days Age ≥12 y: 500 mg PO bid for 3 days	Follow-up stool ova and parasite examination after therapy not essential. Take albendazole with food (bioavailability increases with food, especially fatty meals). Albendazole has theoretical risk of causing seizures in patients coinfected with cysticercosis.

Preferred Therapy for Parasitic Pathogens

9

B. PREFERRED THERAPY FOR SPECIFIC PARASITIC PATHOGENS

Disease/Organism	Treatment (evidence grade)	Comments
Babesiosis (*Babesia* spp)[16–20]	Mild to moderate disease: azithromycin 10 mg/kg/day (max 500 mg/dose) PO on day 1; 5 mg/kg/day from day 2 on (max 250 mg/dose) for 7–10 days PLUS atovaquone 40 mg/kg/day (max 750 mg/dose) PO div bid (this regimen preferred due to fewer adverse events) OR clindamycin 20–40 mg/kg/day IV div tid or qid (max 600 mg/dose), PLUS quinine sulfate 8 mg/kg/dose PO (max 650 mg/dose) tid for 7–10 days Severe disease: azithromycin 10 mg/kg/day 500 mg/dose) IV for 7–10 days PLUS atovaquone 40 mg/kg/day (max 750 mg/dose) PO div bid; OR clindamycin 20–40 mg/kg/day IV div tid or qid (max 600 mg/dose), PLUS quinine sulfate 8 mg/kg/dose PO (max 650 mg/dose) tid for 7–10 days Can transition from IV to PO therapy (at mild to moderate disease doses) when symptoms improve and parasitemia declines	Most asymptomatic infections with *Babesia microti* in immunocompetent individuals do not require treatment. Daily monitoring of hematocrit and percentage of parasitized red blood cells (until <5%) is helpful in guiding management. Exchange blood transfusion may be of benefit for severe disease and *Babesia divergens* infection. Higher doses of medications and prolonged therapy may be needed for asplenic or immunocompromised individuals. Clindamycin and quinine remain the regimen of choice for *B divergens*.
Balantidium coli[21]	Tetracycline (patients >7 y) 40 mg/kg/day PO div qid for 10 days (max 2 g/day) (CII); OR metronidazole 35–50 mg/kg/day PO div tid for 5 days (max 750 mg/dose); OR iodoquinol 30–40 mg/kg/day PO (max 650 mg/dose) div tid for 20 days	Optimal treatment regimen uncertain. Prompt stool examination may increase detection of rapidly degenerating trophozoites. None of these medications have been evaluated by the FDA for this indication. Nitazoxanide may also be effective.
Baylisascaris procyonis (raccoon roundworm)[22–24]	Albendazole 25–50 mg/kg/day PO for 10–20 days given as soon as possible (<3 days) after exposure on an empty stomach (eg, used as a luminal agent for proactive therapy following ingestion of raccoon feces or contaminated soil) might prevent clinical disease (CIII). For clinical disease, administer with food, especially fatty foods, for increased bioavailability.	Therapy generally unsuccessful to prevent fatal outcome or severe neurologic sequelae once CNS disease present. For clinical disease, concurrent steroids are recommended to reduce inflammation.

Blastocystis spp[25,26]	Whether to treat is controversial. If symptoms are significant, treatment trial is appropriate. Metronidazole 35–50 mg/kg/day (max 500–750 mg/dose) PO tid for 5–10 days (CII); OR tinidazole 50 mg/kg (max 2 g) once (age >3 y) (CII).	Pathogenesis debated. Asymptomatic individuals do not need treatment; diligent search for other pathogenic parasites recommended for symptomatic individuals with *Blastocystis* spp. Paromomycin, nitazoxanide (age ≥12 y, 500 mg PO bid; 4–11 y, 200 mg PO bid for 3 days; 1–3 y, 100 mg PO bid for 3 days), and TMP/SMX may also be effective. Combination therapy is another option. Take tinidazole with food; tabs may be crushed and mixed with flavored syrup.
Brugia malayi, timori	See Filariasis later in this table.	
Capillaria	Mebendazole 200 mg PO bid for 20 days OR albendazole 400 mg PO qd for 10 days	Optimal duration of therapy unknown; may treat for up to 30 days
Chagas disease (*Trypanosoma cruzi*)[27-29]	See Trypanosomiasis later in this table.	
Clonorchis sinensis	See Flukes later in this table.	
Cryptosporidiosis (*Cryptosporidium parvum*)[30-33]	Nitazoxanide (ages 1–3 y, 100 mg PO bid; 4–11 y, 200 mg PO bid; ≥12 y, 500 mg PO bid) for minimum 3 days; longer courses may be needed (BII). Paromomycin 25–35 mg/kg/day div bid–qid (CII); OR azithromycin 10 mg/kg/day for minimum 5 days (CII). Combination therapy of either agent with azithromycin may be used for severe disease.	Supportive therapy alone appropriate for immunocompetent patients unless severe or persistent symptoms. Recovery depends largely on immune status of host; medical therapy may have limited efficacy in HIV-infected patients not receiving effective ART. Longer courses (>2 wk) may be needed in immunocompromised patients.

9

B. PREFERRED THERAPY FOR SPECIFIC PARASITIC PATHOGENS

Disease/Organism	Treatment (evidence grade)	Comments
Cutaneous larva migrans or creeping eruption[34,35] (dog and cat hookworm) (*A caninum, braziliense; Uncinaria stenocephala*)	Ivermectin 200 mcg/kg PO qd for 1 day (weight >15 kg) (CII); OR albendazole (age >2 y) 400 mg PO qd for 3 days (CII)	Albendazole bioavailability increased with food, especially fatty meals. The FDA has not reviewed data on the safety and efficacy of ivermectin in children weighing <15 kg, and data on albendazole in children aged <2 y are limited. For individual children, the benefits of treatment are likely to outweigh risks.
Cyclospora spp[36–38] (cyanobacterium-like agent)	TMP/SMX 8–10 mg TMP/kg/day (max 1 DS tab bid) PO div bid for 7–10 days (BIII)	HIV-infected patients may require higher doses/longer therapy. Nitazoxanide may be an alternative for TMP/SMX-allergic patients.
Cysticercosis[39–42] (*Cysticercus cellulosae;* larva of *Taenia solium*)	Neurocysticercosis Patients with 1–2 viable parenchymal cysts: albendazole 15 mg/kg/day PO bid (max 1,200 mg/day) for 10–14 days PLUS steroids (prednisone 1 mg/kg/day or dexamethasone 0.1 mg/kg/day) begun at least 1 day before antiparasitic therapy, continued during antiparasitic treatment followed by rapid taper (to reduce inflammation associated with dying organisms) Patients with >2 viable parenchymal cysts: albendazole 15 mg/kg/day PO bid (max 1,200 mg/day) for 10–14 days PLUS praziquantel 50 mg/kg/day PO div tid (CII) for 10–14 days plus steroids (prednisone 1 mg/kg/day or dexamethasone 0.1 mg/kg/day) begun at least 1 day before antiparasitic therapy, continued during antiparasitic treatment followed by rapid taper (to reduce inflammation associated with dying organisms)	Collaboration with a specialist with experience treating this condition is recommended. See IDSA-ASTMH guidelines.[42] Imaging with both CT and MRI is recommended for classifying disease in patients newly diagnosed with neurocysticercosis. Calcified cysts alone do not require antiparasitic treatment. Management of seizures, cerebral edema, intracranial hypertension, or hydrocephalus may require antiepileptic drugs, neuroendoscopy, or surgical approaches before considering antiparasitic therapy. Optimal dose and duration of steroid therapy are uncertain. Screening for TB infection and *Strongyloides* is recommended for patients likely to require prolonged steroid therapy. Take albendazole with food (bioavailability increases with food, especially fatty meals).

Cystoisospora (formerly *Isospora*) *belli*[43]	Age >2 mo: TMP/SMX 8–10 mg TMP/kg/day PO (or IV) div bid for 7–10 days (max 160 mg TMP/800 mg SMX bid)	Infection often self-limited in immunocompetent hosts; consider treatment if symptoms do not resolve by 5–7 days or are severe. Immunocompromised patients should be treated; longer courses or suppressive therapy may be needed for severely immunocompromised patients. Ciprofloxacin, pyrimethamine plus leucovorin, and nitazoxanide are alternatives.
Dientamoebiasis[44,45] (*Dientamoeba fragilis*)	Paromomycin 25–35 mg/kg/day PO div tid for 7 days; OR metronidazole 35–50 mg/kg/day PO div tid for 10 days (max 750 mg/dose); OR tetracycline 10 mg/kg/day PO div qid (age >7 y) (max 500 mg/dose) or doxycycline 2 mg/kg bid (max 100 mg/dose) for 10 days	Routine treatment of asymptomatic individuals not indicated. Treatment indicated when no other cause except *Dientamoeba* found for abdominal pain or diarrhea lasting >1 wk. Take paromomycin with meals. Tinidazole, secnidazole, ornidazole, and nitazoxanide are potential alternatives. Albendazole and mebendazole have no activity against *Dientamoeba*.
Dibothriocephalus latus	See Tapeworms later in this table.	
Dipylidium caninum	See Tapeworms later in this table.	
Echinococcosis[46,47]		
Echinococcus granulosus	Albendazole 10–15 mg/kg/day PO bid (max 800 mg/day) for 1–6 mo alone (CIII) or as adjunctive therapy with surgery or percutaneous treatment; initiate 1–30 days before and continue for at least 1 mo after surgery (duration has not been studied formally).	Involvement with specialist with experience treating this condition strongly recommended. Surgery is the treatment of choice for management of complicated cysts. PAIR technique effective for appropriate cysts. Mebendazole is an alternative if albendazole is unavailable; if used, continue for 3 mo after PAIR. Praziquantel efficacy variable; may have a role in combination therapy with albendazole. Take albendazole with food (bioavailability increases with food, especially fatty meals).

B. PREFERRED THERAPY FOR SPECIFIC PARASITIC PATHOGENS

Disease/Organism	Treatment (evidence grade)	Comments
Echinococcus multilocularis	Surgical treatment generally the treatment of choice; postoperative albendazole 10–15 mg/kg/day PO div bid (max 800 mg/day) should be administered to reduce relapse; duration uncertain (at least 2 y with long-term monitoring for relapse). Benefit of preoperative albendazole unknown.	Involvement with specialist with experience treating this condition recommended. Take albendazole with food (bioavailability increases with food, especially fatty meals).
Entamoeba histolytica	See Amebiasis earlier in this table.	
Enterobius vermicularis	See Pinworms later in this table.	
Fasciola hepatica	See Flukes later in this table.	
Fasciolopsis buski	See Flukes later in this table.	
Eosinophilic meningitis	See Angiostrongyliasis earlier in this table.	
Filariasis[48-51]		
Loa loa	Symptomatic loiasis with microfilariae (MF) of *L loa*/mL <8,000 (some experts prefer <2,500 MF/mL): DEC (from the CDC) 8–10 mg/kg/day PO tid for 21 days; some use a graded schedule for patients with microfilaremia. Symptomatic loiasis, with MF/mL ≥8,000 (some experts prefer <2,500 MF/mL): apheresis or albendazole 200 mg PO bid for 21 days followed by DEC.	Involvement with specialist with experience treating this condition recommended. Quantification of MF levels is essential before treatment. Apheresis or albendazole may be used to reduce MF levels to <8,000 MF/mL (some experts prefer <2,500 MF/mL) before treatment with DEC. Adverse events with DEC (due to rapid killing of MF) are more likely when level of MF is >2,500 MF/mL. Antihistamines and steroids may be used to limit adverse reactions to treatment. Do not use DEC if onchocerciasis is present. Albendazole is an alternative after 2 failed rounds of DEC.
Mansonella ozzardi	Ivermectin 150 mcg/kg PO once	DEC and albendazole not effective

Mansonella perstans	Combination therapy with DEC and mebendazole may be effective.	Relatively resistant to DEC, ivermectin, albendazole, and mebendazole; doxycycline 4 mg/kg/day PO (max 200 mg/day div bid) for 6 wk beneficial for clearing microfilaria in Mali and Ghana
River blindness (*Onchocerca volvulus*)	For those in areas with ongoing transmission: ivermectin 150 mcg/kg PO once (AIII); repeat q3–6mo until asymptomatic. If no ongoing exposure: ivermectin 150 mcg/kg PO once followed 1 wk later by doxycycline 4 mg/kg/day PO (max 200 mg/day) for 6 wk; may continue ivermectin q3–6mo for persistent symptoms.	Doxycycline targets *Wolbachia*, the endosymbiotic bacteria associated with *O volvulus*. Assess for *L loa* coinfection before using ivermectin if exposure occurred in settings where both *Onchocerca* and *L loa* are endemic. Optimal treatment of onchocerciasis in the setting of *L loa* infection is uncertain; consultation with a specialist familiar with these diseases is recommended. Moxidectin (8 mg PO once) was FDA approved in 2018 for adults and children ≥12 y for treatment of onchocerciasis; not yet available commercially in the United States. Screening for loiasis recommended before use. Safety and efficacy of repeat doses have not been studied. The FDA has not reviewed information on safety and efficacy in children <12 y.
Wuchereria bancrofti; Brugia malayi, timori; Mansonella streptocerca	DEC (from the CDC) 6 mg/kg once	Avoid DEC with *Onchocerca* and *L loa* coinfection. Doxycycline (4 mg/kg/day PO, max 200 mg/day, for 4–6 wk) may be used concurrently with DEC or as an alternative; effectiveness of doxycycline in *M streptocerca* unknown. Albendazole has activity against adult worms. DEC is available from the CDC (404-639-3670).
– Tropical pulmonary eosinophilia[52]	DEC (from the CDC) 6 mg/kg/day PO div tid for 14–21 days; corticosteroids to reduce inflammation; bronchodilators for bronchospasm (CII)	DEC is available from the CDC Drug Service at 404-639-3670. Do not use DEC if onchocerciasis is present.

B. PREFERRED THERAPY FOR SPECIFIC PARASITIC PATHOGENS

Disease/Organism	Treatment (evidence grade)	Comments
Flukes		
– Intestinal fluke (*F buski*)	Praziquantel 75 mg/kg PO div tid for 1 day (BII)	
– Liver flukes[53] (*C sinensis*, *Opisthorchis* spp)	Praziquantel 75 mg/kg PO div tid for 1–2 days (BII); OR albendazole 10 mg/kg/day PO (max 400 mg bid) for 7 days (CIII). Single 30–50 mg/kg dose of praziquantel may be effective in light infection with *Opisthorchis viverrini*.[54]	Take praziquantel with liquids and food. Take albendazole with food (bioavailability increases with food, especially fatty meals).
– Lung fluke[55,56] (*Paragonimus westermani* and other *Paragonimus* lung flukes)	Praziquantel 75 mg/kg/day PO div tid for 2 days (BII) Triclabendazole 10 mg/kg/dose PO bid for 1 day (approved for children ≥6 y for fascioliasis)	Triclabendazole should be taken with food to facilitate absorption. A short course of corticosteroids may reduce inflammatory response around dying flukes in cerebral disease.
– Sheep liver fluke[57] (*F hepatica*, *gigantica*)	Triclabendazole 10 mg/kg/dose PO bid for 1 day (FDA evaluated for age ≥6 y) (BII) OR nitazoxanide PO (take with food), ages 12–47 mo, 100 mg/dose bid for 7 days; 4–11 y, 200 mg/dose bid for 7 days; ≥12 y, 1 tab (500 mg)/dose bid for 7 days (CII)	Responds poorly to praziquantel; albendazole and mebendazole ineffective. Triclabendazole should be taken with food to facilitate absorption.
Giardiasis (*Giardia intestinalis*, or *duodenalis* [formerly *lamblia*][58–60]	Tinidazole 50 mg/kg/day (max 2 g) PO for 1 day (age >3 y) (BII); OR nitazoxanide PO (take with food), ages 1–3 y, 100 mg/dose bid for 3 days; 4–11 y, 200 mg/dose bid for 3 days; ≥12 y, 500 mg/dose bid for 3 days (BII)	Alternatives: metronidazole 15 mg/kg/day (max 250 mg/dose) PO div tid for 5–7 days (BII); albendazole 10–15 mg/kg/day (max 400 mg/dose) PO for 5 days (CII) OR mebendazole 200 mg PO tid for 5 days; OR paromomycin 30 mg/kg/day div tid for 5–10 days; furazolidone 8 mg/kg/day (max 100 mg/dose) in 4 doses for 7–10 days (not available in the United States); quinacrine (refractory cases) 6 mg/kg/day PO div tid (max 100 mg/dose) for 5 days.

	If therapy ineffective, may try a higher dose or longer course of the same agent, or an agent in a different class; combination therapy may be considered for refractory cases. Treatment of asymptomatic carriers not usually indicated unless risk for transmission to vulnerable individuals.
Hookworm[61-63] *Necator americanus,* *Ancylostoma duodenale*	Albendazole 400 mg once (repeat dose may be necessary) (BII); OR mebendazole 100 mg PO for 3 days OR 500 mg PO once; OR pyrantel pamoate 11 mg/kg (max 1 g/day) (BII) PO qd for 3 days	Take albendazole on an empty stomach for this indication.
Hymenolepis nana	See Tapeworms later in this table.
Isospora belli	See *Cystoisospora belli* earlier in this table under Cysticercosis.
Leishmaniasis[64-72] (including kala-azar) *Leishmania* spp	Visceral: L-AmB 3 mg/kg/day on days 1–5, 14, and 21 (AI); OR miltefosine 2.5 mg/kg/day PO (max 150 mg/day) for 28 days (BII) (FDA-approved regimen for children ≥12 y [see IDSA-ASTMH guidelines for these children]: 50 mg PO bid for 28 days for weight 30–44 kg; 50 mg PO tid for 28 days for weight ≥45 kg); other AmB products available but not evaluated by the FDA for this indication. Cutaneous and mucosal disease: there is no generally accepted treatment of choice; treatment decisions should be individualized. Uncomplicated cutaneous: combination of debridement of eschars, cryotherapy, thermotherapy, intralesional, and topical alternative.	Consultation with a specialist familiar with managing leishmaniasis is strongly advised, especially when treating patients with HIV coinfection. Multiple regimens are used globally; we have provided regimens approved by the FDA for use in the United States. See IDSA-ASTMH guidelines for *Leishmania*.[64] Region where infection acquired, spp of *Leishmania*, skill of practitioner with some local therapies, and drugs available in the United States affect therapeutic choices. For immunocompromised patients with visceral disease, FDA-approved dosing of liposomal amphotericin is 4 mg/kg on days 1–5, 10, 17, 24, 31, and 38, with further therapy on an individual basis.

(Continued on next page)

B. PREFERRED THERAPY FOR SPECIFIC PARASITIC PATHOGENS

Disease/Organism	Treatment (evidence grade)	Comments
Leishmaniasis[64–72] (including kala-azar) *Leishmania* spp (continued)	Complicated cutaneous: PO or parenteral systemic therapy with miltefosine 2.5 mg/kg/day PO (max 150 mg/day) for 28 days (FDA-approved regimen for children ≥12 y [see IDSA-ASTMH guidelines for these children]: 50 mg PO bid for 28 days for weight 30–44 kg; 50 mg PO tid for 28 days for weight ≥45 kg) (BII); OR pentamidine isethionate 2–4 mg/day IV or IM qod for 4–7 doses; OR amphotericin (various regimens); OR azoles (fluconazole 200 mg PO qd for 6 wk; or ketoconazole or itraconazole); also intralesional and topical alternatives.

Mucosal: AmB (Fungizone) 0.5–1 mg/kg/day IV qd or qod for cumulative total of about 20–45 mg/kg; OR L-AmB about 3 mg/kg/day IV qd for cumulative total of about 20–60 mg/kg; OR miltefosine 2.5 mg/kg/day PO (max 150 mg/day) for 28 days (FDA-evaluated regimen for children ≥12 y [see IDSA-ASTMH guidelines for these children]: 50 mg PO bid for 28 days for weight 30–44 kg; 50 mg PO tid for 28 days for weight ≥45 kg). | See guidelines for use of pentavalent antimonial drugs for visceral, mucosal, or complicated cutaneous leishmaniasis.

Sodium stibogluconate is unavailable in the United States; information about acquiring meglumine antimoniate is available here: www.astmh.org/blog/blog/ instructions-for-acquiring-glucantime-(meglumine-a

Guideline for the Treatment of Leishmaniasis in the Americas (2022) is available here: www.paho.org/en/ documents/guideline-treatment-leishmaniasis-americas-second-edition |
| **Lice** *Pediculosis capitis, humanus; Phthirus pubis*[73,74] | Follow manufacturer's instructions for topical use: permethrin 1% (≥2 mo) OR pyrethrin (children ≥2 y) (BII); OR ivermectin lotion 0.5% (≥6 mo) (BII); OR spinosad topical suspension 0.9% (≥6 mo) (BII); OR malathion lotion 0.5% (children ≥2 y) (BIII); OR PO ivermectin 200 mcg/kg PO once; repeat 7–10 days later (children >15 kg); OR abametapir lotion 0.74% (children ≥6 mo; contains benzyl alcohol) | Launder bedding and clothing; for eyelash infestation, use petrolatum; for head lice, remove nits with comb designed for that purpose.

Benzyl alcohol can be irritating to skin; systemic absorption may lead to toxicity; parasite resistance unlikely to develop.

Consult specialist before re-treatment with ivermectin lotion; re-treatment with spinosad topical suspension not usually needed unless live lice seen 1 wk after treatment. |

Malaria[75,76]

Plasmodium falciparum, vivax, ovale, malariae	CDC Malaria Hotline 770-488-7788 or 855-856-4713 toll-free (Monday–Friday, 9:00 am–5:00 pm [ET]) or emergency consultation after hours 770-488-7100; online information at www.cdc.gov/malaria/php/public-health-strategy/alternative-drug-prevention.html

Consultation with a specialist familiar with management of malaria is advised, especially for severe malaria.

No antimalarial drug provides absolute protection against malaria; fever after return from an endemic area should prompt an immediate evaluation.

Emphasize personal protective measures (insecticides, bed nets, clothing, and avoidance of dusk–dawn mosquito exposures). |
| **Prophylaxis** | See wwwnc.cdc.gov/travel/yellowbook/2024/infections-diseases/malaria#prevent for current information on travel and prophylaxis. Other drugs not available in the United States are used globally to prevent and treat malaria.[75] |
| For areas with chloroquine-resistant *P falciparum or vivax* | Atovaquone/proguanil (A/P): 5–8 kg, ½ ped tab/day; >8–10 kg, ¾ ped tab/day; >10–20 kg, 1 ped tab (62.5 mg atovaquone/25 mg proguanil); >20–30 kg, 2 ped tabs; >30–40 kg, 3 ped tabs; >40 kg, 1 adult tab (250 mg atovaquone/100 mg proguanil) PO qd begun 1–2 days before travel, continued 7 days after last exposure; for children <5 kg, data on A/P limited (BIII); OR mefloquine: for children <5 kg, 5 mg/kg; ≥5–9 kg, ⅛ tab; ≥10–19 kg, ¼ tab; ≥20–30 kg, ½ tab; ≥31–45 kg, ¾ tab; ≥45 kg (adult dose), 1 tab PO once weekly begun 1 wk before arrival in area, continued for 4 wk after leaving area (BII); OR doxycycline (patients >7 y): 2 mg/kg (max 100 mg) PO qd begun 1–2 days before arrival in area, continued for 4 wk after leaving area (BIII); OR primaquine (check for G6PD deficiency before administering): 0.5-mg/kg base qd begun 1 day before travel, continued for 5 days after last exposure (BI) | Avoid mefloquine for people with a history of seizures or psychosis, active depression, or cardiac conduction abnormalities; see black box warning.

Avoid A/P in severe renal impairment (CrCl <30 mL/min).

P falciparum resistance to mefloquine exists along the borders between Thailand and Myanmar and Thailand and Cambodia, Myanmar and China, and Myanmar and Laos; isolated resistance has been reported in southern Vietnam.

Take doxycycline with adequate fluids to avoid esophageal irritation and food to avoid GI side effects; use sunscreen and avoid excessive sun exposure. |

(Continued on next page)

B. PREFERRED THERAPY FOR SPECIFIC PATHOGENS

Disease/Organism	Treatment (evidence grade)	Comments
For areas with chloroquine-resistant *P falciparum or vivax* (continued)		Tafenoquine FDA approved August 2018 for use in those ≥18 y; must test for G6PD deficiency before use; pregnancy testing recommended before use. Not evaluated by the FDA for those <18 y. LD 200 mg daily for 3 days before travel; 200 mg weekly during travel; after return, 200 mg once 7 days after last maintenance dose; tabs must be swallowed whole. May also be used to prevent malaria in areas with chloroquine-resistant malaria.
For areas without chloroquine-resistant *P falciparum or vivax*	Chloroquine phosphate 5-mg base/kg (max 300-mg base) PO once weekly, beginning 1 wk before arrival in area and continuing for 4 wk after leaving area (available in suspension outside the United States and Canada and at compounding pharmacies) (AII). After return from heavy or prolonged (months) exposure to infected mosquitoes: consider treatment with primaquine (check for G6PD deficiency before administering) 0.5-mg base/kg PO qd with final 2 wk of chloroquine for prevention of relapse with *P ovale* or *vivax*.	
Treatment of disease		See www.cdc.gov/malaria/resources/pdf/Malaria_Treatment_Table_202306.pdf for greater detail about treatment of malaria in the United States. Other drugs not available in the United States are used globally for prevention and treatment of malaria.[75]

– Chloroquine-resistant *P falciparum, vivax*	PO therapy: artemether/lumefantrine 6 doses over 3 days at 0, 8, 24, 36, 48, and 60 h; 5–<15 kg, 1 tab/dose; 15–<25 kg, 2 tabs/dose; 25–<35 kg, 3 tabs/dose; ≥35 kg, 4 tabs/dose (BII); A/P: for children <5 kg, data limited; 5–<8 kg, 2 ped tabs (62.5 mg atovaquone/25 mg proguanil per tab) PO qd for 3 days; 8–<10 kg, 3 ped tabs qd for 3 days; 10–<20 kg, 1 adult tab (250 mg atovaquone/100 mg proguanil) qd for 3 days; 20–<30 kg, 2 adult tabs qd for 3 days; 30–<40 kg, 3 adult tabs qd for 3 days; ≥40 kg, 4 adult tabs qd for 3 days (BII); OR quinine 30 mg/kg/day (max 2 g/day) PO div tid for 3–7 days AND doxycycline 4 mg/kg/day div bid for 7 days OR clindamycin 30 mg/kg/day div tid (max 900 mg tid) for 7 days. Parenteral therapy: artesunate (commercially available, but if not in stock or not available within 24 h, contact the CDC Malaria Hotline). Children >20 kg: 2.4 mg/kg/dose IV at 0, 12, 24, and 48 h. Children <20 kg: 3 mg/kg/dose IV[77] at 0, 12, 24, and 48 h (from the CDC) (BI) AND follow artesunate by one of the following: artemether/lumefantrine, A/P, doxycycline (clindamycin in pregnant women), or, if no other options, mefloquine, all dosed as above. If needed, give interim treatment until artesunate arrives. See the CDC website for details (www.cdc.gov/malaria/resources/pdf/Malaria_Treatment_Table_202306.pdf). For prevention of relapse with *P vivax, ovale*: primaquine (check for G6PD deficiency before administering) 0.5-mg base/kg/day PO (max 30-mg base/day) for 14 days.	Mild disease may be treated with PO antimalarial drugs; severe disease (impaired level of consciousness, convulsion, hypotension, or parasitemia >5%) should be treated parenterally. Avoid mefloquine for treatment of malaria, if possible, given higher dose and increased incidence of adverse events. Take clindamycin and doxycycline with plenty of liquids. Do not use primaquine or tafenoquine during pregnancy. Avoid artemether/lumefantrine and mefloquine in patients with cardiac arrhythmias, and avoid concomitant use of drugs that prolong QT interval. Take A/P and artemether/lumefantrine with food or milk. Artesunate is now available commercially, but if not in stock or not available within 24 hours, contact the CDC Malaria Hotline at 770-488-7788 or 855-856-4713 toll-free, Monday–Friday, 9:00 am to 5:00 pm (ET), and the emergency number is 770-488-7100 for after hours, weekends, and holidays.

B. PREFERRED THERAPY FOR SPECIFIC PARASITIC PATHOGENS

Disease/Organism	Treatment (evidence grade)	Comments
– Chloroquine-susceptible *P falciparum*; chloroquine-susceptible *P vivax, ovale, malariae*	PO therapy: chloroquine 10-mg/kg base (max 600-mg base) PO, then 5 mg/kg at 6, 24, and 48 h after initial dose Parenteral therapy: artesunate, as above For prevention of relapse with *P vivax, ovale*: primaquine (check for G6PD deficiency before administering) 0.5-mg base/kg/day PO (max 30-mg/kg base/day) for 14 days	Alternative if chloroquine not available: hydroxychloroquine 10-mg base/kg PO immediately, followed by 5-mg base/kg PO at 6, 24, and 48 h. Tafenoquine approved July 2018 for prevention of relapse with *P vivax* malaria in those aged ≥16 y. Use only when treatment is with chloroquine or hydroxychloroquine. 300 mg on the first or second day of chloroquine or hydroxychloroquine for acute malaria. Must test for G6PD deficiency before use; pregnancy testing recommended before use. Tabs must be swallowed whole.
Mansonella ozzardi, perstans, streptocerca	See Filariasis earlier in this table.	
Naegleria	See Amebic meningoencephalitis earlier in this table.	
Necator americanus	See Hookworm earlier in this table.	
Onchocerca volvulus	See Filariasis earlier in this table.	
Opisthorchis spp	See Flukes earlier in this table.	
Paragonimus westermani	See Flukes earlier in this table.	
Pinworms (*E vermicularis*)	Mebendazole 100 mg once, repeat in 2 wk; OR albendazole 400 mg PO on an empty stomach once; OR pyrantel pamoate 11 mg/kg (max 1 g) PO once (BIII); repeat in 2 wk.	Treat entire household for recurrent infection (and if this fails, consider treating close child care/school contacts); re-treatment of contacts after 2 wk may be needed to prevent reinfection. Children as young as 1 y may be treated; some pediatric ID practitioners may choose to defer treatment of an exposed but uninfected infant aged <1 y. Launder bedding and clothing.
Plasmodium spp	See Malaria earlier in this table.	

Pneumocystis	See *Pneumocystis jirovecii* pneumonia in Table 5B.
Scabies (*Sarcoptes scabiei*)[78]	Permethrin (5%) cream applied to entire body (including scalp and face of young children), left on for 8–14 h, and then washed off—repeated in 1–2 wk (BII); OR ivermectin 200 mcg/kg PO once weekly for 2 doses (BII); OR crotamiton (10%) applied topically overnight on days 1, 2, 3, and 8 and then washed off in am (BII) OR spinosad (approved for children ≥4 years) applied to skin from neck to toes, allowed to dry 10 minutes before dressing, and left on for at least 6 h	Launder bedding and clothing. Crotamiton treatment failure has been observed. Ivermectin should not be used in children who weigh <15 kg due to lack of safety data. Itching may continue for weeks after successful treatment; can be managed with antihistamines.
Schistosomiasis (*Schistosoma haematobium, intercalatum, japonicum, mansoni, mekongi*)[79–81]	Praziquantel 40 mg/kg/day PO div bid (for *S haematobium, S mansoni,* and *S intercalatum*) or 60 mg/kg/day PO div tid (for *S japonicum* and *S mekongi*) for 1 day (AI)	Take praziquantel with food and liquids. Oxamniquine (not available in the United States) 20 mg/kg PO bid for 1 day (Brazil) or 40–60 mg/kg/day for 2–3 days (most of Africa) (BII). Re-treat with the same dose if eggs still present 6–12 wk after initial treatment.
Strongyloidiasis (*Strongyloides stercoralis*)[82,83]	Ivermectin 200 mcg/kg PO qd for 1–2 days (regimen can be repeated in 2 wk for immunocompromised patients) (BII); OR albendazole 400 mg PO bid for 7 days (BII) Hyperinfection syndrome: optimal duration of treatment unknown; can continue ivermectin until stool and/or sputum examination findings are negative for 2 wk; may add albendazole for dual therapy	Albendazole is less effective but may be adequate if longer courses used. For patients with hyperinfection syndrome, veterinary SUBQ formulations of ivermectin may be lifesaving. The SUBQ formulation may be used under a single-patient IND protocol request to the FDA. Rectal administration may also be used for those unable to tolerate PO administration. Ivermectin should not be used in children who weigh <15 kg due to lack of safety data.

B. PREFERRED THERAPY FOR SPECIFIC PARASITIC PATHOGENS

Disease/Organism	Treatment (evidence grade)	Comments
Tapeworms *Taenia saginata, solium; Hymenolepis nana; Diphyllobothrium latum; Dipylidium caninum*	Praziquantel 5–10 mg/kg PO once (for *H nana*: 25 mg/kg once; may repeat 10 days later) (BII); OR niclosamide (not available in the United States) 50 mg/kg (max 2 g) PO once, chewed thoroughly (for *H nana*: weight 11–34 kg: 1 g in a single dose on day 1, then 500 mg/day PO for 6 days; weight >34 kg: 1.5 g in a single dose on day 1, then 1 g/day PO for 6 days; adults: 2 g in a single dose for 7 days)	Nitazoxanide may be effective (published clinical data limited) at 500 mg PO bid for 3 days for age >11 y; 200 mg PO bid for 3 days for 4–11 y; 100 mg PO bid for 3 days for 1–3 y. Albendazole (400 mg PO daily for 3 days) may be an alternative.
Toxocariasis[84] (*Toxocara canis* [dog roundworm], *cati* [cat roundworm])	Visceral larval migrans: albendazole 400 mg PO bid for 5 days (BII) Ocular larva migrans: prednisone (0.5–1 mg/kg/day with slow taper) plus albendazole 400 mg PO bid for up to 2 wk for sight-threatening inflammation	Mild disease often resolves without treatment; eosinophilia may be prolonged. Corticosteroids may be used for severe symptoms in visceral larval migrans. Mebendazole (100–200 mg/day PO bid for 5 days) is an alternative.
Toxoplasmosis (*Toxoplasma gondii*)[85–87]	See Ch 2 for congenital infection. Severe acute toxoplasmosis: Pyrimethamine 2 mg/kg/day PO div bid for 1 day (max 100 mg), then 1 mg/kg/day (max 50 mg/day) PO qd AND sulfadiazine 100–200 mg/kg/day PO div qid (max 2–4 g/day for severe disease); with supplemental folinic acid (leucovorin) 7.5 PO qd (AI) for 2–4 wk Active toxoplasmic chorioretinitis: Pyrimethamine 2 mg/kg/day PO div bid for 1 day (max 100 mg), then 1 mg/kg/day (max 50 mg/day) PO qd AND sulfadiazine 50 mg/kg PO bid (max 4 g/day) AND folinic acid (leucovorin) 7.5 mg/day PO for 4–6 wk OR TMP/SMX 15–20 mg TMP/kg; 75–100 mg/kg SMX qd div q6–8h for 4–6 wk.	Acute toxoplasmosis in immunocompetent, nonpregnant individuals is typically self-limited and may not require treatment. Consult expert advice for treatment during pregnancy, management of congenital infection, management of chorioretinitis, and management of toxoplasmosis in immunocompromised individuals. For acute disease: clindamycin, azithromycin, or atovaquone plus pyrimethamine may be effective for patients intolerant of sulfa-containing drugs. Experienced ophthalmologic consultation (retinal specialist with experience treating toxoplasmic chorioretinitis) encouraged for treatment of ocular disease.

Organism/Disease	Therapy	Comments
		Steroids may be given concurrently for ocular or CNS infection. Prolonged therapy if HIV positive. Compounded pyrimethamine may be obtained from specialized pharmacies; consult your local pharmacist for information on which pharmacies are approved for creating these products. Take pyrimethamine with food to decrease GI adverse effects; sulfadiazine should be taken on an empty stomach with water.
	For treatment in pregnancy, spiramycin 50–100 mg/kg/day PO div qid (available as investigational therapy through the FDA at 301-796-1400) (CII). Treatment with spiramycin is recommended in general when infections were acquired and diagnosed before 18 wk of gestation and is most effective if initiated within 8 wk of seroconversion. After 18 wk of gestation, treatment with pyrimethamine, sulfadiazine, and leucovorin can be given for new infections or if the fetus is documented or suspected to have infection.	
Travelers diarrhea[38,88-90]	Azithromycin 10 mg/kg qd for 1–3 days (AII); OR rifaximin 200 mg PO tid for 3 days (age ≥12 y) (BII); OR ciprofloxacin (BII)	See 2017 guidelines from International Society of Travel Medicine: https://academic.oup.com/jtm/article/24/suppl_1/S63/3782742 (accessed August 9, 2024). Azithromycin preferable to ciprofloxacin for travelers to Southeast Asia and India given high prevalence of FQ-resistant *Campylobacter*. Do not use rifaximin for *Campylobacter, Salmonella, Shigella,* and other causes of invasive diarrhea or bloody diarrhea that may be associated with bacteremia. Antibiotic regimens may be combined with loperamide (≥2 y). Rifamycin evaluated by the FDA in adults ≥18 y for treatment of TD caused by noninvasive strains of *Escherichia coli* (388 mg [2 tabs] bid for 3 days).
Trichinellosis (*Trichinella spiralis*)[91]	Albendazole 400 mg PO bid for 8–14 days (BII) OR mebendazole 200–400 mg PO tid for 3 days, then 400–500 mg PO tid for 10 days	Therapy ineffective for larvae already in muscles Anti-inflammatory drugs, steroids for CNS or cardiac involvement or severe symptoms
Trichomoniasis (*Trichomonas vaginalis*)[92]	Metronidazole 500 mg PO bid for 7 days for women; 2 g PO in 1 dose for men OR tinidazole 50 mg/kg (max 2 g) PO for 1 dose (BII)	Treat sex partners simultaneously.
Trichuris trichiura	See Whipworm later in this table.	

B. PREFERRED THERAPY FOR SPECIFIC PARASITIC PATHOGENS

Disease/Organism	Treatment (evidence grade)	Comments
Trypanosomiasis		
- Chagas disease[26-28] (*T cruzi*)	Benznidazole PO: age <2 y, 5.0–7.5 mg/kg/day div bid for 60 days; 2–12 y, 5–8 mg/kg/day div bid for 60 days; ≥12 y, 5–7 mg/kg/day div bid for 60 days (BIII); OR nifurtimox PO age birth–<18 y, 2.5–<40 kg: 10–20 mg/kg/day, PO, in 3 div doses for 60 days; ≥17 y, 8–10 mg/kg/day div tid for 60 days (BIII)	Therapy recommended for acute and congenital infection, reactivated infection, and chronic infection in children and teens <18 y; consider in those up to 50 y with chronic infection without advanced cardiomyopathy. Benznidazole has been evaluated by the FDA for use in children aged 2–12 y (www.benznidazoletablets.com; accessed August 9, 2024); data have not been submitted for review in children <2 y. Some experts use 300 mg/day for 60 days for adults regardless of body weight. Nifurtimox has been reviewed and approved by the FDA for children and teens up to 17 y. Side effects are common but occur less often in younger patients; consultation with experts in the management of Chagas disease and adverse drug reactions can be helpful. Both drugs contraindicated in pregnancy.
- Human African trypanosomiasis[93-98] (*Trypanosoma brucei gambiense* [West African], *rhodesiense* [East African])	See CDC guidance (www.cdc.gov/sleeping-sickness/hcp/clinical-care/index.html) or WHO interim guidance for treatment of gambiense HAT; consultation with an ID or subject matter expert recommended when treating patients with HAT.	CDC Drug Service: www.cdc.gov/laboratory/drugservice/formulary.html https://iris.who.int/bitstream/hand le/10665/326178/9789241550567-eng.pdf
Uncinaria stenocephala	See Cutaneous larva migrans earlier in this table.	

Whipworm (trichuriasis) *Trichuris trichiura*	Albendazole 400 mg PO qd for 3 days; OR mebendazole 100 mg PO bid for 3 days; OR ivermectin 200 mcg/kg/day PO qd for 3 days (BII)	Treatment can be given for 5–7 days for heavy infestation. Combination albendazole plus ivermectin is an alternative.
Wuchereria bancrofti	See Filariasis earlier in this table.	
Yaws	Azithromycin 30 mg/kg, max 2 g once (also treats bejel and pinta)	Alternative regimens include IM benzathine penicillin and second-line agents doxycycline, tetracycline, and erythromycin.

10. Choosing Among Antiparasitic Agents: Antimalarial Drugs, Nitroimidazoles, Benzimidazoles, and Neglected Tropical Diseases

Antimalarial Drugs

Prevention of Malaria

Seven drugs are available in the United States for prevention of malaria; one (tafenoquine) is licensed only for adults 18 years and older. Another (doxycycline) is not suitable for children younger than 8 years due to the duration it must be taken. Two (primaquine and tafenoquine) require testing for glucose-6-phosphate dehydrogenase (G6PD) deficiency before use. Five of these drugs are taken weekly (chloroquine, hydroxychloroquine, mefloquine, primaquine, and tafenoquine) and the other 2 are taken daily (atovaquone/proguanil [A/P] and doxycycline). The first consideration in the choice of a drug for prevention of malaria is presence of chloroquine resistance at the destination. If present, neither chloroquine nor hydroxychloroquine can be used. The next factor to consider is preference of caregivers about giving a medication to a child daily or weekly, as antimalarial effectiveness depends primarily on taking the medication, not which medication is prescribed. Potential adverse events factor into the decision families make about antimalarials. Many parents will decline mefloquine as soon as the black box warning about the risk of neuropsychiatric adverse reactions is explained, although taking a weekly medication might increase convenience and adherence, and mefloquine may be less costly. In general, families traveling to destinations where there is chloroquine resistance will be choosing between A/P (daily medication, possibly more costly) and mefloquine (weekly medication, black box warning). Primaquine is used extremely rarely in children; testing for G6PD deficiency is required, and many clinicians are unfamiliar with the use of this drug. Doxycycline needs to be given for a longer period than ideal for children younger than 8 years and is limited by its adverse events profile. Tafenoquine also requires G6PD testing and is limited to those older than 18 years.

For families traveling to areas where there is chloroquine-susceptible malaria, both chloroquine and hydroxychloroquine are options. These medications may be difficult to find, and it is prudent to be sure a family can obtain them; if not, any of the other drugs may be prescribed.

Our preference for the best tolerated and effective agent for prophylaxis in areas of chloroquine resistance is A/P; in areas of chloroquine susceptibility, chloroquine.

Treatment of Malaria

Seven drugs are available in the United States for treatment of acute malaria; choice of drug depends on the severity of illness, location where malaria was acquired, and age of the child. When malaria is acquired in a location without chloroquine resistance, chloroquine or hydroxychloroquine can be used if the patient is able to take medications orally (PO) and it is available. When malaria is acquired in chloroquine-resistant locations, or when it is acquired in chloroquine-susceptible areas but chloroquine or hydroxychloroquine is not available immediately, and when medications can be taken PO, artemether/

lumefantrine is the preferred option, with A/P (if not used for prophylaxis) also being an option. Mefloquine and quinine (in combination with clindamycin or doxycycline) are available but limited by adverse events profiles. When malaria is severe or the patient is unable to take medications PO, intravenous artesunate should be used. Identification of the species of *Plasmodium* may not be available at the time of choosing the antimalarial drug; in general, treating for *Plasmodium falciparum* is appropriate until more information is available.

The Centers for Disease Control and Prevention has detailed treatment decision-tree algorithms and tables available at www.cdc.gov/malaria/hcp/clinical-guidance/index.html.

Choosing Among Nitroimidazoles (Treatment Option for Some Protozoa, Amoebas)

The choice among nitroimidazoles (metronidazole, tinidazole, secnidazole, ornidazole, and triclabendazole) is based primarily on spectrum of activity, availability (ornidazole is not available in the United States), cost, convenience, and adverse events. Tinidazole has a longer half-life and is better tolerated than metronidazole but may be more costly. Triclabendazole has a narrower spectrum confined to *Fasciola hepatica, Fasciola gigantica,* and paragonimiasis. Drugs in this group reportedly produce a disulfiram-like effect when taken with alcohol; this has been called into question recently.[1]

Choosing Among Benzimidazoles (Treatment Option for Some Helminths)

The choice between the benzimidazoles mebendazole and albendazole depends on the specific organism, availability, and cost. Albendazole is a broader-spectrum antihelminth than mebendazole but may be more costly. We have noted when there are data to support recommending one agent over the other.

Need is great for effective, affordable, and easily available drugs for diseases known as *neglected tropical diseases,* which include, but are not limited to, the diseases mentioned previously and Chagas disease, leishmaniasis, lymphatic filariasis, and trypanosomiasis. For many of these diseases, options for treatment are limited, regimens are not standardized, treatment includes drugs with significant adverse events, or it includes drugs with limited availability. Additional funding would accelerate research on drug development and implementation of control measures for these diseases such as mass drug distribution, as it has for treatment and prevention of HIV/AIDS, malaria, and tuberculosis. Until additional focus is put on these neglected tropical diseases, which impose large burdens on the health primarily of those living in low-income countries, the "choosing among" chapter in this book for antiparasitic drugs will continue to be far shorter than those for antibacterial, antiviral, and antifungal drugs.

11. How Antibiotic Dosages Are Determined by Susceptibility Data, Pharmacodynamics, and Treatment Outcomes

Factors Involved in Dosing Recommendations

Our view of assessing the optimal dose of antimicrobials is continually changing as we learn more about drug exposure and how antibiotics kill bacteria at the site of infection. As the published literature and our experience with each drug increase, our recommendations for specific dosages evolve as we compare the efficacy, safety, and cost of each drug in the context of current and previous data from adults and children. Virtually every new antibiotic must first demonstrate some degree of efficacy and safety in adults with antibiotic exposures that occur at specific dosages, which are duplicated in children as closely as possible. We keep track of pediatric pharmacokinetics (PK) in all age-groups, reported toxicities, and unanticipated clinical failures, and on occasion, we may end up modifying our initial recommendations for an antibiotic.

Important considerations in any recommendations we make include (1) the susceptibilities of pathogens to antibiotics, which are always evolving with selective pressure from antibiotic use in communities and hospitals and are different from region to region and hospital to hospital; (2) the antibiotic concentrations achieved at the site of infection over a 24-hour dosing interval; (3) the mechanism of how antibiotics kill bacteria; (4) how often the dose we select produces a clinical and microbiologic cure; (5) how often we encounter toxicity; (6) how likely the antibiotic exposure will lead to antibiotic resistance in the treated child and the general population; and (7) the effect on the child's microbiome.

Susceptibility

Susceptibility data for each bacterial pathogen against a wide range of antibiotics are available from the microbiology laboratory of virtually every hospital. This antibiogram can help guide you in antibiotic selection for empiric therapy while you wait for specific susceptibilities to result from cultures. Many hospitals can separate the inpatient culture results from the outpatient results, and many can give you the data by hospital ward (eg, pediatric ward vs neonatal intensive care unit vs adult intensive care unit). Susceptibility data are also available by region and by country from reference laboratories or public health laboratories. The recommendations made in this book reflect overall susceptibility patterns present in the United States. See Tables 3A and 3B for some overall guidance on susceptibility of gram-positive and gram-negative pathogens, respectively. Wide variations may exist for certain pathogens in different regions of the United States and the world. New techniques for rapid molecular diagnosis of a bacterial, mycobacterial, fungal, or viral pathogen based on polymerase chain reaction or next-generation sequencing may quickly give you the name of the pathogen, but with current molecular technology, complete susceptibility data are not usually available.

11

How Antibiotic Dosages Are Determined

Drug Concentrations at the Site of Infection

With every antibiotic, we can measure the concentration of antibiotic present in the serum. We can also directly measure the concentrations in specific tissue sites, such as spinal fluid or middle ear fluid. Because "free," nonprotein-bound antibiotic is required to inhibit and kill pathogens, it is also important to calculate the amount of free drug available at the site of infection. While traditional methods of measuring antibiotics focused just on the peak concentrations in serum and how rapidly the drugs were excreted (the half-life), newer models of drug distribution in both plasma *and* tissue sites (eg, cerebrospinal fluid, urine, peritoneal fluid) and elimination from both plasma and tissue compartments now exist. Antibiotic exposure to pathogens at the site of infection can be described mathematically in many ways: (1) the percentage of time in a 24-hour dosing interval that the antibiotic concentrations are above the minimum inhibitory concentration (MIC; the antibiotic concentration required for inhibition of growth of an organism) at the site of infection (%T>MIC); (2) area under the curve (AUC; the mathematically calculated area under the serum concentration-versus-time curve); and (3) the maximal concentration of drug achieved in serum and at the tissue site (Cmax). For each of these 3 values, *a ratio of that value to the MIC of the pathogen in question* can be calculated and provides more useful information on specific drug activity against a specific pathogen than a simple look at serum concentrations or the AUC, or an MIC. It allows us to compare the exposure of different antibiotics (that achieve quite different concentrations in tissues) to a pathogen (where the MIC for each drug may be different) and to assess the activity of a single antibiotic that may be used for empiric therapy against the many different pathogens (potentially with many different MICs) that may be causing an infection at that tissue site.

Pharmacodynamics

Pharmacodynamic (PD) descriptions provide the clinician with information on *how* the bacterial pathogens are killed (see Suggested Reading later in this chapter). β-Lactam antibiotics tend to eradicate bacteria following prolonged exposure of relatively low concentrations of the antibiotic to the pathogen at the site of infection, usually expressed as the percentage of time over a dosing interval that the antibiotic is present at the site of infection in concentrations greater than the MIC (%T>MIC). For example, amoxicillin needs to be present at the site of a pneumococcal infection (such as the middle ear) at a concentration above the MIC for only 40% of a 24-hour dosing interval. Remarkably, neither higher concentrations of amoxicillin nor a more prolonged exposure will substantially increase the cure rate. On the other hand, gentamicin's activity against *Escherichia coli* is based primarily on the absolute concentration of free antibiotic at the site of infection, in the context of the MIC of the pathogen (Cmax:MIC). The more antibiotic you can deliver to the site of infection, the more rapidly you can sterilize the tissue; we are limited only by the toxicities of gentamicin. For fluoroquinolones (FQs) such as ciprofloxacin, the antibiotic exposure best linked to clinical and microbiologic success is, as with aminoglycosides, concentration dependent. However, the best mathematical correlate to assess microbiologic (and clinical) outcomes for FQs is the AUC:MIC, rather than the

Cmax:MIC. Each of the 3 PD metrics of antibiotic exposure should be linked to the MIC of the pathogen to best understand how well the antibiotic will eradicate a particular pathogen causing an infection.

Assessment of Clinical and Microbiologic Outcomes

In clinical trials of anti-infective agents, most adults and children will hopefully be cured, but the therapy of a few will fail. For those few, we may note unanticipated treatment failure that, in retrospect, is due to inadequate drug exposure (eg, more rapid drug elimination in a particular patient; the inability of a particular antibiotic to penetrate to the site of infection) or due to a pathogen with a particularly high MIC. By analyzing the successes and the failures based on the appropriate exposure parameters outlined previously (%T>MIC, AUC:MIC, or Cmax:MIC), we can often observe a particular value of exposure, above which we observe a higher rate of cure and below which the cure rate drops quickly. Knowing this target value in adults (the "antibiotic exposure break point") allows us to calculate the dosage that should also predict treatment success in most children. We do not evaluate antibiotics in children with study designs that have failure rates sufficient to calculate a pediatric exposure break point, of course. It is the adult *exposure value* that leads to success that we all (including the US Food and Drug Administration [FDA] and pharmaceutical companies) subsequently share with you, a pediatric health care practitioner, as one likely to cure your patient. US Food and Drug Administration–approved break points that are reported by microbiology laboratories (S, I, and R) are now determined by outcomes linked to drug PK and exposure, the MIC, and the PD parameter for that agent. Recommendations to the FDA for break points for the United States often come from "break point organizations," such as the Clinical and Laboratory Standards Institute Subcommittee on Antimicrobial Susceptibility Testing (www.clsi.org) or the US Committee on Antimicrobial Susceptibility Testing (www.uscast.org).

Physiologic-Based Pharmacokinetic Modeling

Just to keep everyone informed about where the field of antibiotic exposure modeling is going, the next advance has been in physiologic-based pharmacokinetic (PBPK) modeling. Currently, we use PK/PD modeling, in which a Monte Carlo simulation software program uses the overall observed distribution of PK values in a specific pediatric population (eg, neonates, infants, children, adolescents), the range of bacterial MICs observed in the pathogen of interest, and the PD metric for inhibition of bacteria growth for the antibiotic being evaluated to assess predicted outcomes for each antibiotic/pathogen pair. We can find the likelihood that a certain dose will successfully treat a certain pathogen at a certain tissue site. What PBPK adds to the equation is additional information about the physicochemical properties of drugs (some diffuse well into adipose tissues; others, not so well), about ongoing organ function development through childhood, and about blood flow/organ perfusion throughout the entire body, to allow better prediction of how drugs move through tissue compartments of the body during absorption, distribution, metabolism, and excretion for each age-group in pediatrics. In that sense, PK/PD modeling can describe by observation, but PBPK modeling can better predict how an antibiotic will "behave" in a child for both efficacy and toxicity. The FDA is encouraging PBPK modeling, and the more data we have on drug behavior, the better the PBPK models become for children. The Verscheijden review listed next gives a nice overview of PBPK modeling in pediatrics.

Suggested Reading

Le J, et al. *J Clin Pharmacol.* 2018;58(suppl 10):S108–S122 PMID: 30248202

Onufrak NJ, et al. *Clin Ther.* 2016;38(9):1930–1947 PMID: 27449411

Trang M, et al. *Curr Opin Pharmacol.* 2017;36:107–113 PMID: 29128853

Verscheijden LFM, et al. *Pharmacol Ther.* 2020;211:107541 PMID: 32246949

12. Approach to Antibiotic Therapy for Drug-Resistant Gram-Negative Bacilli and Methicillin-Resistant *Staphylococcus aureus*

Multidrug-Resistant Gram-Negative Bacilli

Increasing antibiotic resistance in gram-negative bacilli, primarily the enteric bacilli (eg, *Escherichia coli, Klebsiella, Enterobacter, Serratia, Citrobacter*), *Pseudomonas aeruginosa,* and *Acinetobacter* species, has caused profound difficulties in treatment of patients around the world; some of the pathogens are now resistant to all available agents. *Stenotrophomonas,* with profound intrinsic antibiotic resistance, is increasing as a cause of nosocomial infections and of infection in those with chronic recurrent disease (eg, cystic fibrosis). At this time, only a limited number of pediatric tertiary care centers in North America have reported outbreaks of multidrug-resistant (MDR) pathogens, but *sustained* transmission of completely resistant organisms is quite uncommon in pediatric health care institutions, likely due to the critical infection control strategies in place to identify and prevent the spread of these pathogens. Antibiotic resistance in pathogens, particularly the non-fermenting gram-negative rods, is not new but rather the result of more than 100 million years of exposure to antibiotics elaborated by other organisms in their environment. Inducible enzymes to cleave antibiotics and modify binding sites, efflux pumps, and gram-negative cell wall alterations to prevent antibiotic penetration may all be present. Some mechanisms of resistance, if not intrinsic, can be acquired from other bacilli. By using antibiotics, we "awaken" resistance; therefore, using antibiotics only when appropriate limits the selection or induction of resistance for pathogens in the treated child and for all children (see Chapter 17). Community prevalence, as well as health care institution prevalence, of extended-spectrum β-lactamase (ESBL)–containing enteric bacilli that are resistant to ceftriaxone is increasing. Carbapenemase-containing pathogens that are meropenem resistant are now beginning to spread in neonates, infants, and children. Two major classes of carbapenemases exist: serine β-lactamases (SBLs), named for a serine at the active site, and metallo–β-lactamases (MBLs), having a zinc at the active site. Antibiotic susceptibility patterns differ for the 2 classes. The most prominent carbapenemases in the United States are SBLs, most often *Klebsiella pneumoniae* carbapenemase (KPC)–related enzymes and increasingly OXA-48–like enzymes. Globally, MBLs are often the most prominent classes in circulation (eg, VIM [Verona integron-encoded metallo–β-lactamase], NDM [New Delhi metallo–β-lactamase], IMP [imipenemase metallo–β-lactamase]), with ongoing spread within the United States. Some SBLs and MBLs are now being addressed by new, active antibiotics and new β-lactamase inhibitors (BLIs). However, as we have found in the past, as soon as new drugs are available, resistance develops quickly. We cannot win, but we can usually stay in the fight against these pathogens.

In **Figure 12-1,** we assume that the clinician has the antibiotic susceptibility report in hand (or at least a local antibiogram). Each tier provides increasingly broader-spectrum activity, from the narrowest of the gram-negative agents to the broadest (and most toxic), colistin. Tier 1 is ampicillin, safe and widely available but not active against *Klebsiella, Enterobacter,* or *Pseudomonas* and only active against about half of *E coli* in the community setting. Tier 2 contains antibiotics that have both a broader spectrum against ampicillin-resistant strains of enteric bacilli and are very safe (trimethoprim/sulfamethoxazole [TMP/SMX] and cephalosporins) with decades of experience. In general, use an antibiotic from tier 2 before turning to broader-spectrum agents.

More resistant organisms can be characterized by the presence of AmpC β-lactamases (BLs) that hydrolyze first-, second-, and third-generation cephalosporins but not cefepime, a fourth-generation cephalosporin (Tier 3). Most often the genes that encode these BLs are chromosomal and inducible, clinically most relevant with *Enterobacter* species, *Klebsiella* (formerly *Enterobacter*) *aerogenes,* and *Citrobacter koseri* (formerly *diversus*). Although resistance usually develops after exposure of the pathogen to the

Figure 12-1. Enteric Bacilli: Bacilli (Enterobacterales) and *Pseudomonas aeruginosa* With Known Susceptibilities and Suggested Therapy (See Text for Additional Information)

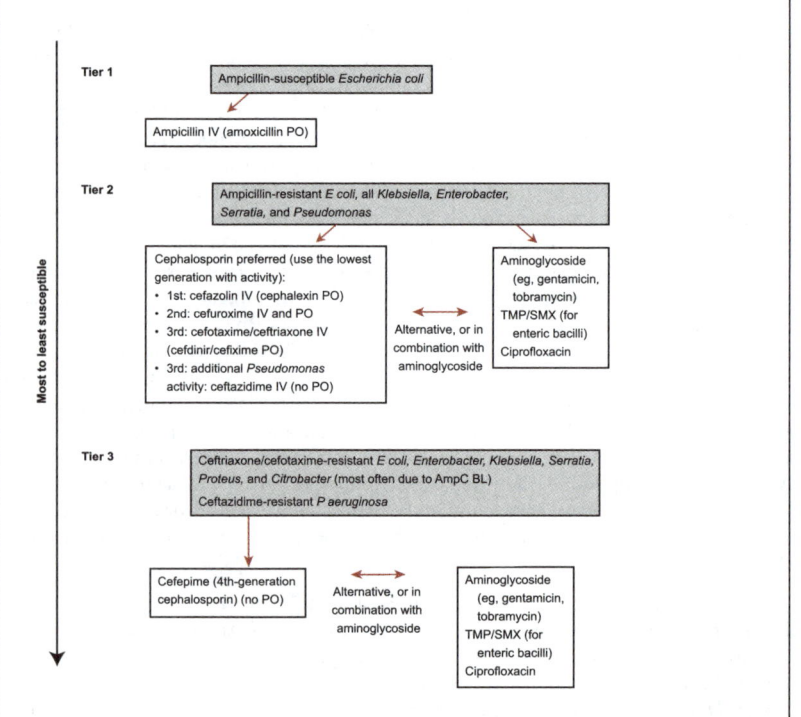

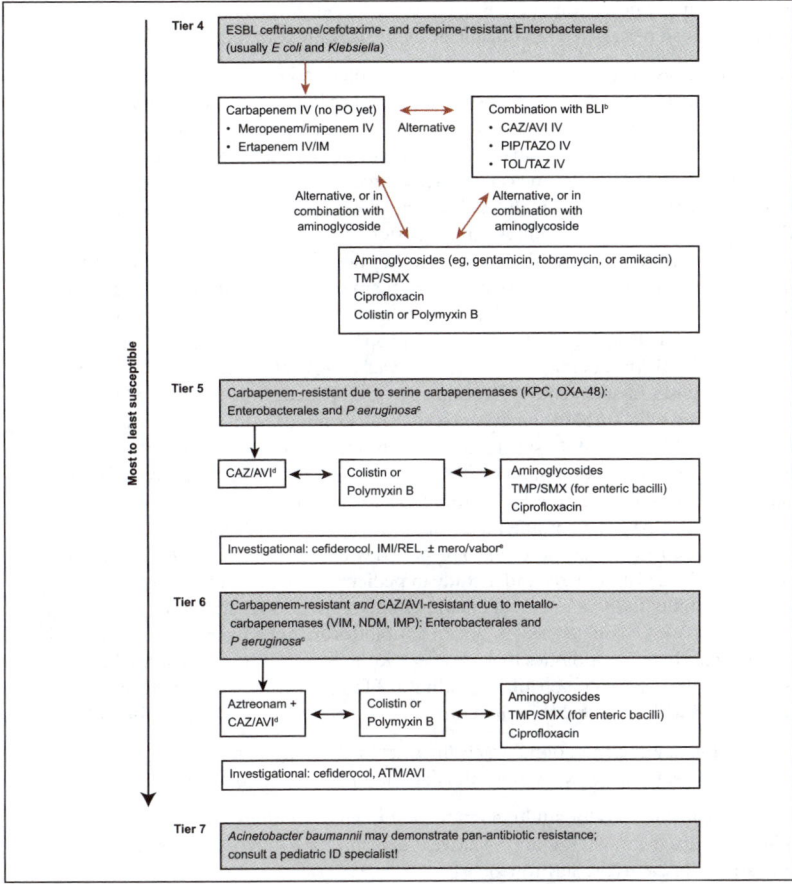

ATM/AVI indicates aztreonam/avibactam; BL, β-lactamase; BLI, β-lactamase inhibitor; CAZ/AVI, ceftazidime/avibactam; ESBL, extended-spectrum β-lactamase; ID, infectious disease; IM, intramuscularly; IMI/REL, imipenem/relebactam; IMP, imipenemase; IV, intravenously; KPC, *Klebsiella pneumoniae* carbapenemase; mero/vabor, meropenem/vaborbactam; NDM, New Delhi; PIP/TAZO, piperacillin/tazobactam; PO, orally; SMX, sulfamethoxazole; TMP, trimethoprim; TOL/TAZ, ceftolozane/tazobactam; and VIM, Verona integron-encoded.

a   *E coli, Klebsiella, Enterobacter, Serratia, Proteus, Citrobacter.*

b   IMI/REL and mero/vabor are not yet approved for children (July 2024): stable to ESBLs.

c   Displays extensive variability in regional susceptibility patterns of circulating clones, with multiple mechanisms of resistance: susceptibility testing advised.

d   Preferred due to safety consideration.

e   Cefiderocol, IMI/REL, and mero/vabor are not yet approved for children (July 2024). IMI/REL and mero/vabor are stable to KPC, but mero/vabor is not always stable to OXA-48–like BLs.

antibiotic, in any population of pathogens some bacteria will be constantly producing AmpC and can be selected out during antibiotic therapy with antibiotics like ceftriaxone.

Additional resistance occurs through ESBLs as noted earlier in this chapter. The first- through fourth-generation cephalosporins are not reliably active against ESBL-containing pathogens. Tier 4 is made up of very broad-spectrum antibiotics stable to most ESBLs (carbapenems, ceftazidime/avibactam [CAZ/AVI], piperacillin/tazobactam, ceftolozane/tazobactam). Ceftolozane is more active against *P aeruginosa* than ceftazidime or piperacillin, and it is paired with tazobactam, allowing for some additional activity against ESBL-producing enteric bacilli. Aminoglycosides remain active against many MDR pathogens with resistance to β-lactams, but they demonstrate significantly more toxicity than β-lactam agents although we have used them safely for decades. Tier 5 is represented by a new broad-spectrum BLI, avibactam, in combination with ceftazidime (CAZ/AVI is US Food and Drug Administration [FDA] approved for children), that demonstrates stability to ESBL-producing enteric bacilli as well as against the KPC and OXA-48 serine carbapenemases (associated with resistance to meropenem/imipenem) but *lacks* stability against the metallo-carbapenemases present most commonly in enteric bacilli (including *E coli*) worldwide.[1] With substantial data on safety with widespread use, CAZ/AVI is preferred over fluoroquinolones (FQs) for treatment of pathogens expressing serine carbapenemases. For treatment of pathogens harboring metallo-carbapenemases, aztreonam with CAZ/AVI is recommended (Tier 6). Remarkably, aztreonam is stable to current metallo-carbapenemases but needs to be paired with avibactam to protect it from AmpC BLs and ESBLs. Cefiderocol, under study in pediatrics, is a new siderophore cephalosporin with stability to metallo-carbapenemases and represents an alternative to aztreonam with CAZ/AVI. Of course, non–β-lactam antibiotics are not affected by BLs, so the clinician may find other antibiotics that are effective, including aminoglycosides, FQs, TMP/SMX, and, if all else fails, colistin. Colistin was FDA approved in 1962 with significant toxicity and with remarkably limited prospective, controlled clinical data for children.

Some of the newer-generation tetracyclines have activity against MBL-producing enteric bacilli (ie, tigecycline, eravacycline, omadacycline) but are not discussed in this book.

Drugs in clinical trials for adults, soon to be studied in children, are discussed next. Many additional drugs for MDR gram-negative organisms have moved from animal models into adult clinical trials. Stay tuned.

Investigational Agents Recently Approved for Adults and Being Studied in Children

Cefiderocol. Represents a new class of β-lactam antibiotics as a siderophore cephalosporin (eg, binding to iron) that defies the "generation" categories with respect to spectrum of activity. The cefiderocol-iron complex allows for pathogens to actively transport the complex across the cell wall into the periplasmic space, thus allowing the antibiotic access to the transpeptidases not as easily achieved for antibiotics that need to diffuse the gram-negative cell wall. It is stable to ESBLs, SBLs and MBLs, AmpC, and OXA-48 enzymes,

12

with activity that includes *Pseudomonas, Acinetobacter,* and *Stenotrophomonas.* Approved for adults in 2019. Pediatric treatment studies are underway.

Imipenem and relebactam. Imipenem was the first carbapenem approved for use in children and is now paired with relebactam, a BLI with similar structure to avibactam, providing stability for the combination against KPC-containing enteric bacilli, thus extending the aerobic/anaerobic broad spectrum of carbapenems that already includes ESBLs and AmpC BLs. Approved for adults in 2019. Pediatric treatment studies are underway.

Meropenem and vaborbactam. Meropenem, a familiar broad-spectrum aerobic/anaerobic coverage carbapenem that is already stable to ESBLs and AmpC BLs, is now paired with vaborbactam, allowing for activity against the KPC serine carbapenemases but not metallo-carbapenemases. Approved for adults in 2017. Pediatric pharmacokinetic (PK) studies are underway.

Sulbactam and durlobactam. Targeted to *Acinetobacter,* including MDR strains. Sulbactam, developed as a BLI, also has direct antibiotic activity against *Acinetobacter.* However, sulbactam is degraded by many of the more broad-spectrum BLs, but when paired with the BLI durlobactam, it is protected from ESBLs and serine carbapenemases (SBLs) as well as AmpC enzymes. Approved for adults in 2023. Pediatric studies are being organized.

Aztreonam and avibactam. This antibiotic is being developed to address metallo-carbapenemases, for which avibactam and relebactam do not provide protection. Aztreonam, a monobactam antibiotic first approved in 1986, is stable to many MBLs but susceptible to cleavage from virtually all the other BLs; *however,* when it is paired with avibactam, the combination becomes stable to a vast array of BLs. Pediatric PK and efficacy studies are underway.

Fosfomycin. An older antibiotic, approved in oral (PO) form for adult women in the United States in 1996 for uncomplicated cystitis, with intravenous (IV) formulations approved in many countries in Europe but never approved in the United States. Interferes with the synthesis of cell walls (inhibits linking of glycan and peptide to form peptido-glycan cross-linked structures that form cell walls) and demonstrates stability to MBLs carried by *E coli.* Clinical trials of the IV formulation are underway for adults; PK studies are underway for children.

Plazomicin. Represents a new aminoglycoside antibiotic that is active against many of the gentamicin-, tobramycin-, and amikacin-resistant enteric bacilli and *Pseudomonas.* Approved for adults in 2018. Not currently available in the United States.

Investigational Agents Under Study in Adults

Cefepime and taniborbactam. Represents another older antibiotic, cefepime, that is now paired with taniborbactam, a broad-spectrum, borate-based BLI, stable against ESBLs, SBLs and MBLs, and AmpC BLs.

Cefepime and enmetazobactam. Another combination with cefepime and a new broad-spectrum BLI, a methylated tazobactam, enmetazobactam is stable against AmpC BLs and ESBLs and SBLs but not MBLs.

Community-Associated Methicillin-Resistant *Staphylococcus aureus*

Community-associated methicillin-resistant *Staphylococcus aureus* (CA-MRSA) is a community pathogen for children (that can also spread from child to child in hospitals) that first emerged in the United States in the mid-1990s and currently represents 10% to 30% of all community isolates in various regions of the United States (check your hospital microbiology laboratory for your local rate); it is present in many areas of the world, with some strain variation documented.[2,3] CA-MRSA resists β-lactam antibiotics, with the notable exception of ceftaroline and ceftobiprole, fifth-generation cephalosporin antibiotics that are FDA approved for pediatrics (see Chapter 1).

There are an undetermined number of pathogenicity factors that make CA-MRSA strains, in general, more aggressive than methicillin-susceptible *Staphylococcus aureus* (MSSA) strains. Response of MRSA to therapy with non–β-lactam antibiotics (eg, vancomycin) seems to be inferior, compared with response of MSSA to oxacillin/nafcillin or cefazolin, but it is unknown whether poorer outcomes are due to a hardier, better-adapted, more aggressive strain of *S aureus* or alternative agents are just not as effective against MRSA as β-lactam agents are against MSSA. In children, studies using ceftaroline to treat skin infections (many caused by MRSA) were conducted by way of a non-inferiority clinical trial design, comparing ceftaroline with vancomycin, with the finding that ceftaroline was equivalent to vancomycin. Guidelines for management of MRSA skin and soft tissue infections have been published by the Infectious Diseases Society of America (IDSA)[4] and are available at www.idsociety.org, as well as in the *AAP Red Book 2024–2027*.

Antimicrobials for CA-MRSA

Ceftaroline, a fifth-generation cephalosporin antibiotic, the first FDA-approved β-lactam antibiotic to be active against MRSA, was approved for children in June 2016. The gram-negative coverage is similar to ceftriaxone, with no activity against *Pseudomonas*. Published data are available for pediatric PK, as well as for prospective, randomized comparative treatment trials of skin and skin-structure infections (SSSIs),[5] community-acquired pneumonia,[6,7] and neonatal sepsis.[8] The efficacy and toxicity profile for adults is what one would expect from most cephalosporins. Based on these published data, ceftaroline should be effective and possibly safer than vancomycin for treatment of MRSA infections for all age-groups, including neonates. Just as β-lactams are preferred over vancomycin for MSSA infections, ceftaroline may be considered by some clinicians to be the preferred treatment of MRSA infections over vancomycin, except for central nervous system infections/endocarditis only due to lack of clinical data for these infections. Neither renal function nor drug levels need to be followed with ceftaroline therapy, in contrast to treatment with vancomycin. Since pediatric approval in mid-2016, there have been no serious postmarketing adverse experiences in children reported; recommendations may change should unexpected clinical data on lack of efficacy or unexpected toxicity beyond what may be expected with β-lactams be presented.

Ceftobiprole, another fifth-generation cephalosporin, was FDA approved in February 2024 for children down to 3 months of age. Its activity and approved indications are similar to those of ceftaroline, with the addition of bacteremia/endocarditis.[9,10] Given the extensive experience with ceftaroline in children, we currently prefer ceftaroline over ceftobiprole until additional safety and efficacy are available from real-world use of ceftobiprole.

Vancomycin (IV) has been the mainstay of parenteral therapy for MRSA infections for the past 4 decades and continues to have activity against more than 98% of strains isolated from children. New guidelines on the use of vancomycin for MRSA infections have been published through a collaboration among the American Society of Health-System Pharmacists, IDSA, Pediatric Infectious Diseases Society, and Society of Infectious Diseases Pharmacists.[11] A few cases of intermediate resistance and "heteroresistance" (transient moderately increased resistance likely to be caused by thickened staphylococcal cell walls) have been reported, most commonly in adults who are receiving long-term therapy or who have received multiple exposures to vancomycin. Unfortunately, the response to therapy using standard vancomycin dosing of 40 mg/kg/day in the treatment of many CA-MRSA strains has not been as predictably successful as in the past with MSSA. For vancomycin efficacy, the ratio of the area under the curve (the mathematically calculated area below the serum concentration-versus-time curve) to minimum inhibitory concentration (AUC:MIC) seems to be the best exposure metric to predict a successful outcome in adults. Better outcomes are likely to be achieved with an AUC:MIC of about 400 or greater, rather than with a serum trough value in the range of 15 to 20 mcg/mL, which is associated with greater renal toxicity (see Chapter 11 for more on the AUC:MIC). This ratio of 400:1 is achievable for CA-MRSA strains with in vitro MIC values of 1 mcg/mL or less but difficult to achieve for strains with values of 2 mcg/mL or greater.[12] Recent data suggest that vancomycin MICs may actually be decreasing in children for MRSA causing bloodstream infections as they increase for MSSA.[13] Strains with MIC values of 4 mcg/mL or greater should be considered resistant to vancomycin. When using "meningitis" treatment dosages of 60 mg/kg/day (or higher) to achieve a 400:1 vancomycin exposure, one needs to follow renal function carefully for the development of toxicity and the possible subsequent need to switch classes of antibiotics.

Dalbavancin is a glycopeptide, structurally very similar to vancomycin but with enhanced in vitro activity against MRSA and a much longer serum half-life, allowing once-weekly dosing, or even just a single dose, to treat skin infections. Approved for pediatrics from birth to age 18 years in 2021, it is an important option for outpatient parenteral therapy once-weekly IV injection, when outpatient *IV* therapy and *PO* therapy are not feasible.

Clindamycin (PO or IV) is active against about 70% to 90% of strains of either MRSA or MSSA, with great geographic variability (again, check with your hospital laboratory).[14] The dosage for moderate to severe infections is 30 to 40 mg/kg/day, in 3 divided doses, with the same milligram per kilogram dose whether PO or IV. Clindamycin is not as bactericidal as vancomycin but achieves higher concentrations in abscesses (because of high intracellular concentrations in neutrophils). Some CA-MRSA strains are susceptible to clindamycin on testing but have inducible clindamycin resistance (methylase-mediated) that is usually assessed by the "D-test" and can now be assessed by multi-well microtiter plates. Within each population of CA-MRSA organisms, a rare organism (between 1 in 10^{11} and 10^{13} organisms) will have a mutation that allows for *constant,* rather than induced, resistance.[15] Although still somewhat controversial, clindamycin should be effective therapy for infections that have a relatively low organism load (eg, cellulitis, small or drained abscesses) and are unlikely to contain a significant population of these constitutive methylase-producing mutants that are truly resistant; in fact, staphylococcal methylase is poorly induced by clindamycin. Infections with a high organism load (empyema) may have a greater risk of failure, as a large population is more likely to have a significant number of truly resistant organisms and clindamycin should not be used as the preferred agent for these infections. Many laboratories do not report D-test results but simply call the organisms "resistant," prompting the clinician to use alternative therapy that may not be needed.

Clindamycin is used to treat most CA-MRSA infections that are not life threatening, and if the child responds, therapy can be switched from IV to PO (although the PO solution is not very well tolerated). *Clostridioides* (formerly *Clostridium*) *difficile* enterocolitis is a concern; however, despite a great increase in the use of clindamycin in children during the past decade, recent published data do not document a clinically significant increase in the rate of this complication in children.

Trimethoprim/sulfamethoxazole (PO, IV), Bactrim/Septra, is active against CA-MRSA in vitro. Prospective, comparative data on treatment of SSSIs in adults and children document efficacy equivalent to clindamycin.[16] There is a lack of prospective, comparative information in the treatment of invasive MRSA infections (eg, bacteremia, pneumonia and osteomyelitis [in contrast to skin infections]) in children, but some experts successfully use TMP/SMX for the treatment of osteomyelitis.[17,18]

Linezolid (PO, IV), active against virtually 100% of CA-MRSA strains, is another reasonable alternative but is considered bacteriostatic as a protein synthesis inhibitor and has relatively frequent hematologic toxicity in adults (ie, neutropenia, thrombocytopenia) and some infrequent neurologic toxicity (ie, peripheral neuropathy, optic neuritis), particularly when used for courses of 2 weeks or longer. A complete blood cell count should be checked every week or two in children receiving prolonged linezolid therapy. Generic linezolid is still substantially more costly than clindamycin or vancomycin.

Daptomycin (IV) is FDA approved for adults with skin infections and bacteremia/endocarditis and was approved for use in children with skin infections in April 2017. It is a unique class of antibiotic, a lipopeptide, and is highly bactericidal. Daptomycin became generic in 2017 and should be considered for treatment of skin infection and bacteremia when other, better-studied antibiotics fail. **Daptomycin should not be used to treat pneumonia,** as it is inactivated by pulmonary surfactant. Pediatric studies for skin infections, bacteremia, and osteomyelitis have been published,[19-21] showing that daptomycin does not differ from comparator standard-of-care antibiotics for *S aureus* infections (including MRSA osteomyelitis). Some newborn animal neurologic toxicity data suggest additional **caution for the use of daptomycin in infants younger than 1 year,** prompting a warning in the package label. Routine pediatric clinical trial investigations in young infants were not pursued due to these concerns.

Tigecycline and fluoroquinolones, both of which may show in vitro activity against MRSA, are not generally recommended for children if other agents are available and are tolerated, due to potential toxicity issues with tetracyclines and FQs as well as emergence of resistance with FQs.

Combination therapy for serious infections, with vancomycin and rifampin (for deep abscesses) or vancomycin and gentamicin (for bacteremia), is often used, but no prospective, controlled human clinical data exist on improved efficacy over single antibiotic therapy. Some experts use vancomycin and clindamycin in combination, particularly for children with a toxic-shock clinical manifestation, considering the protein synthesis inhibition properties of clindamycin. Ceftaroline has also been used in combination therapy with other agents, including daptomycin in adults, but no prospective, controlled clinical data exist to assess benefits (or adverse events) of combinations over single-drug therapy.

Investigational Gram-Positive Agents Recently Approved for Adults and Being Studied in Children

Oritavancin. An IV glycopeptide, structurally very similar to vancomycin but with enhanced in vitro activity against MRSA and a much longer serum half-life, allowing once-weekly dosing. A very similar antibiotic, dalbavancin, was approved for children in 2021.

Telavancin. A glycolipopeptide with mechanisms of activity that include cell wall inhibition and cell membrane depolarization, telavancin is administered once daily. The FDA recently waived the requirement for pediatric investigation; the pediatric PK study has been terminated.

Tedizolid. A second-generation oxazolidinone like linezolid, tedizolid is more potent in vitro against MRSA than linezolid, with somewhat decreased toxicity to bone marrow in adult clinical studies; it is approved for adolescents 12 years and older.

Recommendations for Empiric Therapy for Suspected MRSA Infections

Life-threatening and serious infections. If CA-MRSA is present in your community, empiric therapy for presumed staphylococcal infections that are life threatening, or for infections for which any risk of failure is unacceptable, should follow the recommendations for CA-MRSA and include ceftaroline OR *high-dose* vancomycin, clindamycin, or linezolid, *in addition to nafcillin or oxacillin* (β-lactam antibiotics are considered better than vancomycin or clindamycin for MSSA).

Moderate infections. If you live in a location with greater than 10% methicillin resistance, consider using the CA-MRSA recommendations for hospitalized children with presumed staphylococcal infections of any severity, and start empiric therapy with clindamycin (usually active against >80% of CA-MRSA), ceftaroline, vancomycin, or linezolid IV.

In skin and skin-structure abscess treatment, antibiotics may be unnecessary following incision and drainage, which may, in fact, be curative.

Mild infections. For nonserious, presumed staphylococcal infections in regions with significant CA-MRSA, topical empiric therapy with mupirocin (Bactroban) or retapamulin (Altabax) ointment, or PO therapy with TMP/SMX or clindamycin, is preferred. For older children, doxycycline and minocycline are also options based on data in adults.

13. Antibiotic Therapy for Children With Obesity

NOTE: A list of table abbreviations and acronyms can be found at the start of this publication.

When prescribing an antimicrobial for a child with obesity or overweight, selecting a dose based on milligrams per kilograms of total body weight (TBW) may overexpose the child if the drug does not freely distribute into fat tissue. Conversely, underexposure can occur when a dosage is reduced for obesity for drugs without distribution limitations.

This "distribution-centric" construct does not account for altered drug clearance due to obesity-related pathophysiologic changes, particularly in critical illness. Further, such changes in adults, such as glomerular hyperfiltration, nephron loss, and hepatic steatosis, may not yet be fully developed or present in obese children, making extrapolation of obese adult antibiotic pharmacokinetic (PK) data to children problematic.

In addition to empiric dose adjustment for obesity, we also recommend therapeutic drug monitoring (TDM) of serum or plasma antibiotic concentrations of certain antibiotics to achieve both safe and effective doses for these children.

Table 13-1 lists major antimicrobial classes and our suggestions on appropriate empiric dosing. The evidence to support these recommendations is Level II to III (PK studies in

TABLE 13-1. DOSING RECOMMENDATIONS

Drug Class	By EBW[a]	By Adjusted Body Weight	By TBW[b]
Antibacterials			
β-Lactams			
Aminopenicillins			X (2 g ampicillin/dose max)
Piperacillin/tazobactam			X (4 g PIP/dose max)
Cephalosporins			X
Meropenem			X (2 g/dose max)
Ertapenem	X		
Clindamycin			X (no max)
Vancomycin		1,500–2,000 mg/m²/day	20 mg/kg LD, then 60 mg/kg/day div q6–8h
Aminoglycosides		0.7 × TBW	
Fluoroquinolones		EBW + 0.45 (TBW−EBW)	
Miscellaneous			
TMP/SMX			X
Metronidazole			X
Linezolid			X
Daptomycin			X (See max doses in comments.)

TABLE 13-1 (continued)

Drug Class	By EBW[a]	By Adjusted Body Weight	By TBW[b]
Antifungals			
Amphotericin B			X (max 150 mg for AmB-D, max 500 mg for L-AmB)
Fluconazole			X (max 1,600 mg LD, max 1,200 mg/day)
Flucytosine	X		
Anidulafungin			X (max 250 mg LD, max 125 mg/day)
Caspofungin			X (max 150 mg/day)
Micafungin			X (max 300 mg/day)
Voriconazole	X		
Antivirals (Non-HIV)			
Nucleoside analogues (acyclovir, ganciclovir)	X		
Antimycobacterials			
Isoniazid	X		
Rifampin			X
Pyrazinamide			X
Ethambutol			X

[a] EBW (kg) = BMI 50th percentile for age × actual height (in meters)^2; from Le Grange D, et al. *Pediatrics*. 2012;129(2):e438–e446 PMID: 22218841.

[b] Dose up to adult max (see Ch 18) if not otherwise specified.

13

children, extrapolations from adult studies, and expert opinion). Maximum doses for TBW dosing are given, and, for individual agents, are also found in Chapter 18. For each antibiotic, recommendations for dosing are based on one of the following: expected body weight, the actual or total body weight (ie, TBW), or adjusted body weight.

For **tobramycin and other aminoglycosides,** use the child's fat-free mass, which is an approximate 30% reduction in TBW. Closely following serum or plasma concentrations.

Vancomycin is traditionally dosed based on TBW in adults with obesity due to increases in kidney size and glomerular filtration rate. In children with obesity, weight-adjusted distribution volume and clearance are slightly lower than in their counterparts without obesity. An empiric maximum dose of 60 mg/kg/day based on TBW, or dosing using body surface area, may be more appropriate. Closely follow serum or plasma concentrations.

In the setting of **cefazolin** for surgical prophylaxis (see Chapter 15), adult studies of patients with obesity have generally shown that distribution to the subcutaneous fat tissue target can be subtherapeutic when standard doses are used. Higher single doses are recommended in adults with obesity (eg, 2 g instead of the standard 1 g) with re-dosing at 4-hour intervals for longer cases. In children with obesity, we recommend dosing **cefazolin** for surgical prophylaxis based on TBW up to the adult maximum of 2 g. For treatment of skin infections, dose by TBW up to a maximum of 3 g every 8 hours. The US Food and Drug Administration–approved maximum dose for life-threatening infections is 3 g every 6 hours.

In critically ill adults with obesity treated with **ceftazidime, cefepime, carbapenems,** or **piperacillin/tazobactam,** extended infusion times (over 2–4 hours, instead of 30 minutes) should increase the likelihood of achieving therapeutic bloodstream antibiotic exposures, particularly against bacteria with higher minimum inhibitory concentrations (MICs). Some hospital laboratories perform serum or plasma concentration testing of β-lactam antibiotics in-house, while most offer the service as a send-out.

Daptomycin can be dosed by using TBW, but the maximum dose should be 500 mg for skin infections and 750 mg for bloodstream infections. Bolus administration over 2 minutes can improve the likelihood of achieving target concentrations when the maximum dose is less than the calculated dose in an adolescent with obesity. Serum or plasma concentration testing is not routinely available for daptomycin.

Adult maximum doses of **linezolid** may be inadequate to achieve target plasma concentrations to treat susceptible methicillin-resistant *Staphylococcus aureus* infections with high MICs. Higher doses should be attempted only with the aid of TDM to avoid hematologic toxicity if serum or plasma concentration testing is available.

Bibliography

Camaione L, et al. *Pharmacotherapy*. 2013;33(12):1278–1287 PMID: 24019205

Castro-Balado A, et al. *Antimicrob Agents Chemother*. 2024;68(5):e0171923 PMID: 38526051

Donoso FA, et al. *Arch Argent Pediatr*. 2019;117(2):e121–e130 PMID: 30869490

Gorham J, et al. *Antibiotics*. 2023;12(7):1099 PMID: 37508195

Hall RG. *Curr Pharm Des*. 2015;21(32):4748–4751 PMID: 26112269

Harskamp-van Ginkel MW, et al. *JAMA Pediatr*. 2015;169(7):678–685 PMID: 25961828

Maharaj AR, et al. *Paediatr Drugs*. 2021;23(5):499–513 PMID: 34302290

Meng L, et al. *Pharmacotherapy*. 2023;43(3):226–246 PMID: 36703246

Moffett BS, et al. *Ther Drug Monit*. 2018;40(3):322–329 PMID: 29521784

Natale S, et al. *Pharmacotherapy*. 2017;37(3):361–378 PMID: 28079262

Pai MP. *Clin Ther*. 2016;38(9):2032–2044 PMID: 27524636

Pai MP, et al. *Antimicrob Agents Chemother*. 2011;55(12):5640–5645 PMID: 21930881

Payne KD, et al. *Expert Rev Anti Infect Ther*. 2016;14(2):257–267 PMID: 26641135

Smith MJ, et al. *Antimicrob Agents Chemother*. 2017;61(4):e02014-16 PMID: 28137820

Xie F, et al. *J Antimicrob Chemother*. 2019;74(3):667–674 PMID: 30535122

14. Sequential Parenteral-Oral Antibiotic Therapy (Oral Step-Down Therapy) for Serious Infections

The concept of oral *step-down* or "oral switch" therapy is well established, initially published by Nelson and colleagues more than 40 years ago in the *Journal of Pediatrics*.[1,2] Bone and joint infections,[3–5] complicated bacterial pneumonia with empyema,[6] deep-tissue abscesses, and appendicitis,[7,8] as well as cellulitis or pyelonephritis,[9] may require initial parenteral therapy and surgical drainage if necessary to control the growth and spread of pathogens and minimize injury to tissues. Recent data in adults document the effectiveness of early switch to oral (PO) therapy in uncomplicated gram-negative bacteremia.[10,11] When the signs and symptoms of infection begin to resolve, often within just a few days, with no residual abscess or necrotic tissue noted, intravenous (IV) therapy may no longer be required. A normal host neutrophil response is also capable of clearing the infection as the pathogen load drops below a certain critical density, as has been demonstrated in an animal model.[12] It is likely that the good outcomes seen with PO step-down therapy in normal hosts are based on contributions from both antibiotic and host.

In addition to following the clinical response before PO switch, following objective laboratory markers, such as C-reactive protein (CRP) or procalcitonin (PCT), during the hospitalization may also help the clinician better assess the response to antibacterial therapy, particularly in the infant or child who is difficult to examine.[13,14] The benefits of PO step-down therapy over prolonged parenteral therapy are substantial and well-documented in the treatment of acute osteomyelitis, including a decrease in both emergency department visits and rehospitalizations, with equivalent treatment success outcomes (including for those children with *Staphylococcus aureus* bacteremia).[15,16]

For children with intra-abdominal abscesses who recover quickly after surgical drainage and initial antibiotic therapy, either short-course PO therapy (7 days total) or no additional antibiotic treatment following clinical and laboratory recovery may be appropriate.[17] But differentiating between those who may require ongoing PO step-down therapy and those who will not can be difficult, as the extent of an intra-abdominal abscess, the adequacy of source control (surgical drainage), and the susceptibility of pathogen(s) involved are not always known.[18]

For the β-lactam class of antibiotics, absorption of PO administered antibiotics in *standard* dosages usually studied by pharmaceutical companies for US Food and Drug Administration (FDA) approval for mild to moderate respiratory tract, skin, or urinary tract infections provides peak serum concentrations that are routinely only 5% to 20% of those achieved with IV or intramuscular administration. *High-dose* PO β-lactam therapy, however, provides the tissue antibiotic exposure closer to that achieved with parenteral therapy that is thought to be helpful to eradicate the remaining pathogens at the infection site as the tissue perfusion and antibiotic exposure there improve. For most PO antibiotics, prospectively collected data on safety and efficacy at higher dosages have not been systematically collected and presented by companies or investigators to the FDA for approval; most of the data to support high-dose PO β-lactam often come from retrospectively reviewed data or small prospective studies.

High-dose PO β-lactam antibiotic therapy for osteoarticular infections has been associated with treatment success since 1978.[3] For β-lactams, begin with a dosage 2 to 3 times the normal dosage (eg, 75–100 mg/kg/day of amoxicillin or 100 mg/kg/day of cephalexin) supported by recent pharmacokinetic/pharmacodynamic assessment.[19] High-quality retrospective cohort data have recently confirmed similar outcomes achieved in those treated with PO step-down therapy compared with those treated with IV therapy.[15] High-dose, prolonged PO β-lactam therapy may be associated with reversible neutropenia; checking for hematologic toxicity every few weeks during therapy is suggested.[20]

Clindamycin and many antibiotics of the fluoroquinolone class (eg, ciprofloxacin, levofloxacin) and oxazolidinone class (eg, linezolid, tedizolid) have excellent absorption of their PO formulations and provide virtually the same tissue antibiotic exposure at a particular milligram per kilogram dose, compared with that dose given IV; therefore, for these antibiotic classes, higher dosages are not needed for PO therapy. Trimethoprim/sulfamethoxazole and metronidazole are also very well absorbed and should be effective for PO step-down therapy if appropriate for the pathogen, infection site, and child.

One must also assume that the parent and child are adherent to the administration of each antibiotic dose, that the PO antibiotic will be absorbed from the gastrointestinal tract into the systemic circulation (no vomiting or diarrhea), and that the parent will seek medical care if the clinical course does not continue to improve for their child.

Monitor the child clinically for a continued response during PO therapy; follow CRP or PCT after the switch to PO therapy, and if there are concerns about continued response, make sure the antibiotic and dosage you selected are appropriate and the family is adherent. As John Nelson has pointed out, in one of the first published series of PO step-down therapy for osteoarticular infection from Dallas in 1988, a reported failure of PO therapy was caused by presumed nonadherence.[21]

15. Antimicrobial Prophylaxis/Prevention of Symptomatic Infection

NOTE: A list of table abbreviations and acronyms can be found at the start of this publication.

This chapter summarizes recommendations for prophylaxis of infections, defined as antibiotic therapy before the onset of clinical signs or symptoms of infection in children exposed or at high risk for exposure. Prophylaxis can be considered in several clinical scenarios.

A. Postexposure Antimicrobial Prophylaxis to Prevent Symptomatic New Infection

Given for a relatively short, specified period (days) after a single exposure to specific pathogens/organisms, where the risks of acquiring the infection are felt to justify antimicrobial treatment to prevent symptomatic infection or eradicate a colonizing pathogen when the child (healthy or with increased susceptibility to infection) is likely to have been inoculated/exposed (eg, a child closely exposed to meningococcus; a neonate born to a mother with active genital herpes simplex virus [HSV]) but not yet showing signs or symptoms of infection.

B. Long-Term Antimicrobial Prophylaxis to Prevent Symptomatic New Infection

Given to a particular, defined population of children with relatively high risk of acquiring a severe infection from a single exposure or multiple exposures (eg, a child postsplenectomy; a child with documented rheumatic heart disease to prevent subsequent streptococcal infection), with prophylaxis provided during the period of risk, potentially for months or years.

C. Prophylaxis of Symptomatic Disease in Children Who Have Asymptomatic Infection/Latent Infection

Where a child has a documented infection but is asymptomatic. Targeted antimicrobials are given to prevent the development of symptomatic disease (eg, latent tuberculosis [TB] infection or therapy of a stem cell transplant patient with documented cytomegalovirus viremia but no symptoms of infection or rejection; to prevent reactivation of HSV). Treatment period is usually defined, particularly when the latent infection can be cured (TB, requiring 6 months of therapy), but other circumstances, such as prevention of reactivation of latent HSV, may require months or years of prophylaxis.

D. Surgical/Procedure Prophylaxis

A child receives a surgical/invasive catheter procedure, planned or unplanned, in which the risk for infection postoperatively or post-procedure may justify prophylaxis to prevent an infection from occurring (eg, prophylaxis to prevent infection following spinal rod placement). **Treatment is usually short-term (hours),** beginning just before the procedure and ending at the conclusion of the procedure, or within 24 hours.

E. Travel-Related Exposure Prophylaxis

Not discussed in this chapter; refer to information on specific disease entities (eg, travelers diarrhea, Chapters 1 and 9) or specific pathogens (eg, malaria, Chapter 9). Constantly updated, current information for travelers about prophylaxis (often starting just before travel and continuing until return) and current worldwide infection risks can be found on the Centers for Disease Control and Prevention website at www.cdc.gov/travel (accessed October 21, 2024).

A. POSTEXPOSURE ANTIMICROBIAL PROPHYLAXIS TO PREVENT INFECTION

Prophylaxis Category	Therapy (evidence grade)	Comments
Bacterial		
Bites, animal and human[1-5] (*Pasteurella multocida; Staphylococcus aureus*, including CA-MRSA; *Streptococcus* spp, anaerobes; *Capnocytophaga canimorsus*, particularly in asplenic hosts)	Amox/clav 45 mg/kg/day PO div tid (amox/clav 7:1; see Aminopenicillins in Ch 4 for amox/clav ratio descriptions) for 3–5 days (AII) OR ampicillin and clindamycin OR ceftriaxone and clindamycin (BII), OR, for IV: amp/sul. For penicillin allergy, consider ciprofloxacin (for *Pasteurella*) plus clindamycin (BII).	Recommended for children who (1) have moderate to severe injuries, especially to the hand or face; (2) are immunocompromised; (3) are asplenic; or (4) have injuries that may have penetrated the periosteum or joint capsule (AII).[3] Consider rabies prophylaxis for at-risk animal bites through state and local rabies consultation contacts (AI)[6]; consider tetanus prophylaxis.[7] Human bites have a very high rate of infection (do not close open wounds routinely). Cat bites have a higher rate of infection than dog bites. *S aureus* coverage is only fair with amox/clav and amp/sul, and it provides no coverage for MRSA.

Endocarditis prophylaxis[8,9]: Given that (1) endocarditis is rarely caused by dental/GI procedures and (2) prophylaxis for procedures prevents an exceedingly small number of cases, the risks of antibiotics most often outweigh benefits. However, some "highest-risk" conditions are currently recommended for prophylaxis: (1) prosthetic heart valve (or prosthetic material used to repair a valve); (2) previous endocarditis; (3) cyanotic congenital heart disease that is unrepaired (or palliatively repaired with shunts and conduits); (4) congenital heart disease that is repaired but with defects at the site of repair adjacent to prosthetic material; (5) completely repaired congenital heart disease by using prosthetic material, for the first 6 mo after repair; or (6) cardiac transplant patients with valvulopathy. Routine prophylaxis has not been required for children with native valve abnormalities since updated guidelines were published in 2015.[9] Follow-up data in children suggest that following these new guidelines, no increase in endocarditis has been detected.[10-13]

Prophylaxis Category	Therapy (evidence grade)	Comments
– In highest-risk patients: dental procedures that involve manipulation of the gingival or periodontal region of teeth	Amoxicillin 50 mg/kg (max 2 g) PO 1 h before procedure OR ampicillin or ceftriaxone or cefazolin, all at 50 mg/kg IM/IV 30–60 min before procedure	If penicillin allergy: clindamycin 20 mg/kg PO (1 h before) or IV (30 min before) OR azithromycin 15 mg/kg or clarithromycin 15 mg/kg (1 h before)

Antimicrobial Prophylaxis/Prevention of Symptomatic Infection

Antimicrobial Prophylaxis/Prevention of Symptomatic Infection

15

A. POSTEXPOSURE ANTIMICROBIAL PROPHYLAXIS TO PREVENT INFECTION

Prophylaxis Category	Therapy (evidence grade)	Comments
– Genitourinary and GI procedures	None	No longer recommended
Lyme disease (Borrelia burgdorferi)[14]	Doxycycline 4.4 mg/kg (max 200 mg), once. Dental staining should not occur with a single dose of doxycycline. Amoxicillin prophylaxis is not well studied, and experts recommend a full 14-day course if amoxicillin is used.	ONLY for those in highly Lyme-endemic areas AND the tick has been attached for >36 h (and is engorged) AND prophylaxis started within 72 h of tick removal.
Meningococcus (Neisseria meningitidis)[15,16]	For prophylaxis of close contacts, including household members, child care center contacts, and anyone directly exposed to the child's oral secretions (eg, through kissing, mouth-to-mouth resuscitation, endotracheal intubation/management) in the 7 days before symptom onset **Rifampin** Infants <1 mo: 5 mg/kg PO q12h for 4 doses Children ≥1 mo: 10 mg/kg PO q12h for 4 doses (max 600 mg/dose) OR **Ceftriaxone** Children <15 y: 125 mg IM once Children ≥15 y: 250 mg IM once OR **Ciprofloxacin** Children ≥1 mo: 20 mg/kg PO (max 500 mg) once	A single dose of ciprofloxacin should not present a significant risk of cartilage damage, but no prospective data exist in children for prophylaxis of meningococcal disease. For a child, an exposure for ciprofloxacin equivalent to that in adults would be 15–20 mg/kg as a single dose (max 500 mg). A few ciprofloxacin-resistant strains have been reported. Azithromycin is not recommended routinely, but when used, give 10 mg/kg as a single dose. Meningococcal vaccines that target the specific serogroup may also be recommended in case of an outbreak.
Pertussis[17,18]	PEP uses the same regimen as for treatment of pertussis (see Ch 1) per the AAP[17]: azithromycin 10 mg/kg/day qd for 5 days through age 5 mo; then, for those ≥6 mo, 10 mg/kg/day (max 500 mg) on day 1, followed by 5 mg/kg/day (max 250 mg) for days 2–5 OR clarithromycin (for infants >1 mo) 15 mg/kg/day div bid for 7 days OR erythromycin (estolate preferable) 40 mg/kg/day PO qid for 14 days (AII)	Prophylaxis to family members regardless of immunization status; contacts defined by the CDC: persons within 21 days of exposure to infectious pertussis, who are at high risk for severe illness or will have close contact with a person at high risk for severe illness (including infants, pregnant women in their third trimester, immunocompromised persons, and those who have close contact with infants <12 mo).

Alternative for infants >2 mo:
TMP/SMX 8 mg TMP/kg/day div bid for 14 days (BIII)

Community-wide prophylaxis is not recommended as the CDC attempts to limit unnecessary antibiotic use.
Azithromycin and clarithromycin are better tolerated than erythromycin (see Ch 2); azithromycin is preferred in exposed very young infants to reduce pyloric stenosis risk.

Tetanus
(*Clostridium tetani*)[7,19]

Need for Tetanus Vaccine or TIG[a]

| Number of past tetanus vaccine doses | Clean Wound | | Contaminated Wound | |
	Need for tetanus vaccine	Need for TIG 500 U IM[a]	Need for tetanus vaccine	Need for TIG 500 U IM[a]
<3 doses	Yes	No	Yes	Yes
≥3 doses	No (if <10 y[b]) Yes (if ≥10 y[b])	No	No (if <5 y[b]) Yes (if ≥5 y[b])	No

[a] IV immune globulin should be used when TIG is not available.
[b] Years since last tetanus-containing vaccine dose.

For deep, contaminated wounds, wound debridement is essential. Antimicrobial prophylaxis has not been shown to prevent tetanus, but randomized, controlled studies would be difficult to perform.

15

Antimicrobial Prophylaxis/Prevention of Symptomatic Infection

A. POSTEXPOSURE ANTIMICROBIAL PROPHYLAXIS TO PREVENT INFECTION

Prophylaxis Category	Therapy (evidence grade)	Comments
Tuberculosis (*Mycobacterium tuberculosis*) "Window prophylaxis" of exposed children <4 y, or immunocompromised patient (high risk for dissemination) to prevent infection after exposure, rather than to treat latent asymptomatic infection[20,21] see Tuberculosis in Table 15C. For treatment of latent TB infection,[21,22] see Tuberculosis in Table 15C.	Scenario 1: Previously uninfected child at high risk for serious infection and dissemination becomes exposed to a person with active disease. Exposed children <4 y, or immunocompromised patient (high risk for dissemination): rifampin 15–20 mg/kg/dose PO OR INH 10–20 mg/kg PO qd; for at least 2–3 mo (AIII), at which time cellular immunity is established and PPD/IGRA may be more accurately assessed. If positive, treatment for latent TB should continue. Children ≥4 y may also begin prophylaxis postexposure, but if exposure is questionable, can wait 2–3 mo after exposure to assess for infection; if not given prophylaxis, and PPD/IGRA at 2–3 mo is positive and child remains asymptomatic at that time, see Scenario 2 below.	If PPD or IGRA remains negative at 2–3 mo and child remains well, consider stopping empiric therapy. However, tests at 2–3 mo may not be reliable in immunocompromised patients.
	Scenario 2: An asymptomatic child is found to have a positive skin test/IGRA for TB, documenting latent TB infection; see Tuberculosis in Table 15C. Treat with at least 4 mo of rifampin OR 6 mo of INH, OR 3 mo of combination INH and rifampin, OR, for those ≥2 y, INH and rifapentine.	
Viral		
Herpes simplex virus		
– During pregnancy	For women with recurrent genital herpes, follow ACOG guidelines[23]: acyclovir 400 mg PO tid; valacyclovir 500 mg PO bid from 36 wk of gestation until delivery (CII).	Neonatal HSV disease after unsuccessful maternal suppression has been documented.[24]

– Neonatal: **primary or nonprimary first clinical episode of maternal infection,** neonate exposed at delivery[25]	Asymptomatic, exposed neonate: at 24 h after birth, sample mucosal sites for HSV culture (and PCR if possible) (see Comments), obtain CSF and whole-blood PCR for HSV DNA, obtain ALT, and start preemptive therapeutic acyclovir IV (60 mg/kg/day div q8h) for 10 days (AII). Some experts would evaluate at birth for exposure following presumed maternal primary infection and start preemptive therapy rather than wait 24 h.	*AAP Red Book 2024–2027*[25] provides a management algorithm that determines the type of maternal infection and, thus, the appropriate evaluation and preemptive therapy of the neonate. Mucosal sites for culture: conjunctivae, mouth, nasopharynx, rectum. Infants treated with 10 days of preemptive IV therapy should not subsequently receive PO acyclovir suppression, because their HSV exposure never progressed to infection or disease. Any *symptomatic* baby, at any time, requires a full evaluation for invasive infection and IV acyclovir therapy for 14–21 days, depending on extent of disease.
– Neonatal: **recurrent maternal infection,** neonate exposed at delivery[25]	Asymptomatic, exposed neonate: at 24 h after birth, sample mucosal sites for HSV culture (and PCR if desired) (see Comments) and obtain whole-blood PCR for HSV DNA. Hold on therapy unless diagnostic cultures or PCRs are positive, at which time the diagnostic evaluation should be completed (CSF PCR for HSV DNA, serum ALT) and preemptive therapeutic IV acyclovir (60 mg/kg/day div q8h) should be administered for 10 days (AIII).	*AAP Red Book 2024–2027*[25] provides a management algorithm that determines the type of maternal infection and, thus, the appropriate evaluation and preemptive therapy of the neonate. Mucosal sites for culture: conjunctivae, mouth, nasopharynx, rectum. Infants treated with 10 days of preemptive IV therapy should not subsequently receive PO acyclovir suppression, because their HSV exposure never progressed to infection or disease. Any *symptomatic* baby, at any time, requires a full evaluation for invasive infection and IV acyclovir therapy for 14–21 days, depending on extent of disease.
– Neonatal: following symptomatic disease, to prevent recurrence	See Neonatal in Table 15C under Herpes simplex virus.	
– Keratitis (ocular) in otherwise healthy children	See Keratitis in Table 15C under Herpes simplex virus.	

Antimicrobial Prophylaxis/Prevention of Symptomatic Infection

A. POSTEXPOSURE ANTIMICROBIAL PROPHYLAXIS TO PREVENT INFECTION

Prophylaxis Category	Therapy (evidence grade)	Comments
Influenza virus (A or B)[26]	Oseltamivir prophylaxis (AI) 3–≤8 mo: 3 mg/kg/dose qd for 10 days; 9–11 mo: 3.5 mg/kg/dose PO qd for 10 days[27]; based on body weight for children ≥12 mo: ≤15 kg: 30 mg qd for 10 days; >15–23 kg: 45 mg qd for 10 days; >23–40 kg: 60 mg qd for 10 days; >40 kg: 75 mg qd for 10 days	Not routinely recommended for infants 0–≤3 mo unless exposure judged substantial (single event or ongoing [eg, breastfeeding mother with active influenza]), because of limited reported data on safety/efficacy and variability of drug exposure in this age-group
	Zanamivir prophylaxis (AI) ≥5 y: 10 mg (two 5-mg inhalations) qd for as long as 28 days (community outbreaks) or 10 days (household settings)	
	Baloxavir prophylaxis (AI) ≥5 y: <20 kg: single dose PO of 2 mg/kg 20–79 kg: single dose PO of 40 mg ≥80 kg: single dose PO of 80 mg	
Rabies virus[28]	RIG, 20 IU/kg, infiltrated around wound, with remaining volume injected IM (AII) PLUS Rabies immunization (AII). State and local public health departments and the CDC can provide advice on risk and management (www.cdc.gov/rabies/hcp/prep-pep/index.html; June 20, 2024; accessed October 21, 2024).	For dog, cat, or ferret bite from **symptomatic animal,** immediate RIG and immunization; otherwise, can wait 10 days for observation of animal, if possible, before RIG or vaccine. PLEASE evaluate the context of the bite. A provoked bite from a threatened or annoyed dog (especially a known dog) is not an indication for rabies prophylaxis. Bites of squirrels, hamsters, guinea pigs, gerbils, chipmunks, rats, mice and other rodents, rabbits, hares, and pikas almost never require anti-rabies prophylaxis.

15

If vaccine is not available immediately, RIG should be administered alone, and vaccination should be started as soon as possible. If RIG is not available, vaccine should be administered, and RIG should be administered subsequently if obtained within 7 days after initiating vaccination. If administration of both vaccine and RIG is delayed, both should be used regardless of the interval between exposure and treatment.

For bites of bats, skunks, raccoons, foxes, most other carnivores, and woodchucks, immediate RIG and immunization (regard as rabid unless geographic area is known to be free of rabies or until animal's condition is proven negative by laboratory tests).

Varicella-zoster virus[29]

Varicella vaccine, administered ideally within 3 days but up to 5 days after exposure for those without immunity

VZIG

Acyclovir 20 mg/kg/dose PO qid (max daily dose 3,200 mg) or valacyclovir 20 mg/kg/dose PO tid (max daily dose 3,000 mg) beginning 7 days after exposure and continuing for 7–10 days

Preemptive VZIG or antiviral therapy in those who have been exposed to varicella, during the incubation period, to prevent symptomatic infection: for immunocompromised patients without evidence of immunity from past infection or vaccine or for immunocompetent, susceptible patients for whom varicella may be severe (eg, pregnancy, neonates without significant transplacental varicella antibody, adolescents)

B. LONG-TERM ANTIMICROBIAL PROPHYLAXIS TO PREVENT SYMPTOMATIC NEW INFECTION

Prophylaxis Category	Therapy (evidence grade)	Comments
Bacterial otitis media[30,31]	Amoxicillin or other antibiotics can be used in half the therapeutic dose qd or bid to prevent infections if the benefits outweigh the risks of (1) emergence/selection of resistant organisms for that child (and contacts) and (2) antibiotic side effects.	The AAP and American Academy of Family Physicians recommend that clinicians not prescribe antibiotics for prophylaxis of AOM in children aged 6 mo–12 y. However, the guidance does not apply to children with anatomic abnormalities or genetic conditions that may affect the ears or children with cochlear implants or immunodeficiencies. True, recurrent acute bacterial otitis is far less common in the era of conjugate pneumococcal immunization. To prevent recurrent infections, as an alternative to antibiotic prophylaxis, also consider the risks and benefits of placing tympanostomy tubes to improve middle ear ventilation.[31] Studies have demonstrated that amoxicillin, sulfisoxazole, and TMP/SMX are effective. However, antimicrobial prophylaxis may alter the nasopharyngeal flora and foster colonization with resistant organisms, compromising long-term efficacy of the prophylactic drug. Continuous PO administered antimicrobial prophylaxis should be reserved for control of recurrent AOM, only when defined as ≥3 distinct and well-documented episodes during a period of 6 mo or ≥4 episodes during a period of 12 mo, which is now uncommon in the era of pneumococcal conjugate vaccines.
Impaired splenic function (including splenectomy)	Penicillin V <3 y: 125 mg bid ≥3 y: 250 mg bid OR Amoxicillin 10 mg/kg bid (max 250 mg/dose). Alternative agents: cephalexin 25 mg/kg bid (max 250 mg/dose) OR Azithromycin 5 mg/kg daily (max 250 mg/dose)	Use of antibiotic prophylaxis is generally favored for asplenic and hyposplenic patients who are at highest risk of severe infection (eg, immunocompromised, those in first year post-splenectomy). Patient age, immune status, history of infections with encapsulated organisms, risk of adverse drug reactions, local prevalence of resistant organisms, and other factors are used to determine the need for daily prophylaxis and its duration for individual patients. For most children with anatomic or functional asplenia, daily antibiotic prophylaxis is recommended until age 5 y.

		For children with additional immunocompromising conditions (eg, hematologic malignancy, HIV, transplant), antibiotic prophylaxis is recommended until at least age 18 y and often for life or total duration of immunocompromise.
Rheumatic fever	For >27.3 kg (>60 lb): 1.2 million U penicillin G benzathine, q4wk (q3wk for high-risk children) For ≤27.3 kg: 600,000 U penicillin G benzathine, q4wk (q3wk for high-risk children) OR Penicillin V (phenoxymethyl), 250 mg PO bid	AHA policy statement at www.ahajournals.org/doi/epub/10.1161/CirculationAHA.109.191959 (accessed October 21, 2024). Doses studied many years ago, with no new data; ARF is an uncommon disease currently in the United States, as "rheumatogenic" strains are apparently not circulating widely at this time. Alternatives to penicillin include amoxicillin, sulfisoxazole, or macrolides, including erythromycin, azithromycin, and clarithromycin.
Urinary tract infection, recurrent[32–38]	TMP/SMX 3 mg/kg/dose of TMP PO qhs OR TMP alone, 2 mg/kg/dose (max 100 mg) PO qhs, OR nitrofurantoin 1–2 mg/kg PO qhs; more rapid resistance may develop by using β-lactams (BII).	Amoxicillin is an alternative (although >50% of community-acquired Escherichia coli isolates are resistant). Only used for those with grade III–V reflux or recurrent febrile UTI: prophylaxis no longer recommended for patients with grade I–II (some also exclude grade III) reflux. Prophylaxis prevents infection but may not prevent scarring. Early treatment of new infections is recommended for children not given prophylaxis. Resistance eventually develops to every antibiotic; follow resistance patterns for each patient. Cranberries can, in fact, prevent UTI.[32]

Antimicrobial Prophylaxis/Prevention of Symptomatic Infection

15

B. LONG-TERM ANTIMICROBIAL PROPHYLAXIS TO PREVENT SYMPTOMATIC NEW INFECTION

Prophylaxis Category	Therapy (evidence grade)	Comments
Fungal: For detailed information on prevention on prevention of candidiasis in the neonate, see Ch 2; for detailed information on prevention of fungal infection (*Candida, Aspergillus,* or *Rhizopus* spp) in children undergoing chemotherapy, see Ch 5.		
Pneumocystis jirovecii (formerly *carinii*)[39-42]	Non-HIV infection regimens (stem cell transplants, solid-organ transplants, many malignancies, and T-cell immunodeficiencies [congenital or secondary to treatment]). Duration of prophylaxis depends on the underlying condition. TMP/SMX 5–10 mg/kg/day of TMP PO, in 2 div doses, q12h, either qd or 2×/wk or 3×/wk, on consecutive days or alternating days (AI); OR TMP/SMX 5–10 mg/kg/day of TMP PO as a *single dose*, qd, given daily, 7 days per week (AI) (once-weekly regimens have also been successful); OR dapsone 2 mg/kg (max 100 mg) PO qd, or 4 mg/kg (max 200 mg) once weekly; OR atovaquone 30 mg/kg/day for infants 1–3 mo; 45 mg/kg/day for infants/children 4–24 mo; and 30 mg/kg/day for children ≥24 mo.	Prophylaxis in specific populations based on degree of immunosuppression. For children with HIV, see ClinicalInfo.HIV.gov for information on pediatric opportunistic infections: https://clinicalinfo.hiv.gov/en/guidelines/hiv-clinical-guidelines-pediatric-opportunistic-infections/pneumocystis-jirovecii-pneumonia (updated November 6, 2013; accessed October 21, 2024). Inhaled pentamidine only for those who cannot tolerate the regimens noted above.

C. PROPHYLAXIS OF SYMPTOMATIC DISEASE IN CHILDREN WHO HAVE ASYMPTOMATIC INFECTION/LATENT INFECTION

Prophylaxis Category	Therapy (evidence grade)	Comments
Herpes simplex virus		
Neonatal: following symptomatic disease, to prevent recurrence	Acyclovir 300 mg/m²/dose tid for 6 mo, following cessation of IV acyclovir treatment of acute disease (AIII)	Neonates who recover from early infection may experience relapse and are likely to still be at risk for disseminated infection until out of the neonatal period of immunocompromise. No prospective studies to examine potential benefits of prophylaxis until age 2–3 mo. Follow absolute neutrophil counts at 2 and 4 wk, then monthly during prophylactic/suppressive therapy.
Keratitis (ocular) in otherwise healthy children	Suppressive acyclovir therapy for frequent recurrence (no pediatric data): long-term suppression (≥1 y) of recurrent infection with PO acyclovir 80 mg/kg/day in 3 div doses (max dose 800 mg) (AIII)	Decisions to continue suppressive therapy should be assessed annually. The frequency of dosing may need to be increased to qid or the drug may need to be changed to valacyclovir, if breakthrough ocular infection occurs. Potential risks must balance potential benefits to vision (BIII). Check for acyclovir resistance for those who relapse during appropriate therapy. Suppression oftentimes required for many years. Watch for severe recurrence at conclusion of suppression.
Tuberculosis[20-22] (latent TB infection [asymptomatic, true infection], defined by a positive skin test or IGRA, with no clinical or radiographic evidence of active disease), currently called "TB infection" in contrast to active, symptomatic infection that is now called "TB disease"	Rifampin 15–20 mg/kg/dose qd, preferably the entire daily dose given qd (max 600 mg) for 4 mo, OR For children ≥2 y, once-weekly DOT for 12 wk using BOTH INH 15 mg/kg/dose (max 900 mg) AND rifapentine: 10.0–14.0 kg: 300 mg; 14.1–25.0 kg: 450 mg; 25.1–32.0 kg: 600 mg; 32.1–49.9 kg: 750 mg; ≥50.0 kg: 900 mg (max)	Alternative regimens: INH 10–20 mg/kg PO qd AND rifampin 15–20 mg/kg/dose daily (max 600 mg) for 3 mo, OR INH 10–20 mg/kg PO qd for 6 to 9 mo, OR INH 20–40 mg/kg PO DOT twice weekly for 6–9 mo For exposure to drug-resistant strains, consult with TB specialist.

15

D. SURGICAL/PROCEDURE PROPHYLAXIS[43–48]

The CDC National Healthcare Safety Network uses a classification of surgical procedure-related wound infections based on an estimation of the load of bacterial contamination: Class I, clean; Class II, clean-contaminated; Class III, contaminated; and Class IV, dirty/infected.[44,48] Other major factors creating risk for postoperative surgical site infection include the duration of surgery (a longer-duration operation, defined as one that exceeded the 75th percentile for a given procedure) and the medical comorbidities of the patient, as determined by an American Society of Anesthesiologists score of III, IV, or V (presence of severe systemic disease that results in functional limitations, is life threatening, or is expected to preclude survival from the operation). The virulence/pathogenicity of bacteria inoculated and the presence of foreign debris/devitalized tissue/surgical material in the wound are also considered risk factors for infection.

For all categories of surgical prophylaxis, dosing recommendations are derived from (1) choosing agents likely to be responsible for inoculation of the surgical site; (2) giving the agents at an optimal time (<60 min for cefazolin, or <60–120 min for vancomycin and ciprofloxacin) before starting the operation to achieve appropriate serum and tissue exposures at the time of incision; (3) providing additional doses during the procedure at times based on the standard dosing guideline for that agent (or excessive blood loss during surgery); and (4) stopping the agents at the end of the procedure, even if drains remain.[48] Optimal duration of prophylaxis after delayed sternal or abdominal closure is not well-defined in adults or children.

Topical perioperative use of chlorhexidine or povidone-iodine decreases the risk of surgical site infection.[49,50]

Procedure/Operation	Recommended Agents	Preoperative Dose	Intraoperative Re-Dosing Interval (h) for Prolonged Surgery
Cardiovascular			
Cardiac[48,51]	Cefazolin	30–40 mg/kg	4
Staphylococcus epidermidis,	Vancomycin, if MRSA likely	15 mg/kg	8
Staphylococcus aureus,	Amp/sul if enteric GNB a concern	50 mg/kg ampicillin	3
Corynebacterium spp	Other options: cefuroxime, clindamycin		
Cardiac with CPB[45,52]	Cefazolin	30–40 mg/kg	15 mg/kg at CPB start and also at rewarming. Begin postoperative prophylaxis 30–40 mg/kg 8 h after intraoperative rewarming dose.
	Other antibiotics may be used but should be dosed based on patient's anticipated antibiotic elimination during CPB, with dosing repeated based on antibiotic clearance.		

Vascular	Cefazolin, OR	30–40 mg/kg	4
Staphylococcus epidermidis, *Staphylococcus aureus,* *Corynebacterium* spp, enteric GNB, particularly for procedures in the groin	Vancomycin, if MRSA likely	15 mg/kg	8
	Other option: clindamycin	10 mg/kg	
Thoracic (noncardiac)			
Lobectomy, video-assisted thoracoscopic surgery, thoracotomy (but no prophylaxis needed for simple chest tube placement for pneumothorax)	Cefazolin, OR	30–40 mg/kg	4
	Amp/sul if enteric GNB a concern	50 mg/kg ampicillin	3
	Vancomycin or clindamycin if drug allergy or MRSA likely	15 mg/kg vancomycin	8
		10 mg/kg clindamycin	6
Gastrointestinal			
Gastroduodenal Enteric GNB, respiratory tract gram-positive cocci	Cefazolin	30–40 mg/kg	4
Biliary procedure, open Enteric GNB, enterococci, *Clostridia*	Cefazolin, OR	30–40 mg/kg	4
	Cefoxitin, OR	40 mg/kg	2
	Amp/sul	50 mg/kg ampicillin	3
Appendectomy, non-perforated (no prophylaxis needed postoperatively if appendix is intact)[48,53]	Cefoxitin, OR	40 mg/kg	2
	Cefazolin and metronidazole	30–40 mg/kg cefazolin, 10 mg/kg metronidazole	4 for cefazolin 8 for metronidazole

15

Antimicrobial Prophylaxis/Prevention of Symptomatic Infection

15

Antimicrobial Prophylaxis/Prevention of Symptomatic Infection

D. SURGICAL/PROCEDURE PROPHYLAXIS[43-48]

Complicated appendicitis or other ruptured colorectal viscus[54] Enteric GNB, enterococci, anaerobes	Cefazolin and metronidazole, OR	30–40 mg/kg cefazolin, 10 mg/kg metronidazole	4 for cefazolin 8 for metronidazole
	Cefoxitin, OR	40 mg/kg	2
For complicated appendicitis, antibiotics provided to treat ongoing infection, rather than prophylaxis	Ceftriaxone and metronidazole, OR	50 mg/kg ceftriaxone, 10 mg/kg metronidazole	12 for ceftriaxone 8 for metronidazole
	Meropenem, OR	20 mg/kg	4
	Imipenem	20 mg/kg	4
Genitourinary			
Cystoscopy (requires prophylaxis only for children with suspected active UTI or those having foreign material placed) Enteric GNB, enterococci	Cefazolin, OR	30–40 mg/kg	4
	TMP/SMX (if low local resistance), OR Select a 2nd- (cefuroxime) or 3rd-generation cephalosporin (ceftriaxone) or FQ (ciprofloxacin) if the child is known or suspected to be colonized with cefazolin-resistant, TMP/SMX-resistant strains.	4–5 mg/kg	NA
Open or laparoscopic surgery Enteric GNB, enterococci	Cefazolin	30–40 mg/kg	4

Head and neck surgery

Assuming incision through respiratory tract mucosa (eg, contaminated) Anaerobes, enteric GNB, *Staphylococcus aureus*	Clindamycin, OR	10 mg/kg	6
	Cefazolin and metronidazole, OR	30–40 mg/kg cefazolin, 10 mg/kg metronidazole	4 for cefazolin 8 for metronidazole
	Amp/sul if enteric GNB a concern	50 mg/kg ampicillin	3

Neurosurgery

Craniotomy, ventricular shunt placement *Staphylococcus epidermidis,* *Staphylococcus aureus*	Cefazolin, OR	30–40 mg/kg	4
	Vancomycin or clindamycin, if MRSA likely	15 mg/kg vancomycin	8
		10 mg/kg clindamycin	6

Orthopedic

Internal fixation of fractures, spinal rod placement, prosthetic joints *Staphylococcus epidermidis,* *Staphylococcus aureus*	Cefazolin, OR	30–40 mg/kg	4
	Vancomycin or clindamycin, if MRSA likely	15 mg/kg vancomycin	8
		10 mg/kg clindamycin	6

Antimicrobial Prophylaxis/Prevention of Symptomatic Infection

15

Antimicrobial Prophylaxis/Prevention of Symptomatic Infection

D. SURGICAL/PROCEDURE PROPHYLAXIS[43-48]

15

Trauma

Exceptionally varied; no prospective, comparative data in children; agents should focus on skin flora (S epidermidis, S aureus) as well as flora inoculated into the wound, based on the trauma exposure, that may include enteric GNB, anaerobes (including Clostridium spp), and fungi. Cultures at wound exploration are critical to focus therapy for potential pathogens inoculated into the wound.	Cefazolin (for skin), OR	30–40 mg/kg	4
	Vancomycin or clindamycin (for skin), if MRSA likely, OR	15 mg/kg vancomycin	8
		10 mg/kg clindamycin	6
	Meropenem OR imipenem (for anaerobes, including Clostridium spp, and non-fermenting GNB), OR	20 mg/kg for either	4
	Gentamicin and metronidazole (for non-fermenting GNB and anaerobes, including Clostridium spp), OR	2.5 mg/kg gentamicin, 10 mg/kg metronidazole	6 for gentamicin 8 for metronidazole
	PIP/TAZO	100 mg/kg PIP component	2

16. Approach to Antibiotic Allergies

NOTE: A list of table abbreviations and acronyms can be found at the start of this publication.

Introduction

Antibiotics are a common cause of drug reactions. β-Lactam antibiotics are most commonly implicated, with about 10% of the US population reporting a history of penicillin allergy. However, antibiotic allergies are frequently mislabeled and, even if present, may not persist throughout childhood and into adolescence. In such cases, unnecessary use of alternative broad-spectrum antibiotics may result in suboptimal therapy, medication-related side effects, the development of antibiotic resistance, and increased health care costs. More than 90% of those who report a history of an antibiotic allergy are ultimately able to safely tolerate the antibiotic. Thus, it is important to use a systematic approach to children with reported antibiotic allergies, including the routine evaluation of reported penicillin allergy.

American Academy of Allergy, Asthma and Immunology (AAAAI); American College of Allergy, Asthma, and Immunology; and Joint Council of Allergy, Asthma and Immunology practice parameters provide an excellent overview of drug allergies; the following information summarizes recommendations with respect to antibiotic allergies from these guidelines and other resources listed in Suggested Reading later in this chapter.

Classification of Antibiotic Allergies

Antibiotic allergies are immune-mediated reactions to a drug that occur in a previously sensitized child. More commonly, adverse drug reactions are not immune mediated and do not represent a true antibiotic allergy (but are often mislabeled as such). It is important to distinguish between clinically relevant categories of adverse antibiotic reactions (**Table 16-1**).

Approach to Antibiotic Allergies

16

TABLE 16-1. CLASSIFICATION OF ADVERSE ANTIBIOTIC REACTIONS

Classification	Mechanism	Characteristics	Examples	Future Use of Antibiotic
Immediate hypersensitivity reactions	Type I IgE mediated	Anaphylactic May be life threatening Occur within minutes to <6 h of exposure to the antibiotic Uncommon	Immediate urticaria Angioedema Laryngeal edema/stridor Bronchospasm/wheezing Cardiorespiratory symptoms	If β-lactam, consider repeat skin testing 5–10 y after positive skin test or anaphylactic reaction.[1] If no alternative antibiotic, administer through desensitization protocol (Table 16-3).
Delayed drug-induced exanthems	Type IV Cell mediated	Nonanaphylactic Not life threatening Typically occur after several days of antibiotic exposure More common	Delayed maculopapular rash (typically fixed/nonmobile, non-pruritic) Delayed urticaria	Future use of antibiotic *may be considered.*
Severe cutaneous adverse reactions	Type IV T-cell mediated	Severe delayed hypersensitivity reactions May be life threatening Rare	EM major SJS/TEN DRESS AGEP	Future use of antibiotic *contraindicated* for all cases of SJS, TEN, DRESS, or AGEP. Some allergists may consider supervised PO challenge for children with EM *minor* due to possibility of infection-induced rash (eg, HSV, *Mycoplasma*).

Serum sickness	Type III Immune-complex mediated (drug–antibody complex)	Delayed reaction at 1–3 wk after exposure; May occur earlier if preformed antibody present; Uncommon	Classic symptoms: fever, rash, polyarthralgia, or polyarthritis; May also have urticaria and lymphadenopathy	Future use of antibiotic *contraindicated.*
Serum sickness–like reaction	SSLR immunopathology unclear			Some allergists may recommend PO challenge for *children with a history of* SSLR to β-lactam therapy, given the possibility of infectious (typically viral) etiology.[2,3]
Nonimmune drug reaction	Nonallergic response to a drug	Multiple types; examples include • Drug intolerance • Pseudoallergic reaction Do not require prior sensitization or testing Common, frequently mislabeled as allergy	Drug intolerance • GI symptoms • Headache • Diaper rash/yeast infection • Pseudoallergic reaction • Vancomycin glycopeptide flushing syndrome	Future use of antibiotic *can be considered* by using prevention/management strategies.

Approach to Antibiotic Allergies

16

General Approach

Table 16-2 describes a modified stepwise approach to the workup and management of potential antibiotic allergies.

TABLE 16-2. STEPWISE APPROACH TO REPORTED ANTIBIOTIC ALLERGIES

Steps	Components	Notes
Step 1	Perform a thorough history and physical examination; review available clinical data.	Attempt to classify the reaction. • Timing and duration of symptoms in relation to antibiotic administration • Evaluation for evidence of tolerance of drug in question since adverse reaction, with review of previous antibiotic administration history and other medications • Review of associated signs and symptoms • Physical manifestations (examination and/or review of photos, if available) • Review of imaging/laboratory results (if available) **NOTE:** While the PEN-FAST score has been shown to accurately predict low-risk penicillin allergies among adults, a recent study showed that use of this score was *not* helpful in predicting low-risk penicillin allergies among children aged <12 y.[4]
Step 2	Determine if the adverse reaction is likely due to antibiotic.	If yes, determine type of suspected reaction (eg, immediate hypersensitivity reaction vs delayed drug-induced exanthem vs nonimmune adverse drug reaction). If no, consider removing antibiotic allergy label.
Step 3	If possible immediate hypersensitivity reaction • Perform confirmatory testing (if available); consider referral to allergist.	Testing typically performed ≥4–6 wk after symptom resolution. It is recommended that patients with nonanaphylaxis undergo a direct amoxicillin challenge (without skin testing). Penicillin skin testing can be used to test for IgE-mediated penicillin allergy. Although not standardized, most allergy clinics will also perform ampicillin skin testing.
	If suspected delayed drug-induced exanthem (not SCAR) or nonimmune drug reaction • Consider strategies for evaluation and/or de-labeling.	Depending on type of suspected reaction • Consider management/prevention strategies if nonimmune. • May consider skin testing. • May consider observed challenge. • May be able to remove antibiotic allergy label.

Step 4	Review available results.	Confirmed not allergic
		• OK to give antibiotic.
		• Remove antibiotic allergy label and counsel families to remove in other health care entities.
		Confirmed allergic
		• Choose alternative antibiotic.
		• Consider repeat penicillin skin testing in 5–8 y to determine if child has outgrown allergy.
		• Perform desensitization procedure if need to give antibiotic.
		Possibly allergic
		• Choose alternative antibiotic.
		• Perform observed challenge before giving antibiotic.

Adapted from Khan DA, et al. Drug allergy: a 2022 practice parameter update. *J Allergy Clin Immunol.* 2022;150(6):1333–1393 PMID: 36122788 and The Joint Task Force on Practice Parameters; American Academy of Allergy, Asthma and Immunology; American College of Allergy, Asthma, and Immunology; Joint Council of Allergy, Asthma and Immunology. Drug allergy: an updated practice parameter. *Ann Allergy Asthma Immunol.* 2010;105(4):259–273 PMID: 20934625.

Approach to Antibiotic Allergies

Table 16-3 details protocols.

TABLE 16-3. OBSERVED CHALLENGE AND DESENSITIZATION PROTOCOLS		
Protocol	**Details**	**Notes**
Observed challenge	Test dosing of antibiotic. Perform controlled administration of single dose or divided increasing doses (graded challenge) until full dose reached. Example graded challenge: give 10%–25% of therapeutic dose and observe for 15–30 min (about 75% will react within 20 min), then give rest of dose and observe for another 30–60 min (up to 2 h; about 100% will react within 2 h).	Used when low likelihood of IgE-mediated allergy Can verify child will not have immediate hypersensitivity reaction Does not alter immune response or induce tolerance
Desensitization procedure	Rapid induction of antibiotic tolerance Administration of incremental doses Performed under the guidance of an allergist in a controlled setting	Used when high likelihood of IgE-mediated allergy and no alternative antibiotics available Alters immune response by providing *temporary* tolerance (will need to repeat desensitization protocol if >24 h has elapsed since drug exposure)

Adapted from Khan DA, et al. Drug allergy: a 2022 practice parameter update. *J Allergy Clin Immunol.* 2022;150(6):1333–1393 PMID: 36122788 and The Joint Task Force on Practice Parameters; American Academy of Allergy, Asthma and Immunology; American College of Allergy, Asthma, and Immunology; Joint Council of Allergy, Asthma and Immunology. Drug allergy: an updated practice parameter. *Ann Allergy Asthma Immunol.* 2010;105(4):259–273 PMID: 20934625.

Specific Antibiotic Allergies and Allergic Cross-Reactivity

β-Lactam Antibiotics

Penicillin

Although the AAAAI position statement continues to recommend penicillin skin testing for children with a history of anaphylaxis or recent immediate-onset urticaria following exposure to a penicillin, children with a history of nonserious reactions should forgo penicillin skin testing and instead receive a supervised oral (PO) amoxicillin challenge to test for allergy. For those who require skin testing, the penicillin skin test has a negative predictive value near 100%. If skin testing is negative, the child should then receive a supervised PO challenge to confirm tolerance, ideally in a same-day visit.[5] The positive predictive value of penicillin skin testing appears to be high. If positive, penicillin should be avoided for at least 5 to 8 years; however, repeat testing after this time is recommended, as up to 80% of children will ultimately outgrow penicillin allergy within 10 years.[6] If use of penicillin is indicated before this time (if no acceptable alternatives are available), desensitization should be performed under the care of an allergy specialist. Of note, in vitro serum testing for penicillin-specific IgE has an undefined predictive value and should *not* be used in lieu of skin testing and/or an observed PO challenge.

Penicillin allergic cross-reactivity: The rate of allergic cross-reactivity between penicillin and cephalosporins was traditionally reported to be about 10%, although more recent studies suggest a rate of less than 2%. Cross-reactivity is more common with some PO first-generation cephalosporins (as these antibiotics may have similar R-group side chains; see Cephalosporins discussed next), principally if the reaction to penicillin was anaphylaxis. Most children with a history of penicillin allergy tolerate cephalosporins, particularly if the reaction was not severe. For patients with a history of an unverified nonanaphylactic penicillin allergy, any cephalosporin can be administered routinely without testing or additional precautions. Of children who have a positive penicillin skin test result, about 2% will react to some cephalosporins. **Table 16-4** details various approaches to cephalosporin administration in children with a reported history of penicillin allergy.

TABLE 16-4. APPROACHES TO CEPHALOSPORIN ADMINISTRATION IN CHILDREN WITH REPORTED HISTORY OF PENICILLIN ALLERGY

Skin Test	Options for Cephalosporin Administration
Penicillin skin test	Negative result • OK to give Positive result • Choose alternative (non–β-lactam) antibiotic. • Administer via observed challenge or desensitization (depending on severity of prior reaction).
Cephalosporin skin test (not standardized)	Negative result • Administer via observed challenge. Positive result • Choose alternative (non–β-lactam) antibiotic. • Choose alternative cephalosporin (with dissimilar R-group side chain) and administer via cautious observed challenge or desensitization (depending on severity of prior reaction). • Administer via desensitization if no alternative antibiotic.
Skin testing unavailable	Administer via cautious observed challenge or desensitization (depending on severity of prior reaction).

Adapted from Khan DA, et al. Drug allergy: a 2022 practice parameter update. *J Allergy Clin Immunol.* 2022;150(6):1333–1393 PMID: 36122788 and The Joint Task Force on Practice Parameters; American Academy of Allergy, Asthma and Immunology; American College of Allergy, Asthma, and Immunology; Joint Council of Allergy, Asthma and Immunology. Drug allergy: an updated practice parameter. *Ann Allergy Asthma Immunol.* 2010;105(4):259–273 PMID: 20934625.

Approach to Antibiotic Allergies

16

Cephalosporins

The rate of allergic reactions to cephalosporins is significantly lower than for penicillin. Cephalosporin skin testing is not standardized, although many allergists will perform cefazolin skin testing by using a nonirritating concentration of the antibiotic. While a positive skin test result suggests the presence of specific IgE antibodies, a negative skin test result does not definitively rule out an allergy, and an observed challenge should be considered before administration.

Cephalosporin allergic cross-reactivity: Most immediate hypersensitivity reactions with cephalosporins are directed at the R-group side chains (rather than the core β-lactam ring). Tables are available that detail the β-lactam antibiotics that share similar R-group side chains (see Suggested Reading later in this chapter and **Table 16-5**). If there is a history of an immediate hypersensitivity reaction to a given cephalosporin, β-lactams with similar R-group side chains should be avoided. For those patients with a nonanaphylactic cephalosporin allergy, a direct challenge should be performed to determine tolerance. In contrast, for administration of cephalosporins with similar side chains and for the less common anaphylactic reaction history, a negative cephalosporin skin test to a parenteral cephalosporin should be performed before the challenge to determine tolerance. For patients with a history of a nonanaphylactic cephalosporin allergy, a penicillin can be administered without testing or additional precautions. For example, those with a prior history of skin reactions, including urticaria, to cephalexin can receive amoxicillin without prior testing. But for patients with a history of anaphylaxis to a cephalosporin, penicillin skin testing and a drug challenge should be performed before administration of a penicillin.[1]

TABLE 16-5. CLINICALLY RELEVANT β-LACTAM ANTIBIOTICS WITH SIMILAR R-GROUP SIDE CHAINS

Antibiotics in *italics* are in different classes and/or generations.

Antibiotic	β-Lactam Antibiotics Sharing Similar R-Group Side Chains
Penicillins	Penicillin G, penicillin V (PO phenoxymethyl penicillin)
Aminopenicillins	Amoxicillin, *cefadroxil, cefprozil* Ampicillin, *cefaclor, cephalexin*
First-generation cephalosporins	Cefaclor, cefadroxil, cephalexin, *cefprozil, amoxicillin, ampicillin* Cephalothin, *cefoxitin* **NOTE:** Cefazolin has unique R-group side chains.
Second-generation cephalosporins	Cefoxitin, *cephalothin* Cefuroxime, cefoxitin Cefprozil, *cefaclor, cefadroxil, cephalexin, amoxicillin, ampicillin* **NOTE:** Cefotetan and cefamandole have unique R-group side chains.
Third-, fourth-, and fifth-generation cephalosporins	Ceftriaxone, cefotaxime, cefepime Cefdinir, cefixime Ceftaroline, ceftobiprole, ceftolozane Cefditoren, cefpodoxime Ceftazidime, *aztreonam*
Monobactams	Aztreonam, *ceftazidime*

Adapted from Norton AE, et al. Antibiotic allergy in pediatrics. *Pediatrics.* 2018;141(5):e20172497 PMID: 29700201.

Aminopenicillins

Immediate hypersensitivity reactions to amoxicillin or ampicillin are less common than with penicillin. Skin testing with aminopenicillins is not as standardized as penicillin, although many allergists will perform testing by using a nonirritating concentration of ampicillin along with the major determinants for penicillin. It should be noted that the negative predictive value is unknown, so an observed challenge is recommended in the setting of negative aminopenicillin skin testing results. Children with low-risk histories (eg, nonanaphylactic reactions) may bypass skin testing and proceed directly to an observed challenge with PO amoxicillin.

Delayed drug-induced, non-urticarial exanthems are relatively common with aminopenicillin use in children. The reaction is hypothesized to occur in the setting of a concomitant viral illness, with the classic example being an amoxicillin-induced rash in the setting of a child with acute Epstein-Barr virus infection (occurs in nearly 100%). In such cases, an observed challenge may be conducted before a future course is given.

Aminopenicillin allergic cross-reactivity: Immediate hypersensitivity reactions to aminopenicillins may be directed at either the core penicillin determinants or the R-group side chains. If the reaction is due to IgE antibodies versus the R-group side chains, children will have a negative penicillin skin test result and will be able to tolerate other penicillins. If there is a history of an immediate hypersensitivity reaction to an aminopenicillin, β-lactams with the same R-group side chains should be avoided (see **Table 16-5**). If there is no alternative antibiotic, desensitization should be performed.

Monobactams

Allergic reactions to aztreonam are much less common than those to other β-lactam antibiotics.

Monobactam allergic cross-reactivity: Monobactams do not exhibit allergic cross-reactivity with other β-lactams, which can be given without prior testing, except for ceftazidime, which shares an R-group side chain with aztreonam.

Carbapenems

Immediate hypersensitivity reactions to carbapenems appear to be rare. Carbapenem skin testing is not standardized and has unknown predictive value.

Carbapenem allergic cross-reactivity: Allergic cross-reactivity between other β-lactams and carbapenems is extremely low (<1%). Current recommendations are to administer a carbapenem without testing or additional precautions regardless of whether the previous penicillin or cephalosporin reaction was anaphylactic.

Non–β-Lactam Antibiotics

Immediate hypersensitivity reactions to non–β-lactam antibiotics are uncommon (**Table 16-6**). There are no validated tests to evaluate IgE-mediated reactions for these antibiotic classes (eg, skin testing is not standardized and lacks adequate predictive value). If the prior reaction to a non–β-lactam antibiotic is consistent with an immediate hypersensitivity reaction, that antibiotic should be used only if there is no alternative agent and then only via desensitization.

TABLE 16-6. NON–β-LACTAM ANTIBIOTIC REACTIONS

Antibiotic Class	Frequency of Immediate Hypersensitivity Reactions	Other Antibiotic Reaction Notes
Aminoglycoside	Rare	None
Glycopeptide	Rare	Vancomycin frequently causes non–IgE-mediated histamine release (pseudoallergic reaction), often related to the rapidity of infusion, which is now called "vancomycin glycopeptide flushing syndrome." This syndrome is not a contraindication; premedicate with antihistamines and slow the infusion rate.
Lincosamide	Rare	None
Macrolide	Rare	Delayed drug-induced exanthems more common
Quinolone	Increasingly reported with expanded use	Delayed drug-induced exanthems in about 2%
Sulfonamide	Rare	Delayed drug-induced exanthems more common Severe cutaneous adverse reactions possible
Tetracyclines	Rare	None

Non–β-lactam antibiotics allergic cross-reactivity: Importantly, there is no reported allergic cross-reactivity with β-lactam antibiotics (or with alternative classes of non–β-lactam antibiotics). There may be allergic cross-reactivity within the same antibiotic class (eg, some quinolone or macrolide groups).

Alternative Antibiotic Options for Common Infections

As detailed previously, it is important to identify children who are mislabeled or who have outgrown a reported allergy and can safely receive the antibiotic. For children with confirmed allergies, alternative antibiotic selection should be as narrow in spectrum as possible while balancing the effectiveness, rate of resistance, side effects, and potential allergic cross-reactivity of the medication. **Table 16-7** details alternative antibiotic options for select common infections. Consider the susceptibilities of the pathogens for each infection category, as all alternatives may not cover the required antibacterial spectrum equally well.

TABLE 16-7. ALTERNATIVE ANTIBIOTIC OPTIONS FOR SELECT COMMON INFECTIONS

Infection Category (Antibiotic Allergy)	Alternative Antibiotic Options
Acute otitis media (Amoxicillin allergy)	Third-generation cephalosporin (IV: ceftriaxone, cefotaxime; PO: cefdinir, cefixime, cefpodoxime) Clindamycin (does not cover *Haemophilus influenzae* or *Moraxella*) Levofloxacin
Group A streptococcus pharyngitis (Penicillin/amoxicillin allergy)	Cephalexin if nonanaphylactic reaction Clindamycin, although the CDC has now documented up to 20% resistance to clindamycin Macrolides (eg, azithromycin, erythromycin), although rates of macrolide resistance are increasing globally **NOTE:** *TMP/SMX is not recommended, as it does not reliably prevent rheumatic fever.*
Community-acquired pneumonia (Amoxicillin/ampicillin allergy)	Cephalosporins active against pneumococcus (IV: ceftriaxone, cefotaxime, ceftaroline; PO: cefdinir, cefixime, cefpodoxime) Clindamycin IV or PO (does not cover *H influenzae* or *Moraxella*) Levofloxacin IV or PO Linezolid IV or PO (does not cover *H influenzae* or *Moraxella*) Vancomycin IV (does not cover *H influenzae* or *Moraxella*)
Atypical pneumonia (Macrolide allergy)	Doxycycline IV or PO Levofloxacin IV or PO
Skin and soft tissue/osteoarticular infections (*Staphylococcus aureus*) (β-Lactam allergy)	Clindamycin IV or PO TMP/SMX (skin) IV or PO Linezolid IV or PO Vancomycin IV Daptomycin IV

Suggested Reading

Blumenthal KG, et al. *Lancet*. 2019;393(10167):183–198 PMID: 30558872

Broyles AD, et al. *J Allergy Clin Immunol Pract*. 2020;8(9)(suppl):S16–116 PMID: 33039007

Collins C. *J Pediatr*. 2019;212:216–223 PMID: 31253408

Collins CA, et al. *Ann Allergy Asthma Immunol*. 2019;122(6):663–665 PMID: 30878624

Joint Task Force on Practice Parameters, et al. *Ann Allergy Asthma Immunol*. 2010;105(4):259–273 PMID: 20934625

Khan DA, et al. Drug allergy: a 2022 practice parameter update. *J Allergy Clin Immunol*. 2022;150(6):1333–1393 PMID: 36122788

Norton AE, et al. *Pediatrics*. 2018;141(5):e20172497 PMID: 29700201

Penicillin Allergy in Antibiotic Resistance Workgroup. *J Allergy Clin Immunol Pract*. 2017;5(2):333–334 PMID: 28283158

Approach to Antibiotic Allergies

16

17. Antibiotic Stewardship

NOTE: A list of table abbreviations and acronyms can be found at the start of this publication.

Antibiotic therapy is one of the most important advances in health care, along with the development of vaccines and the improvements in environmental health at the beginning of the 20th century. Appropriate use of antibiotics can be lifesaving. However, the use of antibiotics is also associated with increased microbial resistance, toxicity to the child, and cost. Therefore, antibiotic prescribing should be done carefully and responsibly to maximize benefit while minimizing adverse or unintended consequences. It is this need for balance on which the term *antibiotic stewardship* is based. *Merriam-Webster* defines *stewardship* as "the careful and responsible management of something entrusted to one's care."[1] It is not the purpose of antibiotic stewardship to drive antibiotic use inexorably toward a hypothetical zero, denying the benefit of treatment to those in need. It is, instead, the role of the steward to ensure that the right drug, at the right dose, for the right duration, is administered the right way to the right host for a particular infection caused by the "right" pathogen. In so doing, the steward maximizes the effect of the antibiotic while ensuring its continued availability and efficacy for the patients who follow.

To optimize use, there are 7 principles that should be followed (**Table 17-1**). These include infection prevention, diagnostic stewardship, effective empiric therapy for suspected infections, narrowing or stopping of therapy as additional information becomes available and the infection resolves, avoidance of unnecessary therapy by treating only infections, optimization of administration, and multidisciplinary accountability.

Infection Prevention

Infection prevention is a key component of antibiotic stewardship. Put simply, each infection that does not occur is one less that will require antibiotic treatment. Effective infection prevention strategies vary by site and by pathogen, and a full discussion of infection prevention is beyond the scope of this book. We direct the interested reader to the Centers for Disease Control and Prevention library.[2] The single most effective strategy for infection prevention remains adherence to hand hygiene. Effective hand hygiene can reduce person-to-person spread of pathogens that are spread by contact and droplet transmission, and studies have shown that infection rates correlate closely with hand hygiene performance regardless of other strategies that may be in place.

Diagnostic Stewardship

As discussed later in this chapter, selecting an appropriate antibiotic regimen for a patient depends largely on obtaining the proper test results for infection. Samples for culture or molecular diagnostic tests should be obtained before antibiotic therapy whenever possible, and the samples should be collected in a manner that will maximize the likelihood ratio of a positive or negative test result. For example, it matters if a urine culture that yields *Escherichia coli* was obtained via catheterization or by bag collection, just as it matters if a sterile urine culture was obtained before administering antibiotics or 48 hours after administration. Culture of non-sterile sites, such as the skin, mucous membranes, and trachea,

TABLE 17-1. OPTIMIZING ANTIBIOTIC USE

Facets of Stewardship	Examples for Implementation
Infection prevention	• Effective infection control and prevention • Close attention to hand hygiene
Diagnostic stewardship	• Obtain appropriate cultures before antibiotic therapy. • Avoid culturing non-sterile sites, and interpret cultures from those sites carefully. • Consider molecular diagnostics when appropriate. • Use ancillary laboratory tests for infection, but remember that positive predictive value may be poor.
Empiric therapy	• Use the narrowest-spectrum agents that cover the likely pathogens to achieve the necessary cure rate for your patient, infection site, severity of infection, and underlying comorbid conditions. • Use an antibiotic that penetrates the infected compartment (eg, achieves effective exposure at the site of infection) (see Ch 11). • Use local epidemiology (including antibiogram) and previous patient cultures to guide therapy.
Reevaluation of therapy	• Discontinue empiric antibiotics when infection is no longer suspected. • For proven infection, adjust antibiotics once speciation and susceptibilities are available. • Treat for the shortest effective duration, and follow up to ensure a successful outcome.

Treatment of infections only	• Avoid treating
	  – Colonization
	  – Contaminants
	  – Noninfectious conditions

Optimization of administration	• Closely collaborate with pharmacists. • Use protocols that maximize PD of agent. • Perform therapeutic drug monitoring where appropriate.
Accountability	• Multidisciplinary team • Prospective audit and feedback • Guarantee of representation and buy-in by including "champions"

may be useful in specific scenarios, but positive culture results from non-sterile sites must be interpreted with caution in the context of the pretest probability of infection. Similarly, molecular diagnostic test results from nucleic acid amplification or next-generation sequencing (usually obtained from blood or infected tissue sites) are frequently positive even after antibiotic administration, when sensitivity of cultures decreases quickly.[3] Next-generation sequencing has not been well studied in children; it is likely to pick up a low signal by colonization of commensal organisms that may not represent invasive infection. Those with mucositis may have DNA from multiple organisms detected, which does not necessarily indicate invasive infection by all detected bacteria. Finally, abnormal values of ancillary tests, such as white blood cell count, C-reactive protein (CRP), and procalcitonin, may lead to unnecessary antibiotic use when the likelihood of infection is low. A careful diagnostic approach is needed to optimize antibiotic use.

Empiric Therapy

Appropriate therapy for a suspected infection should be administered once the appropriate diagnostic tests have been obtained. This empiric therapy should be based on a variety of factors, including the organisms most likely to cause the suspected infection, the body compartment(s) infected, host characteristics including renal and hepatic clearance, drug-drug interactions, and local antibiotic susceptibilities. Ideally, empiric therapy is the narrowest-possible regimen that penetrates the infected space and covers the most likely organisms. These parameters may change over time; for example, in the setting of a local methicillin-resistant *Staphylococcus aureus* (MRSA) outbreak, clinicians might consider different empiric therapy for skin and soft tissue infection than they would otherwise. Similarly, prior antibiotic susceptibilities of a recurrent infection should be used to guide empiric treatment. For example, therapy for a child with a first occurrence of *E coli* pyelonephritis will be guided by local rates of susceptibility, but past susceptibility information should guide empiric therapy in the same child experiencing a recurrence. It is also important to assess the need to achieve a certain level of success in selecting empiric antimicrobial therapy. For the child with mild impetigo, perhaps using drugs that provide 70% coverage of the suspected pathogens is acceptable, and the clinician can follow the treatment progress to see if changes need to be made. On the other hand, for the child who has leukemia and neutropenia, with bacterial meningitis associated with gram-negative bacilli on stains of cerebrospinal fluid, we strive to start empiric therapy with antibiotic(s) as close to covering 100% of suspected pathogens as possible, quickly reevaluating therapy (see Reevaluation of Therapy discussed next). Clinicians should assess their willingness to accept some degree of treatment failure for any given infection, acknowledging that 100% coverage is not required for less severe infections.

Reevaluation of Therapy

Empiric therapy is just that, and it should change once additional information is available. In most cases, this means stopping therapy if infection is no longer suspected (eg, if cultures are sterile after 36–48 hours; if molecular tests for pathogens show no significant pathogen signal) or narrowing therapy if an organism is identified (eg, narrowing from ceftriaxone to ampicillin for susceptible *E coli* recovered from urine). However, therapy should also be reevaluated and possibly broadened if the clinical situation dictates (eg, if a child's condition becomes clinically unstable; if new physical examination findings or radiographic changes are seen; if a culture yields an organism that is unlikely to be covered by the empiric antimicrobials).

Treatment of Infections Only

Antibiotics are powerful tools, but they treat *only* fever and other local and systemic signs and symptoms of infection *if* those findings are caused by bacteria, fungi, or mycobacteria. If a stable patient has fever and a careful, systematic evaluation and diagnostic workup have not identified a treatable organism, it is reasonable in many cases to

Antibiotic Stewardship

17

continue to evaluate that patient without prolonged antibiotic therapy. Many noninfectious diseases can develop with signs and symptoms that are consistent with infection, including numerous rheumatologic and oncologic conditions. Anchoring to a diagnosis of infection in the absence of evidence for infection may not only drive unnecessary antibiotic use but also delay time to diagnosis of another significant health condition. Similarly, clinicians should strive to avoid treating organisms that are colonizing commensals or contaminants. For example, prolonged vancomycin therapy for a *Corynebacterium* species recovered from blood culture after 58 hours of incubation is not an appropriate use of antibiotics. Cultures from non-sterile sites are particularly challenging to interpret in this context, and those cultures should be obtained only when the likelihood of infection at those sites is high. Often, tests for inflammation are elevated when true, invasive infection is present. A normal CRP level after 3 to 4 days of high fever suggests a diagnosis other than bacterial infection, particularly when supported by negative culture and negative molecular test results. Next-generation sequencing tests do not require prior knowledge of a specific pathogen to make a diagnosis; they assess the presence of nucleic acid sequences from any of a thousand pathogens in a gene library.

Optimization of Administration

The dose, route, and frequency of antibiotics can be manipulated to optimize their pharmacodynamics (PD) and efficacy and minimize toxicity. Close collaboration with pharmacology is critical to ensure that dosing is optimal. Examples of strategies include continuous infusion of β-lactam antibiotics to maximize time above minimum inhibitory concentration (MIC) for a resistant *Pseudomonas aeruginosa* infection in a child with cystic fibrosis, vancomycin clearance calculations to ensure adequate area under the curve (the mathematically calculated area under the serum concentration-versus-time curve) to MIC ratio for a complex MRSA infection, or therapeutic drug monitoring to minimize toxicity of aminoglycosides or voriconazole. Dosing strategies can be protocolized, but such strategies should be reviewed periodically, as approaches designed to optimize pharmacokinetics and PD are constantly evolving.

Accountability

Effective antibiotic stewardship cannot be accomplished in a vacuum. Effective stewardship programs require multidisciplinary buy-in and support as well as effective and continuous closed-loop communication. At a minimum, these teams usually consist of pharmacists, physicians including infectious disease (ID) specialists, designated clinicians for representative service lines (eg, a "unit champion"), nurses and nursing leadership, and hospital administrators. Clinical microbiologists, infection control and prevention specialists, information technology specialists, and hospital epidemiologists are key resources even if they do not participate directly in stewardship activities. Antibiotic stewardship programs have myriad tools available (**Table 17-2**), including prospective audit and feedback, prior authorization, clinical practice guidelines, electronic decision support, antibiotic time-outs, electronic hard stops, and intravenous-to-oral conversion. Use of some or all of these interventions must be coupled to education and reporting to staff to demonstrate the utility of the program.

TABLE 17-2. ANTIBIOTIC STEWARDSHIP INTERVENTIONS

Intervention	Description	Advantages and Disadvantages
Prospective audit and feedback	Antibiotic use is monitored prospectively, and information about use is shared with clinicians via continuous or intermittent reports. Specific areas of antibiotic misuse and overuse are targeted for education and feedback.	Staple of stewardship Can be time consuming if not automated Should be combined with education to maximize effect
Prior authorization	Specific antibiotics are restricted without prior approval of ID team or stewardship team.	Extremely effective in curtailing specific antibiotic usage but can be unpopular; clinicians may develop work-arounds to circumvent restrictions.
Clinical practice guidelines	Antibiotic use for a given clinical scenario is built into a protocol or guideline.	Can reduce time to effective therapy, but may not allow flexibility if certain aspects of case are different from usual (eg, if patient has a history of ESBL-producing *Escherichia coli* infection but gets ceftriaxone because of UTI guideline)
Electronic decision support	Language built into EMRs to recognize specific conditions (eg, suspected sepsis) and trigger decision support	Can increase awareness of specific conditions, but may contribute to "alert fatigue"
Antibiotic time-outs	Scheduled reevaluation of empiric therapy at a set time point, usually 48 or 72 h after initiation	Important role in ensuring that empiric therapy is reevaluated as new information comes in. Timing may differ based on clinical scenario.
Electronic hard stops	More automated time-out in which antibiotic therapy is automatically discontinued at a set time point	Very effective in limiting empiric therapy, but must be implemented and monitored carefully to ensure antibiotic therapy is not inadvertently discontinued without notice
Intravenous-to-oral conversion	Periodic or automated review by stewardship team to determine if antibiotics can be changed to PO administration	Particularly useful at hospital discharge to avoid unnecessary outpatient parenteral antibiotic therapy. John Nelson first documented success approximately 50 years ago for osteomyelitis.

Antibiotic Stewardship

17

Historically, many of us opposed antibiotic stewardship programs that reported outcomes only in reduced antibiotic costs and volume and did not consider the adverse effects of the inappropriate use of inexpensive narrow-spectrum antibiotics for serious infection (eg, empiric ampicillin treatment of severe pyelonephritis). However, clinicians are generally more concerned with the outcome of their patients than they are on abstract purchasing data. As a result, stewardship programs have moved toward reporting more patient-centered outcomes, including adverse drug reactions, antibiotic resistance rates, length of stay, and failure of initial therapy. Clinicians are also more inclined to participate in and adhere to stewardship program interventions if they have a seat at the table and can contribute to shared decision-making. This is the role of the unit champion. For example, neonatologists, pulmonologists, and ambulatory pediatricians might each designate a faculty member to attend monthly stewardship meetings to ensure that their perspectives are considered. Finally, pediatricians should consider including parents or family members in shared decision-making about antibiotic use.

In conclusion, antibiotics are critically important for treatment of infections. However, overuse or misuse of antibiotics will drive antimicrobial resistance and adverse patient outcomes. We have learned that there is no "new antibiotic" against which bacteria do not develop resistance. It is the role of the antibiotic steward to maximize the benefit of antibiotics, minimize their toxicity, and preserve their use for subsequent children. There are many resources available to achieve these goals—for example, antibiotic stewardship programs, pharmacists, ID physicians, and prescribing guides such as this book. However, at the end of the day, every health care worker who cares for children is also charged with being a steward of antibiotics—to optimize their use for the patient at hand, while safeguarding their efficacy for all the children yet to come.

18. Systemic and Topical Antimicrobial Dosing and Dose Forms

NOTES

- A list of table abbreviations and acronyms can be found at the start of this publication.

- Higher dosages in a dose range are generally indicated for more serious infections.

- Maximum dosages for adult-sized children (≥40 kg) are based on US Food and Drug Administration (FDA)–approved product labeling or postmarketing data.

- See Chapter 7 for HIV and SARS-CoV-2 antiviral agents not listed in this chapter.

- Antiviral monoclonal antibodies and immunomodulators are not listed.

- Dose Levels of Evidence:

  Level I: FDA or European Medicines Agency–approved pediatric dosing, or based on randomized clinical trials

  Level II: data from noncomparative trials or small comparative trials

  Level III: expert or consensus opinion or case reports

- If no oral liquid form is available, round the child's dose to a combination of available solid dosage forms. Consult a pediatric pharmacist for recommendations on the availability of extemporaneously compounded liquid formulations.

- Cost estimates are in US dollars per course, or per month for maintenance regimens. Estimates are based on wholesale acquisition costs at the editor's institution. These may differ from those of the reader. Legend: $ = <$100, $$ = $100–$400, $$$ = $401–$1,000, $$$$ = >$1,000, $$$$$ = >$10,000.

- There are some agents that we do not recommend even though they may be available. We believe they are significantly inferior to those we do recommend in Chapters 1 through 12 and could possibly lead to poor outcomes if used. Such agents are not listed.

Systemic & Topical Antimicrobial Dosing & Dose Forms

18

18

A. SYSTEMIC ANTIMICROBIALS WITH DOSAGE FORMS AND USUAL DOSAGES

Generic and Trade Names	Dosage Form (cost estimate)	Route	Dose (evidence level)	Interval
Acyclovir,[a] Zovirax See also Valacyclovir later in this table.	500-, 1,000-mg vials ($)	IV	15–45 mg/kg/day (I) (See Chs 2 and 7.) Max 1,500 mg/m²/day (III) (See Ch 13.)	q8h
	200-mg/5-mL susp ($) 200-mg cap ($) 400-, 800-mg tab ($)	PO	900 mg/m²/day (I) 60–80 mg/kg/day, max 3,200 mg/day (I) Adult max 4 g/day for VZV (I) See Chs 2 and 7.	q8h q6–8h
Albendazole,[a] Albenza	200-mg tab ($–$$$)	PO	15 mg/kg/day for cysticercosis or echinococcosis (I) See Ch 9 for other indications.	q12h
Amikacin,[a,b] Amikin	500-mg/2-mL, 1,000-mg/4-mL vials ($)	IV, IM	15–22.5 mg/kg/day (I) (See Ch 4.) 30–35 mg/kg/day for CF (II)	q8–24h
		IVesic	50–100 mL of 0.5 mg/mL in NS (III)	q12h
Amoxicillin,[a] Amoxil	125-, 200-, 250-, 400-mg/5-mL susp ($) 125-, 250-mg chew tab ($) 250-, 500-mg cap ($) 500-, 875-mg tab ($)	PO	Standard dosage: 40–45 mg/kg/day (I) High dosage: 80–90 mg/kg/day (I) 150 mg/kg/day for pen-R *Streptococcus pneumoniae* otitis media (III) Max 4,000 mg/day (III)	q8–12h q12h q8h

Amoxicillin/clavulanate,[a] Augmentin NOTE: Only forms likely to be used in children are listed.	14:1 Augmentin ES: 600/42.9-mg/5-mL susp ($)	PO	14:1 formulation ≥3 mo, <40 kg: 90 mg amox/kg/day for AOM (I), max 4,000 mg amox/day (III) ≥40 kg: 90 mg amox/kg/day for AOM or sinusitis div q12h, or aspiration pneumonia div q8h (II)	q12h
	7:1 Augmentin ($): 875/125-mg tab 200/28.5-, 400/57-mg chew tab 200/28.5-, 400/57-mg/5-mL susp	PO	7:1 formulation ≥3 mo, <40 kg: 25 or 45 mg amox/kg/day ≥40 kg and adults: 1,750 mg amox/day (I)	q12h
	4:1 Augmentin: 250/62.5-mg/5-mL susp ($) 125/31.25-mg/5-mL susp ($$$)	PO	4:1 formulation <3 mo: 30 mg amox/kg/day (I) See Ch 2.	q12h
Amphotericin B deoxycholate,[a] Fungizone	50-mg vial ($$)	IV	1–1.5 mg/kg (I), max 150 mg (II) 0.5 mg/kg for *Candida* esophagitis or cystitis (II)	q24h
		IVesic	50–100 mcg/mL in sterile water × 50–100 mL (III)	
Amphotericin B, lipid complex, Abelcet	100-mg/20-mL vial ($$$)	IV	5 mg/kg (I), up to 10 mg/kg or 500 mg for CNS invasive mold disease (II)	q24h
Amphotericin B, liposomal,[a] AmBisome	50-mg vial ($$$)	IV	5 mg/kg (I), up to 10 mg/kg or 500 mg for CNS invasive mold disease (II)	q24h
Ampicillin sodium[a]	125-, 250-, 500-mg vial ($) 1-, 2-, 10-g vial ($)	IV, IM	50–200 mg/kg/day, max 8 g/day (I) 300–400 mg/kg/day, max 12 g/day endocarditis/meningitis (III)	q6h q4–6h
Ampicillin trihydrate[a]	500-mg cap ($) PO susp not available in the United States	PO	50–100 mg/kg/day if <20 kg (I) ≥20 kg and adults: 1–2 g/day (I)	q6h
Ampicillin/sulbactam,[a] Unasyn	1/0.5-, 2/1-, 10/5-g vial ($–$$)	IV, IM	200-mg amp/kg/day (I) ≥40 kg and adults: 4–max 8 g/day (I)	q6h
Anidulafungin, Eraxis	100-mg vial ($$$)	IV	3 mg/kg LD, then 1.5 mg/kg (I) Max 250-mg LD, then 125-mg (not per kg) if obesity (II)	q24h

18

Systemic & Topical Antimicrobial Dosing & Dose Forms

A. SYSTEMIC ANTIMICROBIALS WITH DOSAGE FORMS AND USUAL DOSAGES

Generic and Trade Names	Dosage Form (cost estimate)	Route	Dose (evidence level)	Interval
Artemether and lumefantrine, Coartem	20/120-mg tab ($)	PO	5–<15 kg: 1 tab ≥15–<25 kg: 2 tabs ≥25–<35 kg: 3 tabs ≥35 kg: 4 tabs (l) See Malaria in Table 9B.	6 doses over 3 days at 0, 8, 24, 36, 48, 60 h
Artesunate	110-mg vial ($$$$$)	IV	2.4 mg/kg (l) See Malaria in Table 9B.	q12h × 3, then q24h
Atovaquone,[a] Mepron	750-mg/5-mL susp ($$–$$$)	PO	30 mg/kg/day if 1–3 mo or >24 mo (l) 45 mg/kg/day if >3–24 mo (l) Max 1,500 mg/day (l)	q12h q24h for prophylaxis
Atovaquone/proguanil,[a] Malarone See Malaria in Table 9B.	62.5/25-mg ped tab ($–$$) 250/100-mg adult tab ($)	PO	Prophylaxis (l): 5–8 kg: ½ ped tab >8–10 kg: ¾ ped tab >10–20 kg: 1 ped tab >20–30 kg: 2 ped tabs >30–40 kg: 3 ped tabs >40 kg: 1 adult tab Treatment (l): 5–8 kg: 2 ped tabs >8–10 kg: 3 ped tabs >10–20 kg: 1 adult tab >20–30 kg: 2 adult tabs >30–40 kg: 3 adult tabs >40 kg: 4 adult tabs	q24h

Drug	Dose Forms	Route	Dosage	Interval
Azithromycin,[a] Zithromax	250-, 500-, 600-mg tab ($) 100-, 200-mg/5-mL susp ($) 1-g packet for susp ($)	PO	Otitis: 10 mg/kg/day for 1 day, then 5 mg/kg for 4 days; or 10 mg/kg/day for 3 days; or 30 mg/kg once (I) Pharyngitis: 12 mg/kg/day for 5 days, max 2,500-mg total dose (I) Sinusitis: 10 mg/kg/day for 3 days, max 1.5-g total dose (I) CABP: 10 mg/kg for 1 day, then 5 mg/kg/day for 4 days (max 1.5-g total dose), or 60 mg/kg once of ER (Zmax) susp, max 2 g (I) MAC prophylaxis: 20 mg/kg, max 1.2 g weekly (III) Adult dosing for RTI: 500 mg day 1, then 250 mg daily for 4 days or 500 mg for 3 days Adult and adolescent dosing for STI: Non-gonorrhea: 1 g once Gonorrhea: 2 g once For other indications, see Chs 1, 3, and 9.	q24h
Aztreonam,[a] Azactam	500-mg vial ($) 1-, 2-g vial ($$-$$$)	IV	10 mg/kg, max 500 mg (II)	q24h
		IV, IM	90-120 mg/kg/day, max 8 g/day (I)	q6-8h
Baloxavir, Xofluza	40-, 80-mg tab ($$) 40-mg/20-mL susp ($$)	PO	≥5 y, <20 kg: 2 mg/kg (I) 20-79 kg: 40 mg (I) ≥80 kg: 80 mg (I)	Once
Bedaquiline, Sirturo	20-mg dispersible tab, 100-mg tab Available from Metro Medical specialty distributor: 855-691-0963	PO	≥5 y, ≥15 kg: 200 mg (not per kg), then 100 mg (I) ≥30 kg: 400 mg, then 200 mg (I); in combination with other agents for MDR TB See Table 1F.	q24h for 2 wk, then the lower dose 3×/wk
Benznidazole	12.5-, 100-mg tab Contact: 877-303-7181 or FastAccess@exeltis.com	PO	2-12 y: 5-8 mg/kg/day (I) See Trypanosomiasis in Table 9B.	q12h

A. SYSTEMIC ANTIMICROBIALS WITH DOSAGE FORMS AND USUAL DOSAGES

Generic and Trade Names	Dosage Form (cost estimate)	Route	Dose (evidence level)	Interval
Bezlotoxumab, Zinplava	1-g vial ($$$$)	IV	Adults: 10 mg/kg (I)[c]	One time
Caspofungin,[a] Cancidas	50-, 70-mg vial ($$)	IV	70 mg/m² LD once, then 50 mg/m², max 70 mg (I), max 150 mg if obesity (II)	q24h
Cefaclor,[a] Ceclor	250-, 500-mg cap ($) 500-mg ER tab ($)	PO	20–40 mg/kg/day, max 1 g/day (I)	q12h
Cefadroxil,[a] Duricef	250-, 500-mg/5-mL susp ($) 500-mg cap ($) 1-g tab ($)	PO	30 mg/kg/day, max 2 g/day (I)	q12–24h
Cefazolin,[a] Ancef	0.5-, 1-, 10-g vial ($)	IV, IM	25–100 mg/kg/day (I) 100–150 mg/kg/day for serious infections (III), max 12 g/day	q8h q6h
Cefdinir,[a] Omnicef	125-, 250-mg/5-mL susp ($) 300-mg cap ($)	PO	14 mg/kg/day, max 600 mg/day (I)	q12–24h
Cefepime,[a] Maxipime	1-, 2-g vial ($) 1-g/50-mL IVPB ($$)	IV, IM	100 mg/kg/day, max 4 g/day (I)	q12h
			150 mg/kg/day empiric therapy for fever with neutropenia, max 6 g/day (I)	q8h
Cefiderocol, Fetroja	1-g vial ($$$$)	IV	Adults: 2 g/day (I)[c]	q8h
Cefixime,[a] Suprax	100-, 200-mg/5-mL susp ($) 400-mg cap ($$)	PO	8 mg/kg/day, max 400 mg/day (I)	q24h
			For convalescent PO therapy for serious infections, up to 20 mg/kg/day (III)	q12h
Cefotaxime,[a] Claforan	0.5-, 1-, 2-, 10-g vial Not currently manufactured in the United States	IV, IM	150–180 mg/kg/day, max 8 g/day (I) 200–225 mg/kg/day for meningitis, max 12 g/day (I)	q8h q6h

Cefotetan,[a] Cefotan	1-, 2-g vial ($$)	IV, IM	60–100 mg/kg/day (II), max 6 g/day (I)	q12h
Cefoxitin,[a] Mefoxin	1-, 2-, 10-g vial ($)	IV, IM	80–160 mg/kg/day, max 12 g/day (I)	q6–8h
			40 mg/kg for surgical prophylaxis (I), no max (II)	See Ch 15.
Cefpodoxime,[a] Vantin	100-mg/5-mL susp ($) 100-, 200-mg tab ($)	PO	10 mg/kg/day, max 400 mg/day (I)	q12h
Cefprozil,[a] Cefzil	125-, 250-mg/5-mL susp ($) 250-, 500-mg tab ($)	PO	15–30 mg/kg/day, max 1 g/d (I)	q12h
Ceftaroline, Teflaro	400-, 600-mg vial ($$$$)	IV	0–<2 mo: 18 mg/kg/day (I)	q8h
			≥2 mo–<2 y: 24 mg/kg/day (I)	q8h
			≥2 y: 36 mg/kg/day (I)	q8h
			>33 kg: 1.2 g/day (I)	q12h
			Adults: 1.2 g/day (I)	q12h
			45–60 mg/kg/day, max 3 g/day ± prolonged infusion for CF (II)	q8h
Ceftazidime,[a] Tazicef, Fortaz	0.5-, 1-, 2-, 6-g vial ($)	IV, IM	90–150 mg/kg/day, max 6 g/day (I), max 8 g/day div q6h in children with obesity (II)	q8h
		IV	200–300 mg/kg/day for serious *Pseudomonas* infection, max 12 g/day (II)	q8h
Ceftazidime/avibactam, Avycaz	2-g/0.5-g vial ($$$$)	IV	3–<6 mo: 120 mg ceftazidime/kg/day (I) ≥6 mo: 150 mg ceftazidime/kg/day, max 6 g/day (I)	q8h infused over 2 h
Ceftolozane/tazobactam, Zerbaxa	1.5-g (1-g/0.5-g) vial ($$$$)	IV	60 mg ceftolozane/kg/day, max 3 g ceftolozane/day (I)	q8h
Ceftriaxone,[a] Rocephin	0.25-, 0.5-, 1-, 2-, 10-g vial ($)	IV, IM	50–75 mg/kg/day, max 2 g/day (I)	q24h
			Meningitis: 100 mg/kg/day, max 4 g/day (I)	q12h
			AOM: 50 mg/kg, max 1 g, 1–3 doses (II)	q24h
Cefuroxime,[a] Ceftin	250-, 500-mg tab ($)	PO	20–30 mg/kg/day, max 1 g/day (I)	q12h
			For bone and joint infections, up to 100 mg/kg/day, max 3 g/day (III)	q8h

A. SYSTEMIC ANTIMICROBIALS WITH DOSAGE FORMS AND USUAL DOSAGES

Generic and Trade Names	Dosage Form (cost estimate)	Route	Dose (evidence level)	Interval
Cefuroxime,[a] Zinacef	0.75-, 1.5-g vial ($)	IV, IM	100–150 mg/kg/day, max 6 g/day (I)	q8h
Cephalexin,[a] Keflex	125-, 250-mg/5-mL susp ($) 250-, 500-mg cap, tab ($) 750-mg cap ($–$$)	PO	25–50 mg/kg/day (I)	q12h
			75–100 mg/kg/day for bone and joint, or severe, infections (II); max 4 g/day (I)	q6–8h
Chloroquine phosphate,[a] Aralen	250-, 500-mg (150-, 300-mg base) tabs ($) Dosed by base content	PO	5 mg/kg, max 300 mg for prophylaxis (I) See Malaria in Table 9B.	Weekly
			10 mg/kg, max 600 mg for treatment (I) See Malaria in Table 9B.	One time, then 5 mg/kg at 6, 24, and 36 h later
Cidofovir,[a] Vistide	375-mg vial ($$$)	IV	5 mg/kg (III) See Adenovirus in Table 7C.	Weekly
Ciprofloxacin,[a] Cipro	250-, 500-mg/5-mL susp ($$) 250-, 500-, 750-mg tab ($)	PO	20–40 mg/kg/day, max 1.5 g/day (I). Do not administer susp via feeding tubes.	q12h
	100-mg tab ($)	PO	Adults: 200 mg/day for 3 days (I)	
	200-mg/100-mL, 400-mg/200-mL IVPB ($)	IV	20–30 mg/kg/day, max 1.2 g/day (I)	q12h
Clarithromycin,[a] Biaxin	125-, 250-mg/5-mL susp ($–$$) 250-, 500-mg tab ($)	PO	15 mg/kg/day, max 1 g/day (I)	q12h
Clarithromycin ER,[a] Biaxin XL	500-mg ER tab ($)	PO	Adults: 1 g (I)	q24h

Drug	Dose Form	Route	Dosage	Interval
Clindamycin,[a] Cleocin	75-mg/5-mL soln ($); 75-, 150-, 300-mg cap ($)	PO	10–25 mg/kg/day, max 1.8 g/day (I); 30–40 mg/kg/day for CA-MRSA or AOM (III)	q8h
	150-mg/mL vial in 2-, 4-, 6-, and 60-mL sizes ($); 0.3-, 0.6-, 0.9-g/50-mL IVPB ($$)	IV, IM	20–40 mg/kg/day, max 2.7 g/day (I). Convert 1:1 when switching to PO.	q8h
Clotrimazole,[a] Mycelex	10-mg lozenge ($)	PO	≥3 y: dissolve lozenge in mouth (I).	5 times daily
Colistimethate,[a] Coly-Mycin M	150-mg (colistin base) vial ($). 1-mg base = 2.7 mg colistimethate = 30,000 IU.	IV, IM	2.5- to 5-mg base/kg/day (III); Max 360 mg/day[b] (I)	q8h
Cycloserine, Seromycin	250-mg cap ($$$$)	PO	10–20 mg/kg/day (III); Adults: max 1 g/day (I)	q12h
Dalbavancin, Dalvance	500-mg vial ($$$$)	IV	Birth–<6 y: 22.5 mg/kg (I); ≥6 y: 18 mg/kg, max 1,500 mg (I)	One time
Dapsone[a]	25-, 100-mg tab ($)	PO	2 mg/kg, max 100 mg (I)	q24h
			4 mg/kg, max 200 mg (I)	Once weekly
Daptomycin,[a] Cubicin	350-, 500-mg vial ($$)	IV	For SSSI (I): 1–2 y: 10 mg/kg, 2–6 y: 9 mg/kg, 7–11 y: 7 mg/kg, 12–17 y: 5 mg/kg. For Staphylococcus aureus bacteremia (I): 1–6 y: 12 mg/kg, 7–11 y: 9 mg/kg, 12–17 y: 7 mg/kg. For other indications, see Ch 1. Adults: 4–6 mg/kg TBW (I).	q24h
Delafloxacin, Baxdela	450-mg tab ($$$$)	PO	Adults: 450 mg (I)	q12h
	300-mg vial ($$$)	IV	Adults: 300 mg (I)	q12h
Demeclocycline,[a] Declomycin	150-, 300-mg tab ($)	PO	≥8 y: 7–13 mg/kg/day, max 600 mg/day (I). Dosage differs for SIADH.	q6–12h
Dicloxacillin,[a] Dynapen	250-, 500-mg cap ($)	PO	12–25 mg/kg/day (adults: 0.5–1 g/day) (I); For bone and joint infections, up to 100 mg/kg/day, max 2 g/day (III)	q6h

18 Systemic & Topical Antimicrobial Dosing & Dose Forms

A. SYSTEMIC ANTIMICROBIALS WITH DOSAGE FORMS AND USUAL DOSAGES

Generic and Trade Names	Dosage Form (cost estimate)	Route	Dose (evidence level)	Interval
Doxycycline, Vibramycin	25-mg/5-mL susp[a] ($) 50-mg/5-mL syrup ($$) 20-, 40-, 50-, 75-, 100-, 150-mg tab/cap[a] ($–$$) 200-mg tab[a] ($$$)	PO	4.4 mg/kg/day LD day 1, then 2.2–4.4 mg/kg/day, max 200 mg/day (I) See also Malaria in Table 9B.	q12–24h
	100-mg vial[a] ($$)	IV		
Elbasvir/grazoprevir, Zepatier	50-mg/100-mg tab ($$$$)	PO	Aged ≥12 y or weighing ≥30 kg: 1 tab (I)	q24h
Entecavir, Baraclude See Hepatitis B virus in Ch 7.	0.05-mg/mL soln ($$$) 0.5-, 1-mg tab[a] ($)	PO	2–<16 y (I) (double the following doses if previous 3TC exposure): 10–11 kg: 0.15 mg >11–14 kg: 0.2 mg >14–17 kg: 0.25 mg >17–20 kg: 0.3 mg >20–23 kg: 0.35 mg >23–26 kg: 0.4 mg >26–30 kg: 0.45 mg >30 kg: 0.5 mg ≥16 y: 0.5 mg (I)	q24h
Eravacycline, Xerava	50-mg vial ($$$)	IV	≥18 y: 1 mg/kg	q12h
Ertapenem,[a] Invanz	1-g vial ($$)	IV, IM	30 mg/kg/day, max 1 g/day (I) ≥13 y and adults: 1 g/day (I)	q12h q24h
Erythromycin base[a]	250-, 500-mg tab ($–$$) 250-mg DR cap ($) 250-, 333-, 500-mg DR tab (Ery-Tab) ($$)	PO	50 mg/kg/day, max 4 g/day (I) 12–40 mg/kg/day for GI motility, max 250 mg/dose (II)	q6–8h

Drug	Dose Form (Cost)	Route	Dosage	Interval
Erythromycin ethylsuccinate; EES, EryPed	200-, 400-mg/5-mL susp ($$-$$$) 400-mg tab ($$)	PO	50 mg/kg/day, max 4 g/day (I)	q6–8h
Erythromycin lactobionate, Erythrocin	0.5-g vial ($$-$$$)	IV	20 mg/kg/day, max 4 g/day (I)	q6h
Ethambutol,[a] Myambutol	100-, 400-mg tab ($)	PO	15–25 mg/kg, max 2.5 g (I)	q24h
Ethionamide, Trecator	250-mg tab ($$)	PO	15–20 mg/kg/day, max 1 g/day (I)	q12–24h
Famciclovir,[a] Famvir	125-, 250-, 500-mg tab ($)	PO	Adults: 0.5–2 g/day (I)	q8–12h
Fexinidazole	600-mg tab available from the WHO: neglected.diseases@who.int	PO	≥6 y, ≥20 kg: 2 tabs, then 1 tab (I) ≥35 kg: 3 tabs, then 2 tabs (I) See Trypanosomiasis in Table 9B.	q24h for 4 days, then the lower dose q24h for 6 days
Fidaxomicin, Dificid	200-mg tab ($$$$) 200-mg/5-mL susp ($$$$)	PO	≥6 mo (I) (per dose, not per kg): 4–<7 kg: 80 mg 7–<9 kg: 120 mg 9–<12.5 kg: 160 mg ≥12.5 kg: 200 mg Adults: 200 mg (I)	q12h
Fluconazole,[a] Diflucan	50-, 100-, 150-, 200-mg tab ($) 50-, 200-mg/5-mL susp ($)	PO	6–12 mg/kg, max 800 mg (I). 800–1,000 mg/day may be used for some CNS fungal infections (see Ch 5). See Ch 2 for neonatal dosing.	q24h
	100-mg/50-mL, 200-mg/100-mL, 400-mg/200-mL IVPB ($)	IV		
Flucytosine,[a] Ancobon	250-, 500-mg cap ($$$$)	PO	100 mg/kg/day (I)[b]	q6h
Foscarnet, Foscavir	6-g/250-mL vial ($$$$)	IV	CMV/VZV: 180 mg/kg/day (I)	q8–12h
			CMV suppression: 90–120 mg/kg (I)	q24h
			HSV: 120 mg/kg/day (I)	q8–12h
Fosfomycin, Monurol	3-g granules ($)	PO	Adults: 3 g (I)	Once

18 Systemic & Topical Antimicrobial Dosing & Dose Forms

A. SYSTEMIC ANTIMICROBIALS WITH DOSAGE FORMS AND USUAL DOSAGES

Generic and Trade Names	Dosage Form (cost estimate)	Route	Dose (evidence level)	Interval
Ganciclovir,[a] Cytovene	500-mg vial ($$)	IV	CMV treatment: Non-congenital: 10 mg/kg/day (I). Congenital: See Ch 2.	q12h
			CMV suppression: 5 mg/kg (I)	q24h
			VZV treatment: 10 mg/kg/day (III)	q12h
Gentamicin[a]	10-mg/mL vial ($) 40-mg/mL vial ($)	IV, IM	3–7.5 mg/kg/day (I), CF and oncology 7–10 mg/kg/day (II)[b] See Ch 4 for q24h dosing.	q8–24h
		IVesic	0.5 mg/mL in NS × 50–100 mL (III)	q12h
Glecaprevir/pibrentasvir, Mavyret Doses given in glecaprevir	50-mg/20-mg pellet packet ($$$$) 100-mg/40-mg tab ($$$$$)	PO	≥3 y (I), dosing not in mg/kg <20 kg: 150 mg 20–<30 kg: 200 mg 30–<45 kg: 250 mg ≥45 kg: 300 mg	q24h
Griseofulvin microsize,[a] Grifulvin V	125-mg/5-mL susp ($) 500-mg tab ($$)	PO	20–25 mg/kg (II), max 1 g (I)	q24h
Griseofulvin ultramicrosize,[a] Gris-PEG	125-, 250-mg tab ($$)	PO	10–15 mg/kg (II), max 750 mg (I)	q24h
Hydroxychloroquine sulfate,[a] Plaquenil[a]	100-, 200-, 300-, 400-mg tab ($). 200 mg = 155-mg hydroxychloro-quine base.	PO	10-mg base/kg, max 800-mg base (I) See Malaria in Table 9B.	One time, then 5 mg/kg at 6, 24, and 48 h later
Ibrexafungerp, Brexafemme	150-mg tab ($$$)	PO	Post-menarchal females 300 mg/day (not per kg) (I)	q12h × 2 doses
Imipenem/cilastatin,[a] Primaxin	250/250-, 500/500-mg vial ($)	IV, IM	60–100 mg/kg/day, max 4 g/day (I) IM form not approved for <12 y	q6h

Imipenem/cilastatin/relebactam, Recarbrio	500/500/250-mg vial ($$$$)	IV	Adults: 2 g/day of imipenem (I)[c]	q6h
Interferon-PEG alfa-2a, Pegasys	All ($$$$) 180-mcg vials, prefilled	SUBQ	See Hepatitis B virus and Hepatitis C virus in Ch 7.	Weekly
Isavuconazonium sulfate, Cresemba Dosing in isavuconazole base	74.5-mg cap (40-mg base) ($$$$) 186-mg cap (100-mg base) ($$$$)	PO	16–<18 kg: 80 mg/dose (I) 18–<25 kg: 120 mg/dose (I) 25–<32 kg: 160 mg/dose (I) ≥32 kg: 200 mg/dose (I)	q8h × 6 doses, then q24h
	372-mg vial (200-mg base) ($$$$)	IV	1–<3 y: 15 mg/kg/dose (I) ≥3 y: 10 mg/kg/dose (I) ≥37 kg: 200 mg (not per kg) per dose (I)	q8h × 6 doses, then q24h
Isoniazid,[a] Nydrazid	50-mg/5-mL soln ($$) 100-, 300-mg tab ($) 1,000-mg vial ($$)	PO IV, IM	10–15 mg/kg/day, max 300 mg/day (I)	q12–24h
			With biweekly DOT, dosage is 20–30 mg/kg, max 900 mg/dose (I).	Twice weekly
			In combination with rifapentine (see Rifapentine later in this table): ≥12 y: 15 mg/kg rounded up to the nearest 50 or 100 mg; 900 mg max 2–<12 y: 25 mg/kg; 900 mg max	Once weekly
Itraconazole,[a] Sporanox	50-mg/5-mL soln ($$) (preferred over caps; see Ch 5). 100-mg cap ($).	PO	10 mg/kg/day (II), max 200 mg/day[b]	q12h
			5 mg/kg/day for chronic mucocutaneous *Candida* (II)	q24h
Itraconazole, Tolsura	65-mg cap ($$$$)	PO	Adults: 130 mg/dose (I)	q12h–q24h
Ivermectin,[a] Stromectol	3-mg tab ($)	PO	0.15–0.2 mg/kg, no max (I)	1 dose
Ketoconazole,[a] Nizoral	200-mg tab ($)	PO	≥2 y: 3.3–6.6 mg/kg, max 400 mg (I)	q24h

18

Systemic & Topical Antimicrobial Dosing & Dose Forms

18

A. SYSTEMIC ANTIMICROBIALS WITH DOSAGE FORMS AND USUAL DOSAGES

Generic and Trade Names	Dosage Form (cost estimate)	Route	Dose (evidence level)	Interval
Lefamulin, Xenleta	150-mg vial ($$$) 600-mg tab ($$$$)	IV PO	Adults (I): 300 mg/day IV 1,200 mg/day PO	q12h
Letermovir, Prevymis	240-, 480-mg tab ($$$$) 240-, 480-mg vial ($$$$)	PO, IV	Adults: 480 mg, 240 mg if concomitant cyclosporine therapy (I) See Cytomegalovirus in Ch 7.	q24h
Levofloxacin,[a] Levaquin	125-mg/5-mL soln ($) 250-, 500-, 750-mg tab ($) 500-, 750-mg vial ($) 250-mg/50-mL, 500-mg/100-mL, 750-mg/150-mL IVPB ($)	PO, IV	For postexposure anthrax prophylaxis (I): <50 kg: 16 mg/kg/day, max 500 mg/day ≥50 kg: 500 mg For respiratory infections: <5 y: 20 mg/kg/day (II), ≥5 y: 10 mg/kg/day; max 500 mg/day (II), up to 1,000 mg/dose in children with obesity (III)	q12h q24h q12h q24h
Linezolid,[a] Zyvox	100-mg/5-mL susp ($$$) 600-mg tab ($) 600-mg/300-mL IVPB ($)	PO, IV	Birth–11 y (I): 30 mg/kg/day; 45 mg/kg/day for MIC 2 (II) >11 y (I): 1.2 g/day	q8h q12h
Maribavir, Livtencity	200-mg tab Available through www.livtencity.com	PO	≥12 y: 400 mg (not per kg) (I)	q12h
Mebendazole, Emverm	100-mg chew tab ($$$–$$$$)	PO	≥2 y: 100 mg (not per kg) (I) See parasitic nematodes and helminths (worms) and other indications in Ch 9.	Varies based on indication See Ch 9.
Mefloquine,[a] Lariam	250-mg tab ($)	PO	5 mg/kg (I) See Malaria in Table 9B.	Weekly
Meropenem,[a] Merrem	0.5-, 1-g vial ($) 2-g vial ($$$)	IV	60 mg/kg/day, max 3 g/day (I) 120 mg/kg/day meningitis (I) or PICU sepsis with suspected ARC (II), max 6 g/day	q8h

Drug	Dose form	Route	Dosing	Frequency
Meropenem/vaborbactam,[a] Vabomere	2-g vial (contains 1-g each mero + vabor) ($$$$)	IV	Adults: 6 g mero/day (I)[c]	q8h
Methenamine hippurate,[a] Hiprex	1-g tab ($)	PO	6–12 y: 1–2 g/day (I); >12 y: 2 g/day (I)	q12h
Methenamine mandelate[a]	0.5-, 1-g tab ($)	PO	<6 y: 75 mg/kg/day (I); 6–12 y: 2 g/day (I); >12 y: 4 g/day (I)	q6h
Metronidazole,[a] Flagyl, Likmez (susp)	250-, 500-mg tab ($); 500-mg/5-mL susp ($$); 375-mg cap ($$)	PO	30–50 mg/kg/day, max 2,250 mg/day (I)	q8h
	500-mg/100-mL IVPB ($)	IV	22.5–40 mg/kg/day (II), max 4 g/day (I)	q6–8h
Micafungin,[a] Mycamine	50-, 100-mg vial ($$); 50-mg/50-mL IVPB ($$); 100-mg/100-mL IVPB; 150-mg/150-mL IVPB	IV	Neonates: 10 mg/kg (II) (See Ch 2.); 1–<4 mo (I): 4 mg/kg; ≥4 mo (I): 2 mg/kg, max 100 mg (I); Esophageal candidiasis ≥4 mo (I): ≤30 kg: 3 mg/kg; >30 kg: 2.5 mg/kg, max 150 mg/day; up to 300 mg/day if obesity (II); Prophylaxis: 1 mg/kg q24h (I) or 3 mg/kg q48h (II)	q24h
Miltefosine, Impavido	50-mg cap; Available from www.impavido.com	PO	<12 y: 2.5 mg/kg/day (II); ≥12 y (I): 30–44 kg: 50 mg (not per kg); ≥45 kg: 50 mg (not per kg); See Leishmaniasis and Amebic meningoencephalitis in Table 9B.	bid; bid; tid
Minocycline, Minocin	50-, 75-, 100-mg cap[a] ($); 50-, 75-, 100-mg tab[a] ($$$$); 100-mg vial ($$$$)	PO, IV	≥8 y: 4 mg/kg/day, max 200 mg/day (I)	q12h

18

A. SYSTEMIC ANTIMICROBIALS WITH DOSAGE FORMS AND USUAL DOSAGES

Generic and Trade Names[a]	Dosage Form (cost estimate)	Route	Dose (evidence level)	Interval
Minocycline ER; Solodyn,[a] Ximino	45-, 55-, 65-, 80-, 90-, 105-, 115-, 135-mg ER tab[a] ($–$$) 45-, 90-, 135-mg ER cap ($$$)	PO	≥12 y: 1 mg/kg/day for acne (I). Round dose to nearest strength tab or cap.	q24h
Moxidectin	2-mg tab Available from info@medicines-development.com	PO	≥12 y: 8 mg (I)[c] See River Blindness in Table 9B under Filariasis.	Once
Moxifloxacin,[a] Avelox	400-mg tab ($) 400-mg/250-mL IVPB ($$)	PO, IV	Adults: 400 mg/day (I)	q24h
		IV	Studied in but not FDA approved for children (II): 3 mo–<2 y: 12 mg/kg/day 2–<6 y: 10 mg/kg/day ≥6–<12 y: 8 mg/kg/day, max 400 mg/day ≥12–<18 y (weight <45 kg): 8 mg/kg/day	q12h
		PO, IV	≥12–<18 y (weight >45 kg): 400 mg	q24h
Nafcillin,[a] Nallpen	1-, 2-, 10-g vial ($–$$)	IV, IM	150–200 mg/kg/day (II) Adults: 6 g/day, max 12 g/day (I)	q6h q4h
Neomycin[a]	500-mg tab ($)	PO	50–100 mg/kg/day (II) Adults: 4–12 g/day (I)	q6–8h
Nifurtimox, Lampit	30-, 120-mg tab ($$)	PO	<40 kg: 10–20 mg/kg/day (I) ≥40 kg: 8–10 mg/kg/day (I)	q8h
Nirmatrelvir/ritonavir, Paxlovid	150-mg/100-mg dose pack Distributed by ASPR (https://covid-19-therapeutics-locator-dhhs.hub.arcgis.com)	PO	≥12 y and ≥40 kg: 300 mg nirmatrelvir with 100 mg ritonavir	q12h

Drug	Route	Dosing	Interval
Nirsevimab	IM	50 mg/0.5 mL in 0.5-mL syringe ($$$) 100 mg/1.0 mL in 1.0-mL syringe ($$$) 50 mg/dose (<5 kg) or 100 mg/dose (≥5 kg) once per season (a) at birth for *all* infants born during October–March and (b) when entering first RSV season and <8 mo of age for all infants born during April–September 200 mg/dose for infants at high risk during their second RSV season	1 dose for a 5-mo RSV season
Nitazoxanide, Alinia	PO	100-mg/5-mL susp ($$$) 500-mg tab[a] ($$) 1–3 y: 200 mg/day (l) 4–11 y: 400 mg/day (l) 12 y–adults: 1 g/day (l) See Giardiasis in Table 9B.	q12h
Nitrofurantoin,[a] Furadantin	PO	25-mg/5-mL susp ($$$$) 5–7 mg/kg/day, max 400 mg/day (l) 1–2 mg/kg for UTI prophylaxis (l)	q6h q24h
Nitrofurantoin macrocrystals,[a] Macrodantin	PO	25-, 50-, 100-mg cap ($) Same as susp	
Nitrofurantoin monohydrate and macrocrystalline,[a] Macrobid	PO	100-mg cap ($) >12 y: 200 mg/day (l)	q12h
Nystatin,[a] Mycostatin	PO	500,000-U/5-mL susp ($) 500,000-U tabs ($) Infants 2 mL/dose, children 4–6 mL/dose; to coat PO mucosa (l) Tabs: 3–6 tabs/day	q6h
Obiltoxaximab, Anthim	IV	600-mg/6-mL vial Available from the Strategic National Stockpile ≤15 kg: 32 mg/kg (l) >15–40 kg: 24 mg/kg (l) >40 kg and adults: 16 mg/kg (l)	Once
Omadacycline, Nuzyra	PO	150-mg tab ($$$$) Adults: 450 mg qd for 2 days, then 300 mg (not per kg) (l)	q24h
	IV	100-mg vial ($$$$) Adults: 200 mg once, then 100 mg (not per kg) (l)	q24h

18

A. SYSTEMIC ANTIMICROBIALS WITH DOSAGE FORMS AND USUAL DOSAGES

Generic and Trade Names	Dosage Form (cost estimate)	Route	Dose (evidence level)	Interval
Oritavancin, Orbactiv	400-mg vial ($$$$)	IV	Adults: 1.2 g/day (I)ᶜ	One time
Oseltamivir,ᵃ Tamiflu See Influenza in Chs 2 and 7.	30-mg/5-mL susp ($) 30-, 45-, 75-mg cap ($)	PO	Preterm <38 wk PMA: 2 mg/kg/day Preterm 38–40 wk PMA: 3 mg/kg/day Preterm >40 wk PMA, and full-term, birth–8 mo (I): 6 mg/kg/day 9–11 mo (II): 7 mg/kg/day ≥12 mo (I), dosing by weight bracket: ≤15 kg: 60 mg/day >15–23 kg: 90 mg/day >23–40 kg: 120 mg/day >40 kg: 150 mg/day (I)	q12h
			Prophylaxis: Give half the daily dose (I). Not recommended for infants aged <3 mo.	q24h
Oxacillin,ᵃ Bactocill	1-, 2-, 10-g vial ($–$$)	IV, IM	100 mg/kg/day, max 12 g/day (I) 150–200 mg/kg/day for meningitis (III)	q4–6h
Penicillin G IM				
– Penicillin G benzathine, Bicillin L-A	600,000 U/mL in 1-, 2-, 4-mL prefilled syringes ($$)	IM	Infants: 50,000 U/kg (I) Children (I): <60 lb: 300,000–600,000 U; ≥60 lb: 900,000 U (not per kg) (FDA approved in 1952 for dosing by pounds) Adults: 1.2–2.4 million U (I) See also Syphilis in Chs 1 and 2.	1 dose

Drug	Dose Form	Route	Dose	Interval
- Penicillin G procaine	600,000 U/mL in 1-, 2-mL prefilled syringes ($$)	IM	Infants: 50,000 U/kg (I) See also Syphilis in Ch 2. Children (I): <60 lb: 300,000 U (not per kg); ≥60 lb or >12 y: 600,000 U	q24h
Penicillin G IV				
- Penicillin G potassium,[a] Pfizerpen	5-, 20-million U vial ($)	IV, IM	100,000–300,000 U/kg/day (I) Max daily dose 24 million U	q4–6h
- Penicillin G sodium[a]	5-million U vial ($–$$)	IV, IM	100,000–300,000 U/kg/day (I) Max daily dose 24 million U	q4–6h
Penicillin V PO				
- Penicillin V potassium[a]	125-, 250-mg/5-mL soln ($) 250-, 500-mg tab ($)	PO	25–50 mg/kg/day, max 2 g/day (I)	q6h
Pentamidine; Pentam, Nebupent	300-mg vial[a] ($$$)	IV, IM	4 mg/kg/day (I), max 300 mg	q24h
	300-mg vial ($)	Inhaled	300 mg for prophylaxis (I)	Monthly
Peramivir, Rapivab	200-mg vial Available from 833-964-2956	IV	≥6 mo: 12 mg/kg, max 600 mg (I)	One time
Piperacillin/tazobactam,[a] Zosyn	2/0.25-, 3/0.375-, 4/0.5-, 12/1.5-, 36/4.5-g vial ($)	IV	2–9 mo: 240 or 320 mg PIP/kg/day (I) >9 mo: 300 or 400 mg PIP/kg/day, max 16 g PIP/day (I) Higher dose for HAP	q8h for IAI q6h for HAP
Plazomicin, Zemdri	500-mg vial ($$$$)	IV	Adults: 15 mg/kg (I)	q24h
Polymyxin B[a]	500,000-U vial ($). 1 mg = 10,000 U.	IV	2.5 mg/kg/day (I) Based on TBW, no max (II)	q12h

18

A. SYSTEMIC ANTIMICROBIALS WITH DOSAGE FORMS AND USUAL DOSAGES

Generic and Trade Names	Dosage Form (cost estimate)	Route	Dose (evidence level)	Interval
Posaconazole,[b] Noxafil	300-mg DR susp packet ($$$$)	PO	*Candida* or *Aspergillus* prophylaxis ≥2 y (I), not in mg/kg: 10–<12 kg: 90 mg 12–<17 kg: 120 mg 17–<21 kg: 150 mg 21–<26 kg: 180 mg 26–<36 kg: 210 mg 36–40 kg: 240 mg	q12h × 1 day, then q24h
	200-mg/5-mL susp[a] ($$$)	PO	≥13 y (I): not per kg *Candida* or *Aspergillus* prophylaxis: 600 mg/day	q8h
			OPC treatment: 100 mg/day	q12h × 1 day, then q24h
			Refractory OPC: 800 mg/day	q12h
	100-mg DR tab[a] ($$)	PO, IV	*Candida* or *Aspergillus* prophylaxis ≥2 y (I): ≤40 kg IV: 6 mg/kg >40 kg IV or DR tab (I): 300 mg (not per kg)	q12h × 1 day, then q24h
	300-mg/16.7-mL vial[a] ($$$$)	IV		
Praziquantel,[a] Biltricide	600-mg tab ($$)	PO	20–25 mg/kg/dose, no max (I). Round dose to nearest 200 mg (⅓ tab).	q4–6h for 3 doses
Pretomanid	200-mg tab ($$)	PO	Adults: 200 mg (I) In combination with other agents for MDR TB	q24h
Primaquine phosphate[a]	15-mg base tab ($) (26.3-mg primaquine phosphate)	PO	0.5 mg (base)/kg, max 30 mg (III) See Malaria in Table 9B.	q24h
Pyrantel pamoate[a]	250-mg base/5-mL susp ($) (720-mg pyrantel pamoate/5-mL)	PO	11 mg (base)/kg, max 1 g (I)	Once

Drug	Dose Form (cost)	Route	Dose	Interval
Pyrazinamide[a]	500-mg tab ($)	PO	30 mg/kg/day, max 2 g/day (I)	q24h
			Biweekly DOT, 50 mg/kg (I), no max	Twice weekly
Raxibacumab	1,700-mg/35-mL vial Available from the Strategic National Stockpile	IV	≤15 kg: 80 mg/kg (I); >15–50 kg: 60 mg/kg (I); >50 kg: 40 mg/kg (I)	Once
Remdesivir, Veklury	100-mg and 100-mg/20-mL vial ($$$$)	IV	<28 days of age and ≥1.5 kg OR ≥28 days of age and 1.5–<3 kg: 2.5 mg/kg LD, then 1.25 mg/kg (I); ≥28 days of age and ≥3 kg: 5 mg/kg LD, then 2.5 mg/kg (I); ≥40 kg and adults: 200 mg LD, then 100 mg (not per kg) (I)	q24h
Rezafungin, Rezzayo	200-mg vial ($$$$)	IV	Adults: 400 mg LD, then 200 mg (I)	Weekly
Ribavirin,[a] Rebetol	200-mg cap/tab ($)	PO	<47 kg: 15 mg/kg/day (I); 12–17 y (not per kg) (I): 47–59 kg: 800 mg/day; 60–73 kg: 1,000 mg/day; 74–105 kg: 1,200 mg/day; >105 kg: 1,400 mg/day; Given as combination therapy with other agents (See Hepatitis C virus in Ch 7.)	q12h
Ribavirin,[a] Virazole	6-g vial ($$$$$)	Inhaled	1 vial by SPAG-2; See Respiratory syncytial virus in Table 7C.	q24h
Rifabutin,[a] Mycobutin	150-mg cap ($$)	PO	5 mg/kg for MAC prophylaxis (II); 10–20 mg/kg for MAC or TB treatment (I); Max 300 mg/day	q24h

A. SYSTEMIC ANTIMICROBIALS WITH DOSAGE FORMS AND USUAL DOSAGES

Generic and Trade Names	Dosage Form (cost estimate)	Route	Dose (evidence level)	Interval
Rifampin,[a] Rifadin	150-, 300-mg cap ($) 600-mg vial ($$–$$$)	PO, IV	15–20 mg/kg, max 600 mg for active TB (in combination) (I) or as single-drug therapy for latent TB. Also for non-TB infections (see Ch 3) (II).	q24h
			With biweekly DOT, dosage is still 15–20 mg/kg/dose, max 600 mg.	Twice weekly
			20 mg/kg/day for 2 days for meningococcus prophylaxis, max 1.2 g/day (I)	q12h
Rifampin/isoniazid/pyrazinamide	75-/50-/150-mg dispersible tab available from the Stop TB Partnership global drug facility (www.stoptb.org/buyers; accessed August 15, 2024)	PO	4–7 kg: 1 tab 8–11 kg: 2 tab 12–15 kg: 3 tabs 16–24 kg: 4 tab	q24h
Rifamycin, Aemcolo	194-mg tab ($$)	PO	Adults: 2 tabs for TD (I)	q12h for 3 days
Rifapentine, Priftin	150-mg tab ($$)	PO	≥12 y and adults: 600 mg/dose (I)	Twice weekly
			>2 y, with INH for treatment of latent TB (I): 10–14 kg: 300 mg 14.1–25 kg: 450 mg 25.1–32 kg: 600 mg 32.1–50 kg: 750 mg >50 kg: 900 mg max	Once weekly
Rifaximin, Xifaxan	200-mg tab ($) 550-mg tab ($$$$) used for adults with IBS-D	PO	20–30 mg/kg/day (II) ≥12 y and adults: 600 mg/day (I) for TD	q8h

Drug	Dose Forms	Route	Dose	Interval
Sarecycline, Seysara	60-, 100-, 150-mg tabs ($$$)	PO	For acne (I): ≥9 y: 60 mg (not per kg) 55–84 kg: 100 mg >84 kg: 150 mg	q24h
Secnidazole, Solosec	2-g granules ($$)	PO	≥12 y: 2 g (I) ≥2 y: 30 mg/kg (III)	Once
Sofosbuvir, Sovaldi See Hepatitis C virus in Ch 7.	150-, 200-mg pellet packet 200-, 400-mg tab ($$$$$)	PO	Children ≥3 y (I): <17 kg: 150 mg 17–<35 kg: 200 mg ≥35 kg or ≥12 y: 400 mg	q24h
Sofosbuvir/ledipasvir,[a] Harvoni Doses given in sofosbuvir	150-/33.75-mg pellet packet 200-/45-mg pellet packet 200-/45-mg tab 400-/90-mg tab All forms ($$$$)	PO	Children ≥3 y (I): <17 kg: 37.5 mg ledipasvir with 150 mg sofosbuvir qd 17–<35 kg: 200 mg ≥35 kg: 400 mg (See Hepatitis C virus in Ch 7.)	q24h
Sofosbuvir/velpatasvir,[a] Epclusa Doses given in sofosbuvir	150-/37.5-mg, 200-/50-mg pellet packets ($$$$$) 200-/50-mg tab ($$$$) 400-/100-mg tab ($$$$)	PO	Children ≥3 y (I): <17 kg: 150 mg 17–<30 kg: 200 mg ≥30 kg: 400 mg See Hepatitis C virus in Ch 7.	q24h
Sofosbuvir/velpatasvir/voxilaprevir, Vosevi	400-/100-/100-mg tab ($$$$$)	PO	Adults: 1 tab (I) See Hepatitis C virus in Ch 7.	q24h
Streptomycin[a,b]	1-g vial ($$)	IM, IV	20–40 mg/kg/day, max 1 g/day (I)	q12–24h
Sulbactam/durlobactam, Xacduro	1-g sulbactam/1-g durlobactam vial (not yet commercially available as of May 25, 2023)	IV	≥18 y: 4 g/day (I)	q6h
Sulfadiazine[a]	500-mg tab ($$$)	PO	120–150 mg/kg/day, max 4–6 g/day (I) See Ch 9. Rheumatic fever secondary prophylaxis: 500 mg qd if ≤27 kg, 1,000 mg qd if >27 kg (II)	q6h q24h

A. SYSTEMIC ANTIMICROBIALS WITH DOSAGE FORMS AND USUAL DOSAGES

Generic and Trade Names	Dosage Form (cost estimate)	Route	Dose (evidence level)	Interval
Tafenoquine, Arakoda	100-mg tab ($$)	PO	Adults: 200 mg (I)	q24h for 3 days, then weekly
Tafenoquine, Krintafel	150-mg tab ($)	PO	≥16 y: 300 mg (I) See Malaria in Table 9B.	Once
Tecovirimat, Tpoxx	200-mg vial, cap Available from the Strategic National Stockpile (www.cdc.gov/poxvirus/mpox/clinicians/Tecovirimat.html; 770-488-7100)	IV	<35 kg: 12 mg/kg/day (I) 35–<120 kg: 400 mg/day (I) ≥120 kg: 600 mg/day (I)	q12h infused over 6 h
		PO	<6 kg: 100 mg/day (I) 6–<13 kg: 200 mg/day (I) 13–<25 kg: 400 mg/day (I) 25–<40 kg: 800 mg/day (I) 40–<120 kg: 1,200 mg/day (I) ≥120 kg: 1,800 mg/day (I)	q8h
Tedizolid, Sivextro	200-mg tab, vial ($$$$)	PO, IV	≥12 y and adults: 200 mg (I)[c]	q24h
Telavancin, Vibativ	250-, 750-mg vial ($$$$)	IV	Adults: 10 mg/kg (I)[c]	q24h
Tenofovir alafenamide, Vemlidy	25-mg tab ($$$$)	PO	≥12 y: 25 mg (I) for chronic HBV	q24h
Tenofovir disoproxil fumarate, Viread	40 mg per scoop pwd for mixing with soft food ($$$) 150-, 200-, 250-mg tab ($$$$) 300-mg tab[a] ($)	PO	≥2 y, PO pwd: 8 mg/kg (rounded to nearest 20 mg [½ scoop]) (I) Tab (I): 17–<22 kg: 150 mg (not per kg) 22–<28 kg: 200 mg 28–<35 kg: 250 mg ≥35 kg: 300 mg See Ch 7 for HBV and HIV-HBV coinfection use.	q24h

Drug	Dose Form	Dose	Route	Interval
Terbinafine,[a] Lamisil	250-mg tab ($)	Adults: 250 mg (I)	PO	q24h
Tetracycline[a]	250-, 500-mg cap ($)	≥8 y: 25–50 mg/kg/day (I)	PO	q6h
Tinidazole,[a] Tindamax	250-, 500-mg tab ($)	50 mg/kg, max 2 g (I) See Giardiasis in Table 9B.	PO	q24h
Tobramycin,[a] Nebcin	10-mg/mL vial ($) 40-mg/mL vial ($)	3–7.5 mg/kg/day (CF 7–10 mg/kg/day)[b]	IV, IM	q8–24h
Tobramycin inhalation[a]; Tobi, Bethkis	300-mg ampule ($$$$)	≥6 y: 600 mg/day (I)	Inhaled	q12h
Tobi Podhaler	28-mg cap for inhalation ($$$$)	≥6 y: 224 mg/day via Podhaler device (I)	Inhaled	q12h
Triclabendazole, Egaten	250-mg scored tab available from the WHO fascioliasis partnership (fasciola@who.int)	≥6 y (I): 20 mg/kg/day, given as 2 doses in 1 day See Flukes in Table 9B.	PO	q12h
Trimethoprim/sulfamethoxazole[a]; Bactrim, Septra	80-mg TMP/400-mg SMX tab (single-strength) ($) 160-mg TMP/800-mg SMX tab (DS) ($) 40-mg TMP/200-mg SMX per 5-mL PO susp ($) 16-mg TMP/80-mg SMX per mL injection soln in 5-, 10-, 30-mL vial ($$)	8 mg TMP/kg/day (I) Adults: 2 DS tabs/day (I) 12 mg TMP/kg/day for bacterial MIC 1, max 640 mg TMP/day (II)	PO, IV	q12h
		2 mg TMP/kg/day for UTI prophylaxis (I)		q24h
		15–20 mg TMP/kg/day for PCP treatment (I), no max		q6–8h
		150 mg TMP/m²/day for PCP prophylaxis, max 320 mg TMP/day (I)		q24h OR q12h 3×/wk

Systemic & Topical Antimicrobial Dosing & Dose Forms

18

A. SYSTEMIC ANTIMICROBIALS WITH DOSAGE FORMS AND USUAL DOSAGES

Generic and Trade Names	Dosage Form (cost estimate)	Route	Dose (evidence level)	Interval
Valacyclovir,[a] Valtrex	500-mg, 1-g tab ($) Recipe for preparing susp formulation provided in product labeling	PO	VZV: ≥3 mo: 60 mg/kg/day (I, II) HSV: ≥3 mo: 40 mg/kg/day (II) Max single dose 1 g (I)	q8h q12h
Valganciclovir,[a] Valcyte	250-mg/5-mL soln ($$) 450-mg tab ($$)	PO	Congenital CMV treatment: 32 mg/kg/day (II) (See Ch 2.)	q12h
			CMV prophylaxis (in mg, not mg/kg): 7 mg × BSA (m²) × CrCl (mL/min/1.73 m² with the modified Schwartz formula), max 900 mg (I) (See also Ch 7.)	q24h
Vancomycin, Vancocin	125-, 250-mg/5-mL susp ($–$$) 125-, 250-mg cap[a] ($–$$)	PO	40 mg/kg/day (I), max 500 mg/day (III)	q6h
	0.5-, 0.75-, 1-, 5-, 10-g vial[a] ($) 1.25-, 1.5-g vial ($–$$) 0.5-, 0.75-, 1-, 1.25-, 1.5-, 1.75-, 2-g IVPB ($$)	IV	30–45 mg/kg/day (I) For invasive MRSA infection, 60–80 mg/kg/day adjusted to achieve AUC:MIC 400, max 3,600 mg/day	q6–8h
Voriconazole,[a,b] Vfend See Aspergillosis in Table 5B.	200-mg/5-mL susp ($$$) 50-, 200-mg tab ($)	PO	≥2 y and <50 kg: 18 mg/kg/day, max 700 mg/day (I) ≥50 kg: 400–600 mg/day (I)	q12h
	200-mg vial ($$)	IV	≥2 y and <50 kg: 18 mg/kg/day LD for 1 day, then 16 mg/kg/day (I) ≥50 kg: 12 mg/kg/day LD for 1 day, then 8 mg/kg/day (I)	q12h
Zanamivir, Relenza	5-mg blister cap for inhalation ($)	Inhaled	Prophylaxis: ≥5 y: 10 mg/day (I)	q24h
			Treatment: ≥7 y: 20 mg/day (I)	q12h

[a] Available in a generic formulation.

[b] Monitor serum or plasma concentrations.

[c] Also currently under investigation in children younger than the age given for the listed dosages.

B. TOPICAL ANTIMICROBIALS (SKIN, EYE, EAR, MUCOSA)

Generic and Trade Names	Dosage Form	Route	Dose	Interval
Acyclovir, Sitavig	50-mg tab	Buccal	Adults: 50 mg, for herpes labialis	One time
Azithromycin, AzaSite	1% ophth soln	Ophth	1 drop	bid for 2 days, then qd for 5 days
Bacitracin[a]	Ophth oint	Ophth	Apply to affected eye.	q3–4h
	Oint[b]	Top	Apply to affected area.	bid–qid
Benzyl alcohol, Ulesfia	5% lotion	Top	Apply to scalp and hair.	Once; repeat in 7 days.
Berdazimer, Zelsuvmi	10.3% gel	Top	Apply to lesion.	Daily
Besifloxacin, Besivance	0.6% ophth susp	Ophth	≥1 y: 1 drop to affected eye	tid
Butenafine; Mentax, Lotrimin–Ultra	1% cream	Top	≥12 y: apply to affected area.	qd
Butoconazole, Gynazole-1	2% prefilled cream	Vag	Adults: 1 applicatorful	One time
Ciclopirox[a]; Loprox, Penlac	0.77% cream, gel, lotion	Top	≥10 y: apply to affected area.	bid
	1% shampoo		≥16 y: apply to scalp.	Twice weekly
	8% nail lacquer		≥12 y: apply to infected nail.	qd
Ciprofloxacin,[a] Cetraxal	0.2% otic soln	Otic	≥1 y: apply 3 drops to affected ear.	bid for 7 days
Ciprofloxacin, Ciloxan	0.3% ophth soln[a]	Ophth	Apply to affected eye.	q2h for 2 days, then q4h for 5 days
	0.3% ophth oint			q8h for 2 days, then q12h for 5 days
Ciprofloxacin, Otiprio	6% otic susp	Otic	≥6 mo: 0.1 mL each ear intratympanic, 0.2 mL to external ear canal for otitis externa	One time
Ciprofloxacin + dexamethasone, Ciprodex	0.3% + 0.1% otic soln	Otic	≥6 mo: apply 4 drops to affected ear.	bid for 7 days
Ciprofloxacin + fluocinolone, Otovel	0.3% + 0.025% otic soln	Otic	≥6 mo: instill 0.25 mL to affected ear.	bid for 7 days

B. TOPICAL ANTIMICROBIALS (SKIN, EYE, EAR, MUCOSA)

Generic and Trade Names	Dosage Form	Route	Dose	Interval
Ciprofloxacin + hydrocortisone, Cipro HC	0.2% + 1% otic soln	Otic	≥1 y: apply 3 drops to affected ear.	bid for 7 days
Clindamycin				
– Cleocin	100-mg ovule	Vag	1 ovule	qhs for 3 days
	2% vag cream[a]		1 applicatorful	qhs for 3–7 days
– Cleocin-T[a]	1% soln, gel, lotion	Top	Apply to affected area.	qd–bid
– Clindesse	2% cream	Vag	Adolescents and adults: 1 applicatorful	One time
– Evoclin[a]	1% foam			qd
– Xaciato	2% gel			One time
Clindamycin + adapalene benzoyl peroxide, Cabtreo	1.2%, 0.15% gel	Top	≥12 y: apply to affected area.	qd
Clindamycin + benzoyl peroxide, BenzaClin	1% gel[a]	Top	≥12 y: apply to affected area.	bid
– Acanya	1.2% gel		Apply small amount to face.	q24h
Clindamycin + tretinoin; Ziana, Veltin	1.2% gel	Top	Apply small amount to face.	hs
Clotrimazole,[a,b] Lotrimin	1% cream, lotion, soln	Top	Apply to affected area.	bid
– Gyne-Lotrimin-3[a,b]	2% cream	Vag	≥12 y: 1 applicatorful	qhs for 7–14 days
– Gyne-Lotrimin-7[a,b]	1% cream			qhs for 3 days
Clotrimazole + betamethasone,[a] Lotrisone	1% + 0.05% cream, lotion	Top	≥12 y: apply to affected area.	bid
Colistin + neomycin + hydrocortisone; Coly-Mycin S, Cortisporin TC otic	0.3% otic susp	Otic	Apply 3–4 drops to affected ear canal; may use with wick.	q6–8h
Cortisporin; bacitracin + neomycin + polymyxin B + hydrocortisone	Oint	Top	Apply to affected area.	bid–qid
Cortisporin; neomycin + polymyxin B + hydrocortisone	Otic soln[a]	Otic	3 drops to affected ear	bid–qid
	Cream	Top	Apply to affected area.	bid–qid

Dapsone,[a] Aczone	5% gel	Top	≥9 y: apply to affected area.	bid
	7.5% gel			qd
Econazole,[a] Spectazole	1% cream	Top	Apply to affected area.	qd–bid
Efinaconazole, Jublia	10% soln	Top	Apply to toenail.	qd for 48 wk
Erythromycin[a]	0.5% ophth oint	Ophth	Apply to affected eye.	q4h
– Akne-Mycin	2% oint	Top	Apply to affected area.	bid
– Ery Pads	2% pledgets[a]			
– Eryderm,[a] Erygel[a]	2% soln, gel			
Erythromycin + benzoyl peroxide,[a] Benzamycin	3% gel	Top	≥12 y: apply to affected area.	qd–bid
Ganciclovir, Zirgan	0.15% ophth gel	Ophth	≥2 y: 1 drop in affected eye	q3h while awake (5 times daily) until healed, then tid for 7 days
Gatifloxacin, Zymar	0.3% ophth soln	Ophth	1 drop in affected eye	q2h for 2 days, then q6h
Gatifloxacin,[a] Zymaxid	0.5% ophth soln	Ophth	≥1 y: 1 drop in affected eye	q2h for 1 day, then q6h
Gentamicin,[a] Garamycin	0.1% cream, oint	Top	Apply to affected area.	tid–qid
	0.3% ophth soln, oint	Ophth	Apply to affected eye.	q1–4h (soln) q4–8h (oint)
Gentamicin + prednisolone, Pred-G	0.3% ophth soln, oint	Ophth	Adults: apply to affected eye.	q1–4h (soln) qd–tid (oint)
Imiquimod,[a] Aldara	5% cream	Top	≥12 y: to perianal or external genital warts	3×/wk

B. TOPICAL ANTIMICROBIALS (SKIN, EYE, EAR, MUCOSA)

Generic and Trade Names	Dosage Form	Route	Dose	Interval
Ivermectin, Sklice	0.5% lotion	Top	≥6 mo: thoroughly coat hair and scalp; rinse after 10 minutes.	Once
Ivermectin,[a] Soolantra	1% cream	Top	Adults: apply to face.	qd
Ketoconazole,[a] Nizoral	2% shampoo	Top	≥12 y: apply to affected area.	qd
	2% cream			qd–bid
– Extina, Xolegel	2% foam, gel			bid
– Nizoral A-D	1% shampoo			bid
Levofloxacin[a]; Quixin, Iquix	0.5%, 1.5% ophth soln	Ophth	Apply to affected eye.	q1–4h
Luliconazole, Luzu	1% cream	Top	≥12 y: apply to affected area.	q24h for 1–2 wk
Mafenide, Sulfamylon	8.5% cream	Top	Apply to burn.	qd–bid
	5-g pwd for reconstitution		To keep burn dressing wet	q4–8h as needed
Malathion,[a] Ovide	0.5% soln	Top	≥6 y: apply to hair and scalp.	Once
Maxitrol[a]; neomycin + polymyxin + dexamethasone	Susp, oint	Ophth	Apply to affected eye.	q1–4h (susp) q4h (oint)
Metronidazole[a]	0.75% cream, gel, lotion	Top	Adults: apply to affected area.	bid
	0.75% vag gel	Vag	Adults: 1 applicatorful	qd–bid
	1% gel	Top	Adults: apply to affected area.	qd
Noritate	1% cream	Top	Adults: apply to affected area.	qd
Nuvessa	1.3% vag gel	Vag	≥12 y: 1 applicatorful	Once
Miconazole				
– Fungoid[a,b]	2% tincture	Top	Apply to affected area.	bid

Drug	Dose form	Route	Instructions	Frequency
– Micatin[a,b] and others	2% cream, pwd, oint, spray, lotion, gel	Top	Apply to affected area.	qd–bid
– Monistat-1[a,b]	1.2-g ovule + 2% cream	Vag	≥12 y: insert one ovule (plus cream to external vulva bid as needed).	Once
– Monistat-3[a,b]	200-mg ovule, 4% cream			qhs for 3 days
– Monistat-7[a,b]	100-mg ovule, 2% cream			qhs for 7 days
– Vusion	0.25% oint	Top	To diaper dermatitis	Each diaper change for 7 days
Minocycline, Amzeeq	4% foam	Top	≥9 y: apply to acne.	qd
Moxifloxacin, Vigamox	0.5% ophth soln	Ophth	Apply to affected eye.	tid
Mupirocin,[a] Bactroban	2% oint, cream	Top	Apply to infected skin.	tid
Naftifine,[a] Naftin	1%, 2% cream, gel	Top	Apply to affected area.	qd
Natamycin, Natacyn	5% ophth soln	Ophth	Adults: apply to affected eye.	q1–4h
Neosporin[a]				
– bacitracin + neomycin + polymyxin B	Ophth oint	Ophth	Apply to affected eye.	q4h
	Oint[a,b]	Top	Apply to affected area.	bid–qid
– gramicidin + neomycin + polymyxin B	Ophth soln	Ophth	Apply to affected eye.	q4h
Nystatin,[a] Mycostatin	100,000 U/g cream, oint, pwd	Top	Apply to affected area.	bid–qid
Nystatin + triamcinolone,[a] Mycolog II	100,000 U/g + 0.1% cream, oint	Top	Apply to affected area.	bid
Ofloxacin[a], Floxin Otic, Ocuflox	0.3% otic soln	Otic	5–10 drops to affected ear	qd–bid
	0.3% ophth soln	Ophth	Apply to affected eye.	q1–6h
Oxiconazole, Oxistat	1% cream,[a] lotion	Top	Apply to affected area.	qd–bid
Ozenoxacin, Xepi	1% cream	Top	Apply to affected area.	bid for 5 days

Systemic & Topical Antimicrobial Dosing & Dose Forms

18

18

B. TOPICAL ANTIMICROBIALS (SKIN, EYE, EAR, MUCOSA)

Generic and Trade Names	Dosage Form	Route	Dose	Interval
Permethrin, Nix[a,b]	1% cream	Top	Apply to hair/scalp.	Once for 10 min
– Elimite[a]	5% cream		Apply to all skin surfaces.	Once for 8–14 h
Piperonyl butoxide + pyrethrins,[a,b] Rid	4% + 0.3% shampoo, gel	Top	Apply to affected area.	Once for 10 min
Polysporin,[a] polymyxin B + bacitracin	Ophth oint	Ophth	Apply to affected eye.	qd–tid
	Oint[b]	Top	Apply to affected area.	
Polytrim,[a] polymyxin B + trimethoprim	Ophth soln	Ophth	Apply to affected eye.	q3–4h
Retapamulin, Altabax	1% oint	Top	Apply thin layer to affected area.	bid for 5 days
Selenium sulfide,[a] Selsun	2.5% lotion 2.25% shampoo	Top	Lather into scalp or affected area.	Twice weekly, then q1–2wk
– Selsun Blue[a,b]	1% shampoo			qd
Sertaconazole, Ertaczo	2% cream	Top	≥12 y: apply to affected area.	bid
Silver sulfadiazine,[a] Silvadene	1% cream	Top	Apply to affected area.	qd–bid
Spinosad,[a] Natroba	0.9% susp	Top	Apply to scalp and hair.	Once; may repeat in 7 days
Sulconazole, Exelderm	1% soln, cream	Top	Adults: apply to affected area.	qd–bid
Sulfacetamide sodium[a]	10% soln	Ophth	Apply to affected eye.	q1–3h
	10% ophth oint			q4–6h
	10% lotion, wash, cream	Top	≥12 y: apply to affected area.	bid–qid
Sulfacetamide sodium + prednisolone,[a] Blephamide	10% ophth oint, soln	Ophth	Apply to affected eye.	tid–qid
Tavaborole, Kerydin	5% soln	Top	Adults: apply to toenail.	qd for 48 wk
Terbinafine,[b] Lamisil-AT	1% cream,[a] spray, gel	Top	Apply to affected area.	qd–bid

Terconazole,[a] Terazol	0.4% cream	Vag	Adults:
			1 applicatorful qhs for 7 days
	0.8% cream		1 applicatorful or qhs for 3 days
	80-mg suppository		1 suppository
Tioconazole[a,b]	6.5% oint	Vag	≥12 y: 1 applicatorful One time
Tobramycin, Tobrex	0.3% soln,[a] oint	Ophth	Apply to affected eye. q1–4h (soln)
			q4–8h (oint)
Tobramycin + dexamethasone, Tobradex	0.3% soln,[a] oint	Ophth	Apply to affected eye. q2–6h (soln)
			q6–8h (oint)
Tobramycin + loteprednol, Zylet	0.3% + 0.5% ophth susp	Ophth	Adults: apply to affected eye. q4–6h
Tolnaftate,[a,b] Tinactin	1% cream, soln, pwd, spray	Top	Apply to affected area. bid
Trifluridine,[a] Viroptic	1% ophth soln	Ophth	1 drop (max 9 drops/day) q2h

[a] Generic available.
[b] Over the counter.

Appendix

Nomogram for Determining Body Surface Area

Based on the nomogram shown below, a straight line joining the patient's height and weight will intersect the center column at the calculated body surface area (BSA). For children of normal height for weight, the child's weight in pounds is used, and then the examiner reads across to the corresponding BSA in meters. Alternatively, the Mosteller formula can be used.

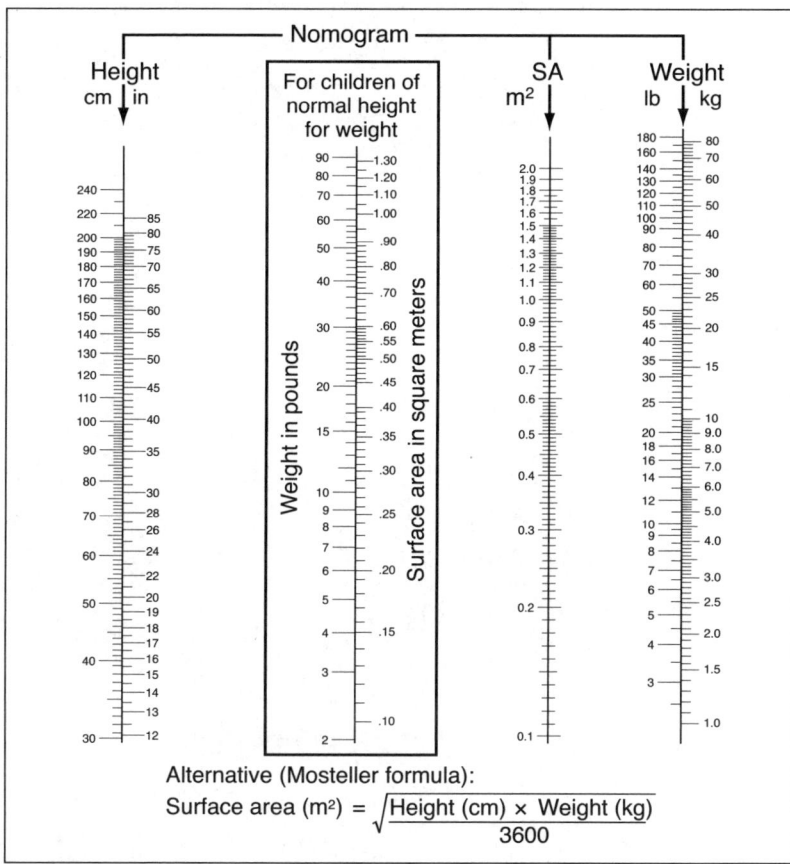

Alternative (Mosteller formula):

$$\text{Surface area (m}^2) = \sqrt{\frac{\text{Height (cm)} \times \text{Weight (kg)}}{3600}}$$

References

Chapter 1

1. Hultén KG, et al. *Pediatr Infect Dis J.* 2018;37(3):235–241 PMID: 28859018
2. Prochaska EC, et al. *Antimicrob Steward Healthc Epidemiol.* 2023;3(1):e12 PMID: 36714287
3. Stevens DL, et al. *Clin Infect Dis.* 2014;59(2):147–159 PMID: 24947530
4. Liu C, et al. *Clin Infect Dis.* 2011;52(3):e18–e55 PMID: 21208910
5. Brown NM, et al. *JAC Antimicrob Resist.* 2021;3(1):dlaa114 PMID: 34223066
6. AAP. *Staphylococcus aureus.* In: Kimberlin DW, et al, eds. *Red Book: 2024–2027 Report of the Committee on Infectious Diseases.* 33rd ed. 2024:767–782
7. AAP. Group A streptococcal infections. In: Kimberlin DW, et al, eds. *Red Book: 2024–2027 Report of the Committee on Infectious Diseases.* 33rd ed. 2024:785–798
8. Klotz SA, et al. *Am Fam Physician.* 2011;83(2):152–155 PMID: 21243990
9. Hatzenbuehler LA, et al. *Pediatr Infect Dis J.* 2014;33(1):89–91 PMID: 24346597
10. Muñoz-Egea MC, et al. *Expert Opin Pharmacother.* 2020;21(8):969–981 PMID: 32200657
11. Zimmermann P, et al. *J Infect.* 2017;74(suppl 1):S136–S142 PMID: 28646953
12. Tebruegge M, et al. *PLoS One.* 2016;11(1):e0147513 PMID: 26812154
13. Aliano D, et al. *Pediatr Infect Dis J.* 2020;39(8):671–677 PMID: 32235244
14. Neven Q, et al. *Eur Arch Otorhinolaryngol.* 2020;277(6):1785–1792 PMID: 32144570
15. Nolt D, et al. *Pediatrics.* 2021;148(6):e2021054663 PMID: 34851422
16. AAP. Tuberculosis. In: Kimberlin DW, et al, eds. *Red Book: 2024–2027 Report of the Committee on Infectious Diseases.* 33rd ed. 2024:888–920
17. Bradley JS, et al. *Pediatrics.* 2014;133(5):e1411–e1436 PMID: 24777226
18. Oehler RL, et al. *Lancet Infect Dis.* 2009;9(7):439–447 PMID: 19555903
19. Thomas N, et al. *Expert Rev Anti Infect Ther.* 2011;9(2):215–226 PMID: 21342069
20. Bula-Rudas FJ, et al. *Pediatr Rev.* 2018;39(10):490–500 PMID: 30275032
21. AAP. Bite wounds. In: Kimberlin DW, et al, eds. *Red Book: 2024–2027 Report of the Committee on Infectious Diseases.* 33rd ed. 2024:202–206
22. Talan DA, et al. *N Engl J Med.* 1999;340(2):85–92 PMID: 9887159
23. Goldstein EJ, et al. *Antimicrob Agents Chemother.* 2012;56(12):6319–6323 PMID: 23027193
24. AAP. Rabies. In: Kimberlin DW, et al, eds. *Red Book: 2024–2027 Report of the Committee on Infectious Diseases.* 33rd ed. 2024:702–711
25. Talan DA, et al. *Clin Infect Dis.* 2003;37(11):1481–1489 PMID: 14614671
26. Miller LG, et al. *N Engl J Med.* 2015;372(12):1093–1103 PMID: 25785967
27. Talan DA, et al. *N Engl J Med.* 2016;374(9):823–832 PMID: 26962903
28. Moran GJ, et al. *JAMA.* 2017;317(20):2088–2096 PMID: 28535235
29. Bradley J, et al. *Pediatrics.* 2017;139(3):e20162477 PMID: 28202770
30. AAP. *Haemophilus influenzae* infections. In: Kimberlin DW, et al, eds. *Red Book: 2024–2027 Report of the Committee on Infectious Diseases.* 33rd ed. 2024:400–409
31. Brindle R, et al. *JAMA Dermatol.* 2019;155(9):1033–1040 PMID: 31188407
32. Koning S, et al. *Cochrane Database Syst Rev.* 2012;(1):CD003261 PMID: 22258953
33. Bridwell R, et al. *Am J Emerg Med.* 2021;41:1–5 PMID: 33383265
34. Vij N, et al. *J Pediatr Orthop.* 2021;41(9):e849–e854 PMID: 34411048
35. Hedetoft M, et al. *BMJ Open.* 2023;13(2):e066117 PMID: 36813488
36. Schröder A, et al. *BMC Infect Dis.* 2019;19(1):317 PMID: 30975101
37. Zundel S, et al. *Eur J Pediatr Surg.* 2017;27(2):127–137 PMID: 27380058
38. Totapally BR. *Pediatr Infect Dis J.* 2017;36(7):641–644 PMID: 28005689
39. Levett D, et al. *Cochrane Database Syst Rev.* 2015;(1):CD007937 PMID: 25879088
40. Stevens DL, et al. *Infect Dis Clin North Am.* 2021;35(1):135–155 PMID: 33303335
41. Daum RS. *N Engl J Med.* 2007;357(4):380–390 PMID: 17652653
42. Sharara SL, et al. *Infect Dis Clin North Am.* 2021;35(1):107–133 PMID: 33303331
43. Elliott SP. *Clin Microbiol Rev.* 2007;20(1):13–22 PMID: 17223620

44. AAP. Rat-bite fever. In: Kimberlin DW, et al, eds. *Red Book: 2024–2027 Report of the Committee on Infectious Diseases*. 33rd ed. 2024:711–713
45. Braunstein I, et al. *Pediatr Dermatol*. 2014;31(3):305–308 PMID: 24033633
46. Liy-Wong C, et al. *Pediatr Dermatol*. 2021;38(1):149–153 PMID: 33283348
47. Woods CR, et al. *J Pediatric Infect Dis Soc*. 2021:10(8):801–844 PMID: 34350458
48. Woods CR, et al. *J Pediatric Infect Dis Soc*. 2024:13(1):1–59 PMID: 37941444
49. Saavedra-Lozano J, et al. *Pediatr Infect Dis J*. 2017;36(8):788–799 PMID: 28708801
50. Keren R, et al. *JAMA Pediatr*. 2015;169(2):120–128 PMID: 25506733
51. McNeil JC, et al. *Pediatr Infect Dis J*. 2017;36(6):572–577 PMID: 28027279
52. Pääkkönen M. *Pediatric Health Med Ther*. 2017;8:65–68 PMID: 29388627
53. Arnold JC, et al. *Pediatrics*. 2012;130(4):e821–e828 PMID: 22966033
54. Chou AC, et al. *J Pediatr Orthop*. 2016;36(2):173–177 PMID: 25929777
55. Delgado-Noguera MF, et al. *Cochrane Database Syst Rev*. 2018;(11):CD012125 PMID: 30480764
56. Workowski KA, et al. *Clin Infect Dis*. 2022;74(suppl 2):S89–S94 PMID: 35416966
57. McDaniel LM, et al. *J Pediatr Infect Dis Soc*. 2023;12(1):534–539 PMID: 37757866
58. McNeil JC, et al. *Pediatr Infect Dis J*. 2021;40(6):518–524 PMID: 33902075
59. Workowski KA, et al. *MMWR Recomm Rep*. 2021;70(4):1–187 PMID: 34292926
60. AAP. Gonococcal infections. In: Kimberlin DW, et al, eds. *Red Book: 2024–2027 Report of the Committee on Infectious Diseases*. 33rd ed. 2024:394–399
61. Peltola H, et al. *N Engl J Med*. 2014;370(4):352–360 PMID: 24450893
62. Funk SS, et al. *Orthop Clin North Am*. 2017;48(2):199–208 PMID: 28336042
63. Messina AF, et al. *Pediatr Infect Dis J*. 2011;30(12):1019–1021 PMID: 21817950
64. Howard-Jones AR, et al. *J Paediatr Child Health*. 2013;49(9):760–768 PMID: 23745943
65. De Marco G, et al. *Front Pediatr*. 2022;10:1043251 PMID: 36601031
66. Chen CJ, et al. *Pediatr Infect Dis J*. 2007;26(11):985–988 PMID: 17984803
67. Volk A, et al. *Pediatr Emerg Care*. 2017;33(11):724–729 PMID: 26785095
68. Kornelsen E, et al. *Cochrane Database Syst Rev*. 2021;(4):CD013535 PMID: 33908631
69. McKenna D, et al. *Clin Case Rep*. 2019;7(3):593–594 PMID: 30899507
70. Seltz LB, et al. *Pediatrics*. 2011;127(3):e566–e572 PMID: 21321025
71. Anosike BI, et al. *J Pediatric Infect Dis Soc*. 2022;11(5):214–220 PMID: 35438766
72. Saltagi MZ, et al. *Allergy Rhinol (Providence)*. 2022;13:21526575221097311 PMID: 35496892
73. McDermott SM, et al. *Otolaryngol Head Neck Surg*. 2020;163(4):814–821 PMID: 32396416
74. Murphy DC, et al. *J Paediatr Child Health*. 2021;57(2):227–233 PMID: 32987452
75. Williams KJ, et al. *Curr Opin Ophthalmol*. 2019;30(5):349–355 PMID: 31261188
76. Chen YY, et al. *Cochrane Database Syst Rev*. 2023;(3):CD001211 PMID: 36912752
77. Johnson D, et al. *JAMA*. 2022;327(22):2231–2237 PMID: 35699701
78. Wilhelmus KR. *Cochrane Database Syst Rev*. 2015;(1):CD002898 PMID: 25879115
79. Sibley D, et al. *Eye (Lond)*. 2020;34(12):2219–2226 PMID: 32843744
80. Wilhelmus KR, et al. *Ophthalmology*. 2020;127(4)(suppl):S5–S18 PMID: 32200827
81. Ali MJ. *Ophthalmic Plast Reconstr Surg*. 2015;31(5):341–347 PMID: 25856337
82. Khan S, et al. *J Pediatr Ophthalmol Strabismus*. 2014;51(3):140–153 PMID: 24877526
83. Slean GR, et al. *Clin Exp Ophthalmol*. 2017;45(5):481–488 PMID: 28013528
84. Birnbaum F, et al. *EyeNet Magazine*. 2016:33–35
85. Pappas PG, et al. *Clin Infect Dis*. 2016;62(4):e1–e50 PMID: 26679628
86. Bragg KJ, et al. Hordeolum. In: StatPearls. StatPearls Publishing; 2023 PMID: 28723014
87. Munro M, et al. *Microorganisms*. 2019;8(1):55 PMID: 31905656
88. Groth A, et al. *Int J Pediatr Otorhinolaryngol*. 2012;76(10):1494–1500 PMID: 22832239
89. Loh R, et al. *J Laryngol Otol*. 2018;132(2):96–104 PMID: 28879826
90. Laulajainen-Hongisto A, et al. *Int J Pediatr Otorhinolaryngol*. 2014;78(12):2072–2078 PMID: 25281339
91. Chong LY, et al. *Cochrane Database Syst Rev*. 2021;(2):CD013053 PMID: 33561891
92. Hussain SZM, et al. *Cureus*. 2022;14(12):e32780 PMID: 36686080
93. Khatri H, et al. *Emerg Med Australas*. 2021;33(6):961–965 PMID: 34569162
94. Rosenfeld RM, et al. *Otolaryngol Head Neck Surg*. 2014;150(1)(suppl):S1–S24 PMID: 24491310
95. Izurieta P, et al. *Hum Vaccin Immunother*. 2022;18(1):2013693 PMID: 35020530

96. Vadlamudi NK, et al. *J Antimicrob Chemother*. 2021;76(9):2419–2427 PMID: 34021757

97. Wald ER, et al. *Pediatr Infect Dis J*. 2018;37(12):1255–1257 PMID: 29570583

98. Lieberthal AS, et al. *Pediatrics*. 2013;131(3):e964–e999 PMID: 23439909

99. Venekamp RP, et al. *Cochrane Database Syst Rev*. 2015;(6):CD000219 PMID: 26099233

100. Shaikh N, et al. *J Pediatr*. 2017;189:54–60.e3 PMID: 28666536

101. Suzuki HG, et al. *BMJ Open*. 2020;10(5):e035343 PMID: 32371515

102. Van Dyke MK, et al. *Pediatr Infect Dis J*. 2017;36(3):274–281 PMID: 27918383

103. Frost HM, et al. *J Pediatr*. 2022;251:98–104.e5 PMID: 35944719

104. Sader HS, et al. *Open Forum Infect Dis*. 2019;6(suppl 1):S14–S23 PMID: 30895211

105. Gregory J, et al. *JAMA Netw Open*. 2021;4(3):e212713 PMID: 33755168

106. Wald ER, et al. *Pediatrics*. 2013;132(1):e262–e280 PMID: 23796742

107. Shaikh N, et al. *Cochrane Database Syst Rev*. 2014;(10):CD007909 PMID: 25347280

108. Chow AW, et al. *Clin Infect Dis*. 2012;54(8):e72–e112 PMID: 22438350

109. Ogle OE. *Dent Clin North Am*. 2017;61(2):235–252 PMID: 28317564

110. Cooper L, et al. *Evid Based Dent*. Published online September 7, 2022 PMID: 36071280

111. AAP. Diphtheria. In: Kimberlin DW, et al, eds. *Red Book: 2024–2027 Report of the Committee on Infectious Diseases*. 33rd ed. 2024:357–361

112. Tibballs J, et al. *J Paediatr Child Health*. 2011;47(3):77–82 PMID: 21091577

113. Sobol SE, et al. *Otolaryngol Clin North Am*. 2008;41(3):551–566 PMID: 18435998

114. Nasser M, et al. *Cochrane Database Syst Rev*. 2008;(4):CD006700 PMID: 18843726

115. Amir J, et al. *BMJ*. 1997;314(7097):1800–1803 PMID: 9224082

116. Kimberlin DW, et al. *Clin Infect Dis*. 2010;50(2):221–228 PMID: 20014952

117. Riordan T. *Clin Microbiol Rev*. 2007;20(4):622–659 PMID: 17934077

118. Correia MS, et al. *J Emerg Med*. 2019;56(6):709–712 PMID: 31229258

119. Ridgway JM, et al. *Am J Otolaryngol*. 2010;31(1):38–45 PMID: 19944898

120. Lee WS, et al. *J Microbiol Immunol Infect*. 2020;53(4):513–517 PMID: 32303484

121. Valerio L, et al. *J Intern Med*. 2021;289(3):325–339 PMID: 32445216

122. Esposito S, et al. *Children (Basel)*. 2022;9(5):618 PMID: 35626793

123. Hur K, et al. *Laryngoscope*. 2018;128(1):72–77 PMID: 28561258

124. Shulman ST, et al. *Clin Infect Dis*. 2012;55(10):e86–e102 PMID: 22965026

125. van Driel ML, et al. *Cochrane Database Syst Rev*. 2021;(3):CD004406 PMID: 33728634

126. Skoog Ståhlgren G, et al. *BMJ*. 2019;367:l5337 PMID: 31585944

127. Altamimi S, et al. *Cochrane Database Syst Rev*. 2012;(8):CD004872 PMID: 22895944

128. Abdel-Haq N, et al. *Pediatr Infect Dis J*. 2012;31(7):696–699 PMID: 22481424

129. Cheng J, et al. *Otolaryngol Head Neck Surg*. 2013;148(6):1037–1042 PMID: 23520072

130. Casazza G, et al. *Otolaryngol Head Neck Surg*. 2019;160(3):546–549 PMID: 30348058

131. de Benedictis FM, et al. *Lancet*. 2020;396(10253):786–798 PMID: 32919518

132. Ramgopal S, et al. *Pediatr Emerg Care*. 2017;33(2):112–115 PMID: 26785088

133. Brook I. *J Chemother*. 2016;28(3):143–150 PMID: 26365224

134. Wardlaw AJ, et al. *J Asthma Allergy*. 2021;14:557–573 PMID: 34079294

135. Mathew JL, et al. *Indian J Pediatr*. 2023;90(7):708–717 PMID: 37264275

136. Agarwal R, et al. *Chest*. 2018;153(3):656–664 PMID: 29331473

137. Meissner HC. *N Engl J Med*. 2016;374(1):62–72 PMID: 26735994

138. Magréault S, et al. *Clin Pharmacokinet*. 2021;60(4):409–445 PMID: 33486720

139. Hahn A, et al. *J Pediatr Pharmacol Ther*. 2018;23(5):379–389 PMID: 30429692

140. Chmiel JF, et al. *Ann Am Thorac Soc*. 2014;11(7):1120–1129 PMID: 25102221

141. Flume PA, et al. *Am J Respir Crit Care Med*. 2009;180(9):802–808 PMID: 19729669

142. Saint GL, et al. *Arch Dis Child*. 2022;107(5):479–485 PMID: 34740877

143. Milinic T, et al. *Semin Respir Crit Care Med*. 2023;44(2):225–241 PMID: 36746183

144. Chmiel JF, et al. *Ann Am Thorac Soc*. 2014;11(8):1298–1306 PMID: 25167882

145. Waters V, et al. *Cochrane Database Syst Rev*. 2020;(6):CD010004 PMID: 32521055

146. Cogen JD, et al. *Ann Am Thorac Soc*. 2020;17(12):1590–1598 PMID: 32726564

147. Smith S, et al. *Cochrane Database Syst Rev*. 2020;(5):CD006961 PMID: 32412092

148. Langton Hewer SC, et al. *Cochrane Database Syst Rev*. 2023;(6):CD004197 PMID: 37268599

149. Smith S, et al. *Cochrane Database Syst Rev.* 2022;(11):CD001021 PMID: 36373968
150. Flume PA, et al. *J Cyst Fibros.* 2016;15(6):809–815 PMID: 27233377
151. Mogayzel PJ Jr, et al. *Am J Respir Crit Care Med.* 2013;187(7):680–689 PMID: 23540878
152. Southern KW, et al. *Cochrane Database Syst Rev.* 2012;(11):CD002203 PMID: 23152214
153. Li D, et al. *Antibiotics (Basel).* 2023;12(3):484 PMID: 36978351
154. Nichols DP, et al. *Thorax.* 2022;77(6):581–588 PMID: 34706982
155. AAP. Pertussis. In: Kimberlin DW, et al, eds. *Red Book: 2024–2027 Report of the Committee on Infectious Diseases.* 33rd ed. 2024:656–667
156. Kilgore PE, et al. *Clin Microbiol Rev.* 2016;29(3):449–486 PMID: 27029594
157. Wang K, et al. *Cochrane Database Syst Rev.* 2014;(9):CD003257 PMID: 25243777
158. Jain S, et al. *N Engl J Med.* 2015;372(9):835–845 PMID: 25714161
159. Bradley JS, et al. *Clin Infect Dis.* 2011;53(7):e25–e76 PMID: 21880587
160. Blumer JL, et al. *Pediatr Infect Dis J.* 2016;35(7):760–766 PMID: 27078119
161. Ambroggio L, et al. *Pediatr Pulmonol.* 2016;51(5):541–548 PMID: 26367389
162. Williams DJ, et al. *JAMA Pediatr.* 2017;171(12):1184–1191 PMID: 29084336
163. Bielicki JA, et al. *JAMA.* 2021;326(17):1713–1724 PMID: 34726708
164. Same RG, et al. *J Pediatric Infect Dis Soc.* 2021;10(3):267–273 PMID: 32525203
165. Dorman RM, et al. *J Pediatr Surg.* 2016;51(6):885–890 PMID: 27032611
166. Islam S, et al. *J Pediatr Surg.* 2012;47(11):2101–2110 PMID: 23164006
167. Redden MD, et al. *Cochrane Database Syst Rev.* 2017;(3):CD010651 PMID: 28304084
168. Pacilli M, et al. *Paediatr Resp Rev.* 2019;30:42–48 PMID: 31130425
169. Derderian SC, et al. *J Pediatr Surg.* 2020;55(11):2356–2361 PMID: 31973927
170. Dworsky ZD, et al. *Hosp Pediatr.* 2022;12(4):377–384 PMID: 35233619
171. Randolph AG, et al. *Clin Infect Dis.* 2019;68(3):365–372 PMID: 29893805
172. Bradley JS, et al. *Pediatr Infect Dis J.* 2007;26(10):868–878 PMID: 17901791
173. Hidron AI, et al. *Lancet Infect Dis.* 2009;9(6):384–392 PMID: 19467478
174. Frush JM, et al. *J Hosp Med.* 2018;13(12):848–852 PMID: 30379141
175. Wunderink RG, et al. *Clin Infect Dis.* 2012;54(5):621–629 PMID: 22247123
176. Lehrnbecher T, et al. *J Clin Oncol.* 2023;41(9):1774–1785 PMID: 36689694
177. Kalil AC, et al. *Clin Infect Dis.* 2016;63(5):e61–e111 PMID: 27418577
178. Chang I, et al. *Paediatr Respir Rev.* 2016;20:10–16 PMID: 26527358
179. Sweeney DA, et al. *Clin Microbiol Infect.* 2019;25(10):1195–1199 PMID: 31035015
180. AAP. Chlamydial infections. In: Kimberlin DW, et al, eds. *Red Book: 2024–2027 Report of the Committee on Infectious Diseases.* 33rd ed. 2024:298–308
181. AAP. Cytomegalovirus infection. In: Kimberlin DW, et al, eds. *Red Book: 2024–2027 Report of the Committee on Infectious Diseases.* 33rd ed. 2024:344–352
182. Balani SS, et al. *Front Pediatr.* 2023;11:1098434 PMID: 36891229
183. Limaye AP, et al. *Clin Microbiol Rev.* 2020;34(1):e00043-19 PMID: 33115722
184. Danziger-Isakov L, et al. *J Pediatric Infect Dis Soc.* 2018;7(suppl 2):S72–S74 PMID: 30590625
185. AAP. Tularemia. In: Kimberlin DW, et al, eds. *Red Book: 2024–2027 Report of the Committee on Infectious Diseases.* 33rd ed. 2024:929–932
186. Galgiani JN, et al. *Clin Infect Dis.* 2016;63(6):e112–e146 PMID: 27470238
187. AAP. Coccidioidomycosis. In: Kimberlin DW, et al, eds. *Red Book: 2024–2027 Report of the Committee on Infectious Diseases.* 33rd ed. 2024:320–324
188. AAP. Histoplasmosis. In: Kimberlin DW, et al, eds. *Red Book: 2024–2027 Report of the Committee on Infectious Diseases.* 33rd ed. 2024:478–482
189. Barros N, et al. *J Fungi (Basel).* 2023;9(2):236 PMID: 36836350
190. Arrieta AC, et al. *Infect Dis Ther.* 2023;12(6):1465–1485 PMID: 37209297
191. Salmanton-García J, et al. *J Antimicrob Chemother.* 2019;74(11):3315–3327 PMID: 31393591
192. Uyeki TM, et al. *Clin Infect Dis.* 2019;68(6):895–902 PMID: 30834445
193. AAP Committee on Infectious Disease. *Pediatrics.* 2022;150(4):e2022059274 PMID: 36065749
194. Kimberlin DW, et al. *J Infect Dis.* 2013;207(5):709–720 PMID: 23230059
195. Stewart AG, et al. *Open Forum Infect Dis.* 2021;8(8):ofab387 PMID: 34395716
196. Lu B, et al. *J Antimicrob Chemother.* 2023;78(4):1009–1014 PMID: 36879495

197. Daley CL, et al. *Clin Infect Dis.* 2020;71(4):905–913 PMID: 32797222
198. Gardiner SJ. *Cochrane Database Syst Rev.* 2015;(1):CD004875 PMID: 25566754
199. Lee H, et al. *Expert Rev Anti Infect Ther.* 2018;16(1):23–34 PMID: 29212389
200. Panel on Opportunistic Infections in Children With and Exposed to HIV. Guidelines for the prevention and treatment of opportunistic infections in children with and exposed to HIV. *Pneumocystis jirovecii* pneumonia. Updated November 6, 2013. Accessed October 29, 2024. https://clinicalinfo.hiv.gov/en/guidelines/hiv-clinical-guidelines-pediatric-opportunistic-infections/pneumocycstis-jirovecii-pneumonia
201. Caselli D, et al. *J Pediatr.* 2014;164(2):389–392.e1 PMID: 24252793
202. Karruli A, et al. *Antibiotics (Basel).* 2023;12(2):399 PMID: 36830309
203. Reynolds D, et al. *Drugs.* 2021;81(18):2117–2131 PMID: 34743315
204. AAP. Respiratory syncytial virus. In: Kimberlin DW, et al, eds. *Red Book: 2024–2027 Report of the Committee on Infectious Diseases.* 33rd ed. 2024:713–721
205. Nahid P, et al. *Am J Respir Crit Care Med.* 2019;200(10):e93–e142 PMID: 31729908
206. Jaganath D, et al. *Infect Dis Clin North Am.* 2022;36(1):49–71 PMID: 35168714
207. Sterling TR, et al. *MMWR Recomm Rep.* 2020;69(1):1–11 PMID: 32053584
208. Pantell RH, et al. *Pediatrics.* 2021;148(2):e2021052228 PMID: 34281996
209. Aronson PL, et al. *Pediatrics.* 2018;142(6):e20181879 PMID: 30425130
210. Aronson PL, et al. *Pediatrics.* 2019;144(1):e20183604 PMID: 31167938
211. Greenhow TL, et al. *Pediatrics.* 2017;139(4):e20162098 PMID: 28283611
212. Yaeger JP, et al. *J Hosp Med.* 2022;17(11):893–900 PMID: 36036211
213. Kuppermann N, et al. *JAMA Pediatr.* 2019;173(4):342–351 PMID: 30776077
214. McMullan BJ, et al. *JAMA Pediatr.* 2016;170(10):979–986 PMID: 27533601
215. Ruiz J, et al. *Minerva Pediatr (Torino).* 22;74(5):525–529 PMID: 29651827
216. Russell CD, et al. *J Med Microbiol.* 2014;63(pt 6):841–848 PMID: 24623637
217. Ligon J, et al. *Pediatr Infect Dis J.* 2014;33(5):e132–e134 PMID: 24732394
218. Arrieta AC, et al. *Pediatr Infect Dis J.* 2018;37(9):893–900 PMID: 29406465
219. Baddour LM, et al. *Circulation.* 2015;132(15):1435–1486 PMID: 26373316
220. Baltimore RS, et al. *Circulation.* 2015;132(15):1487–1515 PMID: 26373317
221. Eleyan L, et al. *Eur J Pediatr.* 2021;180(10):3089–3100 PMID: 33852085
222. Abdelghani M, et al. *J Am Heart Assoc.* 2018;7(13):e008163 PMID: 29934419
223. Dixon G, et al. *Curr Opin Infect Dis.* 2017;30(3):257–267 PMID: 28319472
224. Wilson WR, et al. *Circulation.* 2021;143(20):e963–e978 PMID: 33853363
225. Williams ML, et al. *Ther Adv Cardiovasc Dis.* 2021;15:1753944721002687 PMID: 33784909
226. Radovanovic M, et al. *J Cardiovasc Dev Dis.* 2022;9(4):103 PMID: 35448079
227. Abdel-Haq N, et al. *Int J Pediatr.* 2018;2018:5450697 PMID: 30532791
228. Shane AL, et al. *Clin Infect Dis.* 2017;65(12):1963–1973 PMID: 29194529
229. Denno DM, et al. *Clin Infect Dis.* 2012;55(7):897–904 PMID: 22700832
230. Freedman SB, et al. *Clin Infect Dis.* 2016;62(10):1251–1258 PMID: 26917812
231. Bennish ML, et al. *Clin Infect Dis.* 2006;42(3):356–362 PMID: 16392080
232. Smith KE, et al. *Pediatr Infect Dis J.* 2012;31(1):37–41 PMID: 21892124
233. Imdad A, et al. *Cochrane Database Syst Rev.* 2021;(7):CD012997 PMID: 34219224
234. Florez ID, et al. *Curr Infect Dis Rep.* 2020;22(2):4 PMID: 31993758
235. Ashkenazi S, et al. *Pediatr Infect Dis J.* 2016;35(6):698–700 PMID: 26986771
236. Taylor DN, et al. *J Travel Med.* 2017;24(suppl 1):S17–S22 PMID: 28520998
237. Riddle MS, et al. *J Travel Med.* 2017;24(suppl 1):S57–S74 PMID: 28521004
238. Williams PCM, et al. *Paediatr Int Child Health.* 2018;38(suppl 1):S50–S65 PMID: 29790845
239. *Med Lett Drugs Ther.* 2019;61(1582):153–160 PMID: 31599872
240. Adler AV, et al. *J Travel Med.* 2022;29(1):taab099 PMID: 34230966
241. Kantele A, et al. *Clin Infect Dis.* 2015;60(6):837–846 PMID: 25613287
242. Riddle MS, et al. *Clin Infect Dis.* 2008;47(8):1007–1014 PMID: 18781873
243. Janda JM, et al. *Clin Microbiol Rev.* 2010;23(1):35–73 PMID: 20065325
244. AAP. *Campylobacter* infections. In: Kimberlin DW, et al, eds. *Red Book: 2024–2027 Report of the Committee on Infectious Diseases.* 33rd ed. 2024:283–286

245. Same RG, et al. *Pediatr Rev.* 2018;39(11):533–541 PMID: 30385582
246. Kanungo S, et al. *Lancet.* 2022;399(10333):1429–1440 PMID: 35397865
247. Connor BA, et al. *J Travel Med.* 2019;26(8):taz085 PMID: 31804684
248. AAP. *Clostridioides difficile* (formerly *Clostridium difficile*). In: Kimberlin DW, et al, eds. *Red Book: 2024–2027 Report of the Committee on Infectious Diseases.* 33rd ed. 2024:313–319
249. McDonald LC, et al. *Clin Infect Dis.* 2018;66(7):987–994 PMID: 29562266
250. Adams DJ, et al. *J Pediatric Infect Dis Soc.* 2021;10(suppl 3):S22–S26 PMID: 34791398
251. O'Gorman MA, et al. *J Pediatric Infect Dis Soc.* 2018;7(3):210–218 PMID: 28575523
252. Weng MK, et al. *Epidemiol Infect.* 2019;147:e172 PMID: 31063097
253. Mühlen S, et al. *Antimicrob Agents Chemother.* 2020;64(4):e02159-19 PMID: 32015030
254. Jones NL, et al. *J Pediatr Gastroenterol Nutr.* 2017;64(6):991–1003 PMID: 28541262
255. Crowe SE. *N Engl J Med.* 2019;380(12):1158–1165 PMID: 30893536
256. AAP. *Helicobacter pylori* infections. In: Kimberlin DW, et al, eds. *Red Book: 2024–2027 Report of the Committee on Infectious Diseases.* 33rd ed. 2024:412–417
257. Helmbold L, et al. *Pathogens.* 2022;11(2):178 PMID: 35215122
258. AAP. *Giardia duodenalis* (formerly *Giardia lamblia* and *Giardia intestinalis*) infections. In: Kimberlin DW, et al, eds. *Red Book: 2024–2027 Report of the Committee on Infectious Diseases.* 33rd ed. 2024:390–393
259. Ordóñez-Mena JM, et al. *J Antimicrob Chemother.* 2018;73(3):596–606 PMID: 29186570
260. Leinert JL, et al. *Antibiotics (Basel).* 2021;10(10):1187 PMID: 34680768
261. AAP. *Salmonella* infections. In: Kimberlin DW, et al, eds. *Red Book: 2024–2027 Report of the Committee on Infectious Diseases.* 33rd ed. 2024:742–750
262. Frenck RW Jr, et al. *Clin Infect Dis.* 2004;38(7):951–957 PMID: 15034826
263. Trivedi NA, et al. *J Postgrad Med.* 2012;58(2):112–118 PMID: 22718054
264. Kuehn R, et al. *Cochrane Database Syst Rev.* 2022;(11):CD010452 PMID: 36420914
265. Begum B, et al. *Mymensingh Med J.* 2014;23(3):441–448 PMID: 25178594
266. Akram J, et al. *Biomed Res Int.* 2020;2020:6432580 PMID: 32462008
267. CDC. National Antimicrobial Resistance Monitoring System for Enteric Bacteria (NARMS). Accessed October 29, 2024. www.cdc.gov/narms/data/index.html
268. Kotloff KL, et al. *Lancet.* 2018;391(10122):801–812 PMID: 29254859
269. AAP. *Shigella* infections. In: Kimberlin DW, et al, eds. *Red Book: 2024–2027 Report of the Committee on Infectious Diseases.* 33rd ed. 2024:756–760
270. Abdel-Haq NM, et al. *Pediatr Infect Dis J.* 2000;19(10):954–958 PMID: 11055595
271. Abdel-Haq NM, et al. *Int J Antimicrob Agents.* 2006;27(5):449–452 PMID: 16621458
272. El Qouqa IA, et al. *Int J Infect Dis.* 2011;15(1):e48–e53 PMID: 21131221
273. Yousef Y, et al. *J Pediatr Surg.* 2018;53(2):250–255 PMID: 29223673
274. Marino NE, et al. *Surg Infect (Larchmt).* 2017;18(8):894–903 PMID: 29064344
275. Anandalwar SP, et al. *JAMA Surg.* 2018;153(11):1021–1027 PMID: 30046808
276. Solomkin JS, et al. *Clin Infect Dis.* 2010;50(2):133–164 PMID: 20034345
277. Sawyer RG, et al. *N Engl J Med.* 2015;372(21):1996–2005 PMID: 25992746
278. Felber J, et al. *Front Cell Infect Microbiol.* 2023;13:1027769 PMID: 37228669
279. Kronman MP, et al. *Pediatrics.* 2016;138(1):e20154547 PMID: 27354453
280. Bradley JS, et al. *Pediatr Infect Dis J.* 2019;38(8):816–824 PMID: 31306396
281. Hurst AL, et al. *J Pediatric Infect Dis Soc.* 2017;6(1):57–64 PMID: 26703242
282. Theodorou CM. *J Pediatr Surg.* 2021;56(10):1826–1830 PMID: 33223225
283. Hamdy RF, et al. *Surg Infect (Larchmt).* 2019;20(5):399–405 PMID: 30874482
284. Wang C, et al. *BMC Pediatr.* 2019;19(1):407 PMID: 31684906
285. Scott C, et al. *Clin Infect Dis.* 2016;63(5):594–601 PMID: 27298329
286. Sartoris G, et al. *J Pediatric Infect Dis Soc.* 2020;9(2):218–227 PMID: 31909804
287. Soni H, et al. *Infection.* 2019;47(3):387–394 PMID: 30324229
288. Lin CA, et al. *J Pediatr Surg.* 2023;58(7):1274–1280 PMID: 36894443
289. Sethna CB, et al. *Clin J Am Soc Nephrol.* 2016;11(9):1590–1596 PMID: 27340282
290. Warady BA, et al. *Perit Dial Int.* 2012;32(suppl 2):S32–S86 PMID: 22851742
291. Preece ER, et al. *ANZ J Surg.* 2012;82(4):283–284 PMID: 22510192

292. Gkentzis A, et al. *Ann R Coll Surg Engl.* 2014;96(3):181–183 PMID: 24780779
293. George CRR, et al. *PLoS One.* 2019;14(4):e0213312 PMID: 30943199
294. Radovanovic M, et al. *Pathogens.* 2022;11(11):1230 PMID: 36364980
295. Hammad WAB, et al. *Eur J Obstet Gynecol Reprod Biol.* 2021;259:38–45 PMID: 33581405
296. *Obstet Gynecol.* 2020;135(5):e193–e202 PMID: 32332414
297. Savaris RF, et al. *Sex Transm Infect.* 2019;95(1):21–27 PMID: 30341232
298. Peeling RW, et al. *Nat Rev Dis Primers.* 2017;3:17073 PMID: 29022569
299. Jordan SJ, et al. *Sex Transm Infect.* 2020;96(4):306–311 PMID: 31515293
300. Abbe C, et al. *Front Reprod Health.* 2023;5:1100029 PMID: 37325243
301. Matheson A, et al. *Aust N Z J Obstet Gynaecol.* 2017;57(2):139–145 PMID: 28299777
302. Baka S, et al. *Eur J Pediatr.* 2022;181(12):4149–4155 PMID: 36163515
303. Beyitler İ, et al. *World J Pediatr.* 2017;13(2):101–105 PMID: 28083751
304. Hansen MT, et al. *J Pediatr Adolesc Gynecol.* 2007;20(5):315–317 PMID: 17868900
305. Brouwer MC, et al. *N Engl J Med.* 2014;371(5):447–456 PMID: 25075836
306. Mameli C, et al. *Childs Nerv Syst.* 2019;35(7):1117–1128 PMID: 31062139
307. Boucher A, et al. *Med Mal Infect.* 2017;47(3):221–235 PMID: 28341533
308. Dalmau J, et al. *N Engl J Med.* 2018;378(9):840–851 PMID: 29490181
309. Abzug MJ, et al. *J Pediatric Infect Dis Soc.* 2016;5(1):53–62 PMID: 26407253
310. Cheng H, et al. *BMC Infect Dis.* 2020;20(1):886 PMID: 33238935
311. Matthews E, et al. *Curr Trop Med Rep.* 2022;9(3):92–100 PMID: 36186545
312. Ajibowo AO, et al. *Cureus.* 2021;13(4):e14579 PMID: 34036000
313. Iro MA, et al. *Cochrane Database Syst Rev.* 2017;(10):CD011367 PMID: 28967695
314. Brouwer MC, et al. *Cochrane Database Syst Rev.* 2015;(9):CD004405 PMID: 26362566
315. Tunkel AR, et al. *Clin Infect Dis.* 2017;64(6):e34–e65 PMID: 28203777
316. Jhaveri R. *J Pediatric Infect Dis Soc.* 2019;8(1):92–93 PMID: 30380088
317. Bradley JS, et al. *Pediatr Infect Dis J.* 1991;10(11):871–873 PMID: 1749702
318. Prasad K, et al. *Cochrane Database Syst Rev.* 2016;(4):CD002244 PMID: 27121755
319. Konrad E, et al. *Arch Dis Child.* 2022;108(9):693–697 PMID: 36450441
320. Cies JJ, et al. *J Pediatr Pharmacol Ther.* 2020;25(4):336–339 PMID: 32461749
321. Bradley JS. *Pediatrics.* 2022;150(1):e2022056219 PMID: 35734947
322. National Institute for Health and Care Excellence. Urinary tract infection in under 16s: diagnosis and management. July 27, 2022. Accessed October 29, 2024. www.nice.org.uk/guidance/ng224
323. Tullus K, et al. *Lancet.* 2020;395(10237):1659–1668 PMID: 32446408
324. Meesters K, et al. *Antimicrob Agents Chemother.* 2018;62(9):e00517-18 PMID: 29987142
325. Chen WL, et al. *Pediatr Neonatal.* 2015;56(3):176–182 PMID: 25459491
326. Fujita Y, et al. *Pediatr Infect Dis J.* 2021;40(7):e278–e280 PMID: 34097665
327. Strohmeier Y, et al. *Cochrane Database Syst Rev.* 2014;(7):CD003772 PMID: 25066627
328. Fox MT, et al. *JAMA Netw Open.* 2020;3(5):e203951 PMID: 32364593
329. Tamma PD, et al. *Clin Infect Dis.* 2015;60(9):1319–1325 PMID: 25586681
330. National Institute for Health and Care Excellence. Urinary tract infection (recurrent): antimicrobial prescribing; treatment for children and young people under 16 years with recurrent UTI. October 31, 2018. Accessed October 29, 2024. www.nice.org.uk/guidance/ng112/chapter/Recommendations#treatment-for-children-and-young-people-under-16-years-with-recurrent-uti
331. AAP Subcommittee on Urinary Tract Infection and Steering Committee on Quality Improvement and Management. *Pediatrics.* 2011;128(3):595–610 PMID: 21873693
332. Williams G, et al. *Cochrane Database Syst Rev.* 2019;(4):CD001534 PMID: 30932167
333. Williams G, et al. *Cochrane Database Syst Rev.* 2023;(4):CD001321 PMID: 37068952
334. Hoberman A, et al. *N Engl J Med.* 2014;370(25):2367–2376 PMID: 24795142
335. Craig JC. *J Pediatr.* 2015;166(3):778 PMID: 25722276
336. Hewitt IK, et al. *Pediatrics.* 2017;139(5):e20163145 PMID: 28557737
337. AAP. Actinomycosis. In: Kimberlin DW, et al, eds. *Red Book: 2024–2027 Report of the Committee on Infectious Diseases.* 33rd ed. 2024:221–222
338. Chew SJ, et al. *J Paediatr Child Health.* 2023;59(6):833–839 PMID: 37017147
339. Wacharachaisurapol N, et al. *Pediatr Infect Dis J.* 2017;36(3):e76–e79 PMID: 27870811

340. Biggs HM, et al. *MMWR Recomm Rep.* 2016;65(2):1–44 PMID: 27172113
341. Dixon DM, et al. *Ticks Tick Borne Dis.* 2021;12(6):101823 PMID: 34517150
342. AAP. Brucellosis. In: Kimberlin DW, et al, eds. *Red Book: 2024–2027 Report of the Committee on Infectious Diseases.* 33rd ed. 2024:277–280
343. Bukhari EE. *Saudi Med J.* 2018;39(4):336–341 PMID: 29619483
344. Shorbatli LA, et al. *Int J Clin Pharm.* 2018;40(6):1458–1461 PMID: 30446895
345. Zangwill KM. *Adv Exp Med Biol.* 2013;764:159–166 PMID: 23654065
346. Chang CC, et al. *Paediatr Int Child Health.* 2016;36(3):232–234 PMID: 25940800
347. Mogg M, et al. *Vector Borne Zoonotic Dis.* 2020;20(7):547–550 PMID: 32077809
348. Mukkada S, et al. *Infect Dis Clin North Am.* 2015;29(3):539–555 PMID: 26188606
349. Ruhayel SD, et al. *Pediatr Infect Dis J.* 2021;40(9):832–834 PMID: 34285167
350. Taplitz RA, et al. *J Clin Oncol.* 2018;36(14):1443–1453 PMID: 29461916
351. Alali M, et al. *J Pediatr Hematol Oncol.* 2020;42(6):e445–e451 PMID: 32404688
352. Haeusler GM, et al. *EClinicalMedicine.* 2020;23:100394 PMID: 32637894
353. Miedema KG, et al. *Eur J Cancer.* 2016;53:16–24 PMID: 26700076
354. Payne JR, et al. *J Pediatr.* 2018;193:172–177 PMID: 29229452
355. Son MBF, et al. *Pediatr Rev.* 2018;39(2):78–90 PMID: 29437127
356. Green J, et al. *Cochrane Database Syst Rev.* 2022;(5):CD011188 PMID: 35622534
357. Friedman KG, et al. *Arch Dis Child.* 2021;106(3):247–252 PMID: 32943389
358. McCrindle BW, et al. *Circulation.* 2017;135(17):e927–e999 PMID: 28356445
359. Broderick C, et al. *Cochrane Database Syst Rev.* 2023;(1):CD014884 PMID: 36695415
360. Yang J, et al. *J Pediatr.* 2022;243:173–180.e8 PMID: 34953816
361. AAP. Leprosy. In: Kimberlin DW, et al, eds. *Red Book: 2024–2027 Report of the Committee on Infectious Diseases.* 33rd ed. 2024:539–532
362. Haake DA, et al. *Curr Top Microbiol Immunol.* 2015;387:65–97 PMID: 25388133
363. AAP. Leptospirosis. In: Kimberlin DW, et al, eds. *Red Book: 2024–2027 Report of the Committee on Infectious Diseases.* 33rd ed. 2024:542–545
364. AAP. Lyme disease. In: Kimberlin DW, et al, eds. *Red Book: 2024–2027 Report of the Committee on Infectious Diseases.* 33rd ed. 2024:549–556
365. Nguyen CT, et al. *JAMA.* 2022;327(8):772–773 PMID: 35191942
366. Wiersinga WJ, et al. *Nat Rev Dis Primers.* 2018;4:17107 PMID: 29388572
367. Chetchotisakd P, et al. *Lancet.* 2014;383(9919):807–814 PMID: 24284287
368. Haworth CS, et al. *BMJ Open Respir Res.* 2017;4(1):e000242 PMID: 29449949
369. Griffith DE, et al. *Chest.* 2022;161(1):64–75 PMID: 34314673
370. Pasipanodya JG, et al. *Antimicrob Agents Chemother.* 2017;61(11):e01206-17 PMID: 28807911
371. Traxler RM, et al. *Clin Microbiol Rev.* 2022;35(4):e0002721 PMID: 36314911
372. AAP. Nocardiosis. In: Kimberlin DW, et al, eds. *Red Book: 2024–2027 Report of the Committee on Infectious Diseases.* 33rd ed. 2024:620–622
373. Kugeler KJ, et al. *Clin Infect Dis.* 2020;70(suppl 1):S20–S26 PMID: 32435801
374. Barbieri R, et al. *Clin Microbiol Rev.* 2020;34(1):e00024-19 PMID: 33298527
375. Apangu T, et al. *Emerg Infect Dis.* 2017;23(3):553–555 PMID: 28125398
376. Cherry CC, et al. *Curr Infect Dis Rep.* 2020;22(4) PMID: 34135692
377. Anderson A, et al. *MMWR Recomm Rep.* 2013;62(RR-03):1–30 PMID: 23535757
378. AAP. Rocky Mountain spotted fever. In: Kimberlin DW, et al, eds. *Red Book: 2024–2027 Report of the Committee on Infectious Diseases.* 33rd ed. 2024:727–730
379. Jay R, et al. *J Vector Borne Dis.* 2020;57(2):114–120 PMID: 34290155
380. AAP. Tetanus. In: Kimberlin DW, et al, eds. *Red Book: 2024–2027 Report of the Committee on Infectious Diseases.* 33rd ed. 2024:848–854
381. CDC. Clinical overview of tetanus. August 15, 2024. Accessed October 29, 2024. www.cdc.gov/tetanus/hcp/clinical-overview/index.html
382. Gaensbauer JT, et al. *Pediatr Infect Dis J.* 2018;37(12):1223–1226 PMID: 29601458
383. Cook A, et al. *Emerg Infect Dis.* 2020;26(6):1077–1083 PMID: 32442091
384. Harik NS. *Pediatr Ann.* 2013;42(7):288–292 PMID: 23805970

Chapter 2

1. Allegaert K, et al. *Acta Clin Belg*. 2019;74(3):157–163 PMID: 29745792
2. Keij FM, et al. *BMJ Open*. 2019;9(7):e026688 PMID: 31289068
3. Gifford A, et al. *Arch Dis Child*. 2024;109(8):681–687 PMID: 38307705
4. Arnold CJ, et al. *Pediatr Infect Dis J*. 2015;34(9):964–968 PMID: 26376308
5. Martin E, et al. *Eur J Pediatr*. 1993;152(6):530–534 PMID: 8335024
6. Hile GB, et al. *J Pediatr Pharmacol Ther*. 2021;26(1):99–103 PMID: 33424507
7. Bradley JS, et al. *Pediatrics*. 2009;123(4):e609–e613 PMID: 19289450
8. Zikic A, et al. *J Pediatric Infect Dis Soc*. 2018;7(3):e107–e115 PMID: 30007329
9. AAP. Chlamydial infections. In: Kimberlin DW, et al, eds. *Red Book: 2024–2027 Report of the Committee on Infectious Diseases*. 33rd ed. 2024:298–308
10. Honein MA, et al. *Lancet*. 1999;354(9196):2101–2105 PMID: 10609814
11. Hammerschlag MR, et al. *Pediatr Infect Dis J*. 1998;17(11):1049–1050 PMID: 9849993
12. Abdellatif M, et al. *Eur J Pediatr*. 2019;178(3):301–314 PMID: 30470884
13. Laga M, et al. *N Engl J Med*. 1986;315(22):1382–1385 PMID: 3095641
14. Workowski KA, et al. *MMWR Recomm Rep*. 2015;64(RR-3):1–137 PMID: 26042815
15. Newman LM, et al. *Clin Infect Dis*. 2007;44(suppl 3):S84–S101 PMID: 17342672
16. MacDonald N, et al. *Adv Exp Med Biol*. 2008;609:108–130 PMID: 18193661
17. AAP. Gonococcal infections. In: Kimberlin DW, et al, eds. *Red Book: 2024–2027 Report of the Committee on Infectious Diseases*. 33rd ed. 2024:394–399
18. Cimolai N. *Am J Ophthalmol*. 2006;142(1):183–184 PMID: 16815280
19. Marangon FB, et al. *Am J Ophthalmol*. 2004;137(3):453–458 PMID: 15013867
20. AAP. Coagulase-negative staphylococcal infections. In: Kimberlin DW, et al, eds. *Red Book: 2024–2027 Report of the Committee on Infectious Diseases*. 33rd ed. 2024:782–785
21. Brito DV, et al. *Braz J Infect Dis*. 2003;7(4):234–235 PMID: 14533982
22. Chen CJ, et al. *Am J Ophthalmol*. 2008;145(6):966–970 PMID: 18378213
23. Shah SS, et al. *J Perinatol*. 1999;19(6, pt 1):462–465 PMID: 10685281
24. Kimberlin DW, et al. *J Pediatr*. 2003;143(1):16–25 PMID: 12915819
25. Kimberlin DW, et al. *J Infect Dis*. 2008;197(6):836–845 PMID: 18279073
26. AAP. Cytomegalovirus infection. In: Kimberlin DW, et al, eds. *Red Book: 2024–2027 Report of the Committee on Infectious Diseases*. 33rd ed. 2024:344–352
27. Kimberlin DW, et al. *N Engl J Med*. 2015;372(10):933–943 PMID: 25738669
28. Kimberlin DW, et al. *J Pediatr*. 2024;268:113934 PMID: 38309519
29. Marsico C, et al. *J Infect Dis*. 2019;219(9):1398–1406 PMID: 30535363
30. Chung PK, et al. *J Pediatr*. 2024;268:113945 PMID: 38336204
31. AAP. Candidiasis. In: Kimberlin DW, et al, eds. *Red Book: 2024–2027 Report of the Committee on Infectious Diseases*. 33rd ed. 2024:286–293
32. Hundalani S, et al. *Expert Rev Anti Infect Ther*. 2013;11(7):709–721 PMID: 23829639
33. Saez-Llorens X, et al. *Antimicrob Agents Chemother*. 2009;53(3):869–875 PMID: 19075070
34. Ericson JE, et al. *Clin Infect Dis*. 2016;63(5):604–610 PMID: 27298330
35. Smith PB, et al. *Pediatr Infect Dis J*. 2009;28(5):412–415 PMID: 19319022
36. Wurthwein G, et al. *Antimicrob Agents Chemother*. 2005;49(12):5092–5098 PMID: 16304177
37. Heresi GP, et al. *Pediatr Infect Dis J*. 2006;25(12):1110–1115 PMID: 17133155
38. Kawaguchi C, et al. *Pediatr Int*. 2009;51(2):220–224 PMID: 19405920
39. Hsieh E, et al. *Early Hum Dev*. 2012;88(suppl 2):S6–S10 PMID: 22633516
40. Pappas PG, et al. *Clin Infect Dis*. 2016;62(4):e1–e50 PMID: 26679628
41. Hwang MF, et al. *Antimicrob Agents Chemother*. 2017;61(12):e01352-17 PMID: 28893774
42. Watt KM, et al. *Antimicrob Agents Chemother*. 2015;59(7):3935–3943 PMID: 25896706
43. Ascher SB, et al. *Pediatr Infect Dis J*. 2012;31(5):439–443 PMID: 22189522
44. Swanson JR, et al. *Pediatr Infect Dis J*. 2016;35(5):519–523 PMID: 26835970
45. Santos RP, et al. *Pediatr Infect Dis J*. 2007;26(4):364–366 PMID: 17414408
46. Frankenbusch K, et al. *J Perinatol*. 2006;26(8):511–514 PMID: 16871222
47. Thomas L, et al. *Expert Rev Anti Infect Ther*. 2009;7(4):461–472 PMID: 19400765

48. Mehler K, et al. *Pediatr Infect Dis J.* 2022;41(4):352–357 PMID: 34817413
49. Fatemizadeh R, et al. *Pediatr Infect Dis J.* 2020;39(4):310–312 PMID: 32084112
50. Verweij PE, et al. *Drug Resist Updat.* 2015;21–22:30–40 PMID: 26282594
51. Shah D, et al. *Cochrane Database Syst Rev.* 2012;(8):CD007448 PMID: 22895960
52. Cohen-Wolkowiez M, et al. *Clin Infect Dis.* 2012;55(11):1495–1502 PMID: 22955430
53. Knell J, et al. *Curr Probl Surg.* 2019;56(1):11–38 PMID: 30691547
54. Smith MJ, et al. *Pediatr Infect Dis J.* 2021;40(6):550–555 PMID: 33902072
55. Commander SJ, et al. *Pediatr Infect Dis J.* 2020;39(9):e245–e248 PMID: 32453198
56. Blakely ML, et al. *Ann Surg.* 2021;274(4):e370–e380 PMID: 34506326
57. Morgan RL, et al. *Gastroenterology.* 2020;159(2):467–480 PMID: 32592699
58. Gray KD, et al. *J Pediatr.* 2020;222:59–64.e1 PMID: 32418818
59. AAP. *Salmonella* infections. In: Kimberlin DW, et al, eds. *Red Book: 2024–2027 Report of the Committee on Infectious Diseases.* 33rd ed. 2024:742–750
60. Pinninti SG, et al. *Pediatr Clin North Am.* 2013;60(2):351–365 PMID: 23481105
61. AAP. Herpes simplex. In: Kimberlin DW, et al, eds. *Red Book: 2024–2027 Report of the Committee on Infectious Diseases.* 33rd ed. 2024:467–478
62. Jones CA, et al. *Cochrane Database Syst Rev.* 2009;(3):CD004206 PMID: 19588350
63. Downes KJ, et al. *J Pediatr.* 2020;219:126–132 PMID: 32037154
64. Kimberlin DW, et al. *N Engl J Med.* 2011;365(14):1284–1292 PMID: 21991950
65. Grondin A, et al. *Neuropediatrics.* 2020;51(3):221–224 PMID: 31887772
66. Sampson MR, et al. *Pediatr Infect Dis J.* 2014;33(1):42–49 PMID: 24346595
67. Panel on Antiretroviral Therapy and Medical Management of Children Living with HIV. Guidelines for the use of antiretroviral agents in pediatric HIV infection. What's new in the guidelines? Updated June 27, 2024. Accessed October 29, 2024. https://clinicalinfo.hiv.gov/en/guidelines/pediatric-arv/whats-new
68. Panel on Treatment of HIV During Pregnancy and Prevention of Perinatal Transmission. Recommendations for the use of antiretroviral drugs in pregnant women with HIV infection and interventions to reduce perinatal HIV transmission in the United States. Updated January 31, 2024. Accessed October 29, 2024. https://clinicalinfo.hiv.gov/en/guidelines/perinatal/whats-new
69. Luzuriaga K, et al. *N Engl J Med.* 2015;372(8):786–788 PMID: 25693029
70. AAP Committee on Infectious Diseases. *Pediatrics.* 2019;144(4):e20192478 PMID: 31477606
71. Acosta EP, et al. *J Infect Dis.* 2010;202(4):563–566 PMID: 20594104
72. McPherson C, et al. *J Infect Dis.* 2012;206(6):847–850 PMID: 22807525
73. Kamal MA, et al. *Clin Pharmacol Ther.* 2014;96(3):380–389 PMID: 24865390
74. Kimberlin DW, et al. *J Infect Dis.* 2013;207(5):709–720 PMID: 23230059
75. Bradley JS, et al. *Pediatrics.* 2017;140(5):e20162727 PMID: 29051331
76. Hayden FG, et al. *N Engl J Med.* 2018;379(10):913–923 PMID: 30184455
77. Fraser N, et al. *Acta Paediatr.* 2006;95(5):519–522 PMID: 16825129
78. Ulloa-Gutierrez R, et al. *Pediatr Emerg Care.* 2005;21(9):600–602 PMID: 16160666
79. Sawardekar KP. *Pediatr Infect Dis J.* 2004;23(1):22–26 PMID: 14743041
80. Bingol-Kologlu M, et al. *J Pediatr Surg.* 2007;42(11):1892–1897 PMID: 18022442
81. Brook I. *J Perinat Med.* 2002;30(3):197–208 PMID: 12122901
82. Kaplan SL. *Adv Exp Med Biol.* 2009;634:111–120 PMID: 19280853
83. Korakaki E, et al. *Jpn J Infect Dis.* 2007;60(2–3):129–131 PMID: 17515648
84. Dessi A, et al. *J Chemother.* 2008;20(5):542–550 PMID: 19028615
85. Berkun Y, et al. *Arch Dis Child.* 2008;93(8):690–694 PMID: 18337275
86. Greenberg D, et al. *Paediatr Drugs.* 2008;10(2):75–83 PMID: 18345717
87. Ismail EA, et al. *Pediatr Int.* 2013;55(1):60–64 PMID: 23039834
88. Megged O, et al. *J Pediatr.* 2018;196:319 PMID: 29428272
89. Engle WD, et al. *J Perinatol.* 2000;20(7):421–426 PMID: 11076325
90. Brook I. *Microbes Infect.* 2002;4(12):1271–1280 PMID: 12467770
91. Darville T. *Semin Pediatr Infect Dis.* 2005;16(4):235–244 PMID: 16210104
92. Eberly MD, et al. *Pediatrics.* 2015;135(3):483–488 PMID: 25687145
93. Waites KB, et al. *Semin Fetal Neonatal Med.* 2009;14(4):190–199 PMID: 19109084

94. Morrison W. *Pediatr Infect Dis J*. 2007;26(2):186–188 PMID: 17259889
95. AAP. Pertussis. In: Kimberlin DW, et al, eds. *Red Book: 2024–2027 Report of the Committee on Infectious Diseases*. 33rd ed. 2024:656–667
96. Foca MD. *Semin Perinatol*. 2002;26(5):332–339 PMID: 12452505
97. AAP Committee on Infectious Diseases and Bronchiolitis Guidelines Committee. *Pediatrics*. 2014;134(2):e620–e638 PMID: 25070304
98. Banerji A, et al. *CMAJ Open*. 2016;4(4):E623–E633 PMID: 28443266
99. Borse RH, et al. *J Pediatric Infect Dis Soc*. 2014;3(3):201–212 PMID: 26625383
100. Vergnano S, et al. *Pediatr Infect Dis J*. 2011;30(10):850–854 PMID: 21654546
101. Nelson MU, et al. *Semin Perinatol*. 2012;36(6):424–430 PMID: 23177801
102. Lyseng-Williamson KA, et al. *Paediatr Drugs*. 2003;5(6):419–431 PMID: 12765493
103. AAP. Group B streptococcal infections. In: Kimberlin DW, et al, eds. *Red Book: 2024–2027 Report of the Committee on Infectious Diseases*. 33rd ed. 2024:799–806
104. Schrag S, et al. *MMWR Recomm Rep*. 2002;51(RR-11):1–22 PMID: 12211284
105. AAP. *Ureaplasma urealyticum* and *Ureaplasma parvum* infections. In: Kimberlin DW, et al, eds. *Red Book: 2024–2027 Report of the Committee on Infectious Diseases*. 33rd ed. 2024:936–938
106. Merchan LM, et al. *Antimicrob Agents Chemother*. 2015;59(1):570–578 PMID: 25385115
107. Viscardi RM, et al. *Arch Dis Child Fetal Neonatal Ed*. 2020;105(6):615–622 PMID: 32170033
108. Viscardi RM, et al. *Pediatr Res*. 2022;91(1):178–187 PMID: 33658655
109. AAP. *Escherichia coli* diarrhea. In: Kimberlin DW, et al, eds. *Red Book: 2024–2027 Report of the Committee on Infectious Diseases*. 33rd ed. 2024:376–382
110. Venkatesh MP, et al. *Expert Rev Anti Infect Ther*. 2008;6(6):929–938 PMID: 19053905
111. Aguilera-Alonso D, et al. *Antimicrob Agents Chemother*. 2020;64(3):e02183-19 PMID: 31844014
112. Nakwan N, et al. *Pediatr Infect Dis J*. 2019;38(11):1107–1112 PMID: 31469781
113. Abzug MJ, et al. *J Pediatric Infect Dis Soc*. 2016;5(1):53–62 PMID: 26407253
114. AAP. *Listeria monocytogenes* infections. In: Kimberlin DW, et al, eds. *Red Book: 2024–2027 Report of the Committee on Infectious Diseases*. 33rd ed. 2024:545–549
115. Workowski KA, et al. *MMWR Recomm Rep*. 2021;70(4):1–187 PMID: 34292926
116. van der Lugt NM, et al. *BMC Pediatr*. 2010;10:84 PMID: 21092087
117. Fortunov RM, et al. *Pediatrics*. 2006;118(3):874–881 PMID: 16950976
118. Fortunov RM, et al. *Pediatrics*. 2007;120(5):937–945 PMID: 17974729
119. Riccobene TA, et al. *J Clin Pharmacol*. 2017;57(3):345–355 PMID: 27510635
120. Stauffer WM, et al. *Pediatr Emerg Care*. 2003;19(3):165–166 PMID: 12813301
121. Kaufman DA, et al. *Clin Infect Dis*. 2017;64(10):1387–1395 PMID: 28158439
122. Dehority W, et al. *Pediatr Infect Dis J*. 2006;25(11):1080–1081 PMID: 17072137
123. AAP. Syphilis. In: Kimberlin DW, et al, eds. *Red Book: 2024–2027 Report of the Committee on Infectious Diseases*. 33rd ed. 2024:825–841
124. AAP. Tetanus. In: Kimberlin DW, et al, eds. *Red Book: 2024–2027 Report of the Committee on Infectious Diseases*. 33rd ed. 2024:848–854
125. AAP. *Toxoplasma gondii* infections. In: Kimberlin DW, et al, eds. *Red Book: 2024–2027 Report of the Committee on Infectious Diseases*. 33rd ed. 2024:867–875
126. Petersen E. *Semin Fetal Neonatal Med*. 2007;12(3):214–223 PMID: 17321812
127. Beetz R. *Curr Opin Pediatr*. 2012;24(2):205–211 PMID: 22227782
128. RIVUR Trial Investigators, et al. *N Engl J Med*. 2014;370(25):2367–2376 PMID: 24795142
129. Williams G, et al. *Cochrane Database Syst Rev*. 2019;(4):CD001534 PMID: 30932167
130. van Donge T, et al. *Antimicrob Agents Chemother*. 2018;62(4):e02004-17 PMID: 29358294
131. Sahin L, et al. *Clin Pharmacol Ther*. 2016;100(1):23–25 PMID: 27082701
132. Roberts SW, et al. Placental transmission of antibiotics. In: *Glob Libr Women's Med*. Updated June 2008. Accessed October 29, 2024. www.glowm.com/section_view/heading/Placental%20Transmission%20of%20Antibiotics/item/174
133. Zhang Z, et al. *Drug Metab Dispos*. 2017;45(8):939–946 PMID: 28049636
134. Pacifici GM. *Int J Clin Pharmacol Ther*. 2006;44(2):57–63 PMID: 16502764
135. Sachs HC, et al. *Pediatrics*. 2013;132(3):e796–e809 PMID: 23979084

136. Hale TW. *Medication and Mothers' Milk 2021: A Manual of Lactational Pharmacology*. 19th ed. 2021
137. Briggs GG, et al. *Briggs Drugs in Pregnancy and Lactation*. 12th ed. 2021
138. Ito S, et al. *Am J Obstet Gynecol*. 1993;168(5):1393–1399 PMID: 8498418

Chapter 3

1. Shields RK, et al. *Clin Infect Dis*. 2023;76(suppl 2):S179–S193 PMID: 37125467
2. Watkins RR, et al. *Clin Infect Dis*. 2023;76(suppl 2):S163–S165 PMID: 37125465
3. Viale P, et al. *Ann Intensive Care*. 2023;13(1):52 PMID: 37322293
4. Chiotos K, et al. *J Pediatric Infect Dis Soc*. 2020;9(1):56–66 PMID: 31872226
5. Aguilera-Alonso D, et al. *Antimicrob Agents Chemother*. 2020;64(3):e02183-19 PMID: 31844014
6. Mantzana P, et al. *Antibiotics (Basel)*. 2023;12(1):93 PMID: 36671295
7. Mohd Sazlly Lim S, et al. *Int J Antimicrob Agents*. 2019;53(6):726–745 PMID: 30831234
8. Wacharachaisurapol N, et al. *Pediatr Infect Dis J*. 2017;36(3):e76–e79 PMID: 27870811
9. Gandhi K, et al. *Ann Otol Rhinol Laryngol*. 2021:34894211021273 PMID: 34060325
10. Pessoa RBG, et al. *Front Microbiol*. 2022;13:868890 PMID: 35711774
11. Sharma K, et al. *Ann Clin Microbiol Antimicrob*. 2017;16(1):12 PMID: 28288638
12. Maraki S, et al. *J Microbiol Immunol Infect*. 2016;49(1):119–122 PMID: 24529567
13. Sigurjonsdottir VK, et al. *Diagn Microbiol Infect Dis*. 2017;89(3):230–234 PMID: 29050793
14. Dixon DM, et al. *Ticks Tick Borne Dis*. 2021;12(6):101823 PMID: 34517150
15. Alrwashdeh AM, et al. *IDCases*. 2022;31:e01645 PMID: 36579145
16. Bradley JS, et al. *Pediatrics*. 2014;133(5):e1411–e1436 PMID: 24777226
17. AAP. *Bacillus cereus* infections and intoxications. In: Kimberlin DW, et al, eds. *Red Book: 2024–2027 Report of the Committee on Infectious Diseases*. 33rd ed. 2024:256–258
18. Lotte R, et al. *Clin Microbiol Rev*. 2022;35(2):e0008821 PMID: 35138121
19. Zafar H, et al. *Gut Microbes*. 2021;13(1):1–20 PMID: 33535896
20. Snydman DR, et al. *Anaerobe*. 2017;43:21–26 PMID: 27867083
21. Shorbatli LA, et al. *Int J Clin Pharm*. 2018;40(6):1458–1461 PMID: 30446895
22. Zangwill KM. *Adv Exp Med Biol*. 2013;764:159–166 PMID: 23654065
23. Angelakis E, et al. *Int J Antimicrob Agents*. 2014;44(1):16–25 PMID: 24933445
24. Kilgore PE, et al. *Clin Microbiol Rev*. 2016;29(3):449–486 PMID: 27029594
25. AAP. Pertussis. In: Kimberlin DW, et al, eds. *Red Book: 2024–2027 Report of the Committee on Infectious Diseases*. 33rd ed. 2024:656–667
26. Nguyen CT, et al. *JAMA*. 2022;327(8):772–773 PMID: 35191942
27. AAP. Lyme disease. In: Kimberlin DW, et al, eds. *Red Book: 2024–2027 Report of the Committee on Infectious Diseases*. 33rd ed. 2024:549–556
28. AAP. *Borrelia* infections other than Lyme disease. In: Kimberlin DW, et al, eds. *Red Book: 2024–2027 Report of the Committee on Infectious Diseases*. 33rd ed. 2024:274–277
29. Rodino KG, et al. *Infect Dis Clin North Am*. 2022;36(3):689–701 PMID: 36116843
30. AAP. Brucellosis. In: Kimberlin DW, et al, eds. *Red Book: 2024–2027 Report of the Committee on Infectious Diseases*. 33rd ed. 2024:277–280
31. Bukhari EE. *Saudi Med J*. 2018;39(4):336–341 PMID: 29619483
32. Yagupsky P. *Adv Exp Med Biol*. 2011;719:123–132 PMID: 22125040
33. AAP. *Burkholderia* infections. In: Kimberlin DW, et al, eds. *Red Book: 2024–2027 Report of the Committee on Infectious Diseases*. 33rd ed. 2024:280–283
34. Massip C, et al. *J Antimicrob Chemother*. 2019;74(2):525–528 PMID: 30312409
35. Mazer DM, et al. *Antimicrob Agents Chemother*. 2017;61(9):e00766-17 PMID: 28674053
36. Lord R, et al. *Cochrane Database Syst Rev*. 2020;(4):CD009529 PMID: 32239690
37. Wiersinga WJ, et al. *N Engl J Med*. 2012;367(11):1035–1044 PMID: 22970946
38. Wiersinga WJ, et al. *Nat Rev Dis Primers*. 2018;4:17107 PMID: 29388572
39. Chetchotisakd P, et al. *Lancet*. 2014;383(9919):807–814 PMID: 24284287
40. Same RG, et al. *Pediatr Rev*. 2018;39(11):533–541 PMID: 30385582
41. Wagenaar JA, et al. *Clin Infect Dis*. 2014;58(11):1579–1586 PMID: 24550377

42. AAP. *Campylobacter* infections. In: Kimberlin DW, et al, eds. *Red Book: 2024–2027 Report of the Committee on Infectious Diseases.* 33rd ed. 2024:283–286
43. Schiaffino F, et al. *Antimicrob Agents Chemother.* 2019;63(2):e01911-18 PMID: 30420482
44. Bula-Rudas FJ, et al. *Pediatr Rev.* 2018;39(10):490–500 PMID: 30275032
45. Butler T. *Eur J Clin Microbiol Infect Dis.* 2015;34(7):1271–1280 PMID: 25828064
46. Wang HK, et al. *J Clin Microbiol.* 2007;45(2):645–647 PMID: 17135428
47. Alhifany AA, et al. *Am J Case Rep.* 2017;18:674–667 PMID: 28620153
48. Rivero M, et al. *BMC Infect Dis.* 2019;19(1):816 PMID: 31533642
49. Kohlhoff SA, et al. *Expert Opin Pharmacother.* 2015;16(2):205–212 PMID: 25579069
50. AAP. Chlamydial infections. In: Kimberlin DW, et al, eds. *Red Book: 2024–2027 Report of the Committee on Infectious Diseases.* 33rd ed. 2024:298–308
51. Workowski KA, et al. *Clin Infect Dis.* 2022;74(suppl 2):S89–S94 PMID: 35416966
52. Blasi F, et al. *Clin Microbiol Infect.* 2009;15(1):29–35 PMID: 19220337
53. Hogerwerf L, et al. *Epidemiol Infect.* 2017;145(15):3096–3105 PMID: 28946931
54. Campbell JI, et al. *BMC Infect Dis.* 2013;13:4 PMID: 23286235
55. Alisjahbana B, et al. *Int J Gen Med.* 2021;14:3259–3270 PMID: 34267544
56. Richard KR, et al. *Am J Case Rep.* 2015;16:740–744 PMID: 26477750
57. Paterson DL, et al. *Curr Opin Infect Dis.* 2020;33(2):214–223 PMID: 32068644
58. Harris PN, et al. *J Antimicrob Chemother.* 2016;71(2):296–306 PMID: 26542304
59. National Institute for Health and Care Excellence. *Clostridioides difficile* infection: antimicrobial prescribing. July 23, 2021. Accessed October 29, 2024. www.nice.org.uk/guidance/ng199
60. AAP. *Clostridioides difficile* (formerly *Clostridium difficile*). In: Kimberlin DW, et al, eds. *Red Book: 2024–2027 Report of the Committee on Infectious Diseases.* 33rd ed. 2024:313–319
61. McDonald LC, et al. *Clin Infect Dis.* 2018;66(7):987–994 PMID: 29562266
62. O'Gorman MA, et al. *J Pediatric Infect Dis Soc.* 2018;7(3):210–218 PMID: 28575523
63. Carrillo-Marquez MA. *Pediatr Rev.* 2016;37(5):183–192 PMID: 27139326
64. AAP. Botulism and infant botulism. In: Kimberlin DW, et al, eds. *Red Book: 2024–2027 Report of the Committee on Infectious Diseases.* 33rd ed. 2024:308–312
65. Hill SE, et al. *Ann Pharmacother.* 2013;47(2):e12 PMID: 23362041
66. AAP. Clostridial myonecrosis. In: Kimberlin DW, et al, eds. *Red Book: 2024–2027 Report of the Committee on Infectious Diseases.* 33rd ed. 2024:312–313
67. AAP. *Clostridium perfringens* foodborne illness. In: Kimberlin DW, et al, eds. *Red Book: 2024–2027 Report of the Committee on Infectious Diseases.* 33rd ed. 2024:319–320
68. AAP. Tetanus. In: Kimberlin DW, et al, eds. *Red Book: 2024–2027 Report of the Committee on Infectious Diseases.* 33rd ed. 2024:848–854
69. Yen LM, et al. *Lancet.* 2019;393(10181):1657–1668 PMID: 30935736
70. Rhinesmith E, et al. *Pediatr Rev.* 2018;39(8):430–432 PMID: 30068747
71. AAP. Diphtheria. In: Kimberlin DW, et al, eds. *Red Book: 2024–2027 Report of the Committee on Infectious Diseases.* 33rd ed. 2024:357–361
72. Fernandez-Roblas R, et al. *Int J Antimicrob Agents.* 2009;33(5):453–455 PMID: 19153032
73. Gupta R, et al. *Cardiol Rev.* 2021;29(5):259–262 PMID: 32976125
74. Forouzan P, et al. *Cureus.* 2020;12(9):e10733 PMID: 33145138
75. Dalal A, et al. *J Infect.* 2008;56(1):77–79 PMID: 18036665
76. Eldin C, et al. *Clin Microbiol Rev.* 2017;30(1):115–190 PMID: 27856520
77. Cherry CC, et al. *Curr Infect Dis Rep.* 2020;22(4):10.1007/s11908-020-0719-0 PMID: 34135692
78. Mayslich C, et al. *Microorganisms.* 2021;9(2):303 PMID: 33540667
79. Lin ZX, et al. *Orthopedics.* 2020;43(1):52–61 PMID: 31958341
80. Dixon DM, et al. *Ticks Tick Borne Dis.* 2021;12(6):101823 PMID: 34517150
81. Xu G, et al. *Emerg Infect Dis.* 2018;24(6):1143–1144 PMID: 29774863
82. Paul K, et al. *Clin Infect Dis.* 2001;33(1):54–61 PMID: 11389495
83. Tricard T, et al. *Arch Pediatr.* 2016;23(11):1146–1149 PMID: 27663465
84. Huang YC, et al. *Int J Antimicrob Agents.* 2018;51(1):47–51 PMID: 28668676

85. Dziuban EJ, et al. *Clin Infect Dis.* 2018;67(1):144–149 PMID: 29211821
86. Siedner MJ, et al. *Clin Infect Dis.* 2014;58(11):1554–1563 PMID: 24647022
87. Tamma PD, et al. *Clin Infect Dis.* 2013;57(6):781–788 PMID: 23759352
88. Tamma PD, et al. IDSA 2024 guidance on the treatment of antimicrobial resistant gram-negative infections. Infectious Diseases Society of America. June 12, 2024. Accessed October 29, 2024. www.idsociety.org/practice-guideline/amr-guidance
89. Iovleva A, et al. *Clin Lab Med.* 2017;37(2):303–315 PMID: 2845735290
90. Arias CA, et al. *Nat Rev Microbiol.* 2012;10(4):266–278 PMID: 22421879
91. Yim J, et al. *Pharmacotherapy.* 2017;37(5):579–592 PMID: 28273381
92. Beganovic M, et al. *Clin Infect Dis.* 2018;67(2):303–309 PMID: 29390132
93. Shah NH, et al. *Open Forum Infect Dis.* 2021;8(4):ofab102 PMID: 34805443
94. Principe L, et al. *Infect Dis Rep.* 2016;8(1):6368 PMID: 27103974
95. AAP. Tularemia. In: Kimberlin DW, et al, eds. *Red Book: 2024–2027 Report of the Committee on Infectious Diseases.* 33rd ed. 2024:929–932
96. Mittal S, et al. *Pediatr Rev.* 2019;40(4):197–201 PMID: 30936402
97. Van TT, et al. *J Clin Microbiol.* 2018;56(12):e00487-18 PMID: 30482869
98. Riordan T. *Clin Microbiol Rev.* 2007;20(4):622–659 PMID: 17934077
99. Valerio L, et al. *J Intern Med.* 2021;289(3):325–339 PMID: 32445216
100. Abou Chacra L, et al. *Front Cell Infect Microbiol.* 2022;11:672429 PMID: 35118003
101. Butler DF, et al. *Infect Dis Clin North Am.* 2018;32(1):119–128 PMID: 29233576
102. AAP. *Helicobacter pylori* infections. In: Kimberlin DW, et al, eds. *Red Book: 2024–2027 Report of the Committee on Infectious Diseases.* 33rd ed. 2024:412–417
103. Jones NL, et al. *J Pediatr Gastroenterol Nutr.* 2017;64(6):991–1003 PMID: 28541262
104. Crowe SE. *N Engl J Med.* 2019;380(12):1158–1165 PMID: 30893536
105. Yagupsky P. *Clin Microbiol Rev.* 2015;28(1):54–79 PMID: 25567222
106. Gouveia C, et al. *Pediatr Infect Dis J.* 2021;40(7):623–627 PMID: 33657599
107. Livermore DM, et al. *Clin Infect Dis.* 2020;71(7):1776–1782 PMID: 32025698
108. Mesini A, et al. *Clin Infect Dis.* 2018;66(5):808–809 PMID: 29020309
109. Bradley JS, et al. *Pediatr Infect Dis J.* 2019;38(9):920–928 PMID: 31335570
110. van Duin D, et al. *Clin Infect Dis.* 2018;66(2):163–171 PMID: 29020404
111. Viasus D, et al. *Infect Dis Ther.* 2022;11(3):973–986 PMID: 35505000
112. Jiménez JIS, et al. *J Crit Care.* 2018;43:361–365 PMID: 29129539
113. Janow G, et al. *Am J Perinatol.* 2009;26(1):89–91 PMID: 19031357
114. Schlech WF. *Microbiol Spectr.* 2019;7(3) PMID: 31837132
115. Dickstein Y, et al. *Eur J Clin Microbiol Infect Dis.* 2019;38(12):2243–2251 PMID: 31399915
116. Murphy TF, et al. *Clin Infect Dis.* 2009;49(1):124–131 PMID: 19480579
117. Shi H, et al. *J Clin Lab Anal.* 2022;36(5):e24399 PMID: 35349730
118. Milligan KL, et al. *Clin Pediatr (Phila).* 2013;52(5):462–464 PMID: 22267858
119. AAP. Nontuberculous mycobacteria. In: Kimberlin DW, et al, eds. *Red Book: 2024–2027 Report of the Committee on Infectious Diseases.* 33rd ed. 2024:920–929
120. Daley CL, et al. *Clin Infect Dis.* 2020;71(4):905–913 PMID: 32797222
121. Koh WJ, et al. *Clin Infect Dis.* 2017;64(3):309–316 PMID: 28011608
122. Waters V, et al. *Cochrane Database Syst Rev.* 2020;(6):CD010004 PMID: 32521055
123. Haworth CS, et al. *BMJ Open Respir Res.* 2017;4(1):e000242 PMID: 29449949
124. Adelman MH, et al. *Curr Opin Pulm Med.* 2018;24(3):212–219 PMID: 29470253
125. Griffith DE, et al. *Chest.* 2022;161(1):64–75 PMID: 34314673
126. Muñoz-Egea MC. *Expert Opin Pharmacother.* 2020;21(8):969–981 PMID: 32200657
127. AAP. Tuberculosis. In: Kimberlin DW, et al, eds. *Red Book: 2024–2027 Report of the Committee on Infectious Diseases.* 33rd ed. 2024:888–920
128. Scott C, et al. *Clin Infect Dis.* 2016;63(5):594–601 PMID: 27298329
129. Sartoris G, et al. *J Pediatric Infect Dis Soc.* 2020;9(2):218–227 PMID: 31909804129
130. Brown-Elliott BA, et al. *J Clin Microbiol.* 2016;54(6):1586–1592 PMID: 27053677
131. CDC. Clinical overview of Hansen's disease (leprosy). May 8, 2024. Accessed November 18, 2024. www.cdc.gov/leprosy/hcp/clinical-overview

132. Johnson MG, et al. *Infection*. 2015;43(6):655–662 PMID: 25869820
133. Jaganath D, et al. *Infect Dis Clin North Am*. 2022;36(1):49–71 PMID: 35168714
134. Scaggs Huang FA, et al. *Pediatr Infect Dis J*. 2019;38(7):749–751 PMID: 30985508
135. Watt KM, et al. *Pediatr Infect Dis J*. 2012;31(2):197–199 PMID: 22016080
136. Waites KB, et al. *Clin Microbiol Rev*. 2017;30(3):747–809 PMID: 28539503
137. Gardiner SJ, et al. *Cochrane Database Syst Rev*. 2015;(1):CD004875 PMID: 25566754
138. Oishi T, et al. *J Clin Med*. 2022;11(7):1782 PMID: 35407390
139. St Cyr S, et al. *MMWR Morb Mortal Wkly Rep*. 2020;69(50):1911–1916 PMID: 33332296
140. Brady RC. *Adv Pediatr*. 2020;67:29–46 PMID: 32591062
141. Nadel S, et al. *Front Pediatr*. 2018;6:321 PMID: 30474022
142. Traxler RM, et al. *Clin Microbiol Rev*. 2022;35(4):e0002721 PMID: 36314911
143. AAP. Nocardiosis. In: Kimberlin DW, et al, eds. *Red Book: 2024–2027 Report of the Committee on Infectious Diseases*. 33rd ed. 2024:620–622
144. Wilson BA, et al. *Clin Microbiol Rev*. 2013;26(3):631–655 PMID: 23824375
145. Mogilner L, et al. *Pediatr Rev*. 2019;40(2):90–92 PMID: 30709978
146. Badri M, et al. *Clin Microbiol Infect*. 2019;25(6):760.e1–760.e6 PMID: 30217761
147. Ozdemir O, et al. *J Microbiol Immunol Infect*. 2010;43(4):344–346 PMID: 20688296
148. Janda JM, et al. *Clin Microbiol Rev*. 2016;29(2):349–374 PMID: 26960939
149. Brook I, et al. *Clin Microbiol Rev*. 2013;26(3):526–546 PMID: 23824372
150. Schaffer JN, et al. *Microbiol Spectr*. 2015;3(5) PMID: 26542036
151. Abdallah M, et al. *New Microbes New Infect*. 2018;25:16–23 PMID: 29983987
152. Kunz Coyne AJ, et al. *Infect Dis Ther*. 2022;11(2):661–682 PMID: 35150435
153. Kalil AC, et al. *Clin Infect Dis*. 2016;63(5):e61–e111 PMID: 27418577
154. Alali M, et al. *J Pediatr Hematol Oncol*. 2020;42(6):e445–e451 PMID: 32404688
155. Jiao Y, et al. *Antimicrob Agents Chemother*. 2019;63(7):e00425-19 PMID: 30988147
156. McCarthy KL, et al. *Infect Dis (Lond)*. 2018;50(5):403–406 PMID: 29205079
157. Kim HS, et al. *BMC Infect Dis*. 2017;17(1):500 PMID: 28716109
158. Milinic T, et al. *Semin Respir Crit Care Med*. 2023;44(2):225–241 PMID: 36746183
159. Epps QJ, et al. *Pediatr Pulmonol*. 2021;56(6):1784–1788 PMID: 33524241
160. Langton Hewer SC, et al. *Cochrane Database Syst Rev*. 2023;(6):CD004197 PMID: 37268599
161. Mogayzel PJ Jr, et al. *Ann Am Thorac Soc*. 2014;11(10):1640–1650 PMID: 25549030
162. Ryan MP, et al. *Eur J Clin Microbiol Infect Dis*. 2014;33(3):291–304 PMID: 24057141
163. Lin WV, et al. *Clin Microbiol Infect*. 2019;25(3):310–315 PMID: 29777923
164. AAP. Rickettsial diseases. In: Kimberlin DW, et al, eds. *Red Book: 2024–2027 Report of the Committee on Infectious Diseases*. 33rd ed. 2024:723–725
165. Blanton LS. *Infect Dis Clin North Am*. 2019;33(1):213–229 PMID: 30712763
166. AAP. *Salmonella* infections. In: Kimberlin DW, et al, eds. *Red Book: 2024–2027 Report of the Committee on Infectious Diseases*. 33rd ed. 2024:742–750
167. Leinert JL, et al. *Antibiotics (Basel)*. 2021;10(10):1187 PMID: 34680768
168. Onwuezobe IA, et al. *Cochrane Database Syst Rev*. 2012;(11):CD001167 PMID: 23152205
169. Karkey A, et al. *Curr Opin Gastroenterol*. 2018;34(1):25–30 PMID: 29059070
170. Manesh A, et al. *J Travel Med*. 2021;28(3):taab012 PMID: 33550411
171. Yousfi K, et al. *Eur J Clin Microbiol Infect Dis*. 2017;36(8):1353–1362 PMID: 28299457
172. Janda JM, et al. *Crit Rev Microbiol*. 2014;40(4):293–312 PMID: 23043419
173. Baker S, et al. *Nat Rev Microbiol*. 2023;21(7):409–410 PMID: 37188805
174. AAP. *Shigella* infections. In: Kimberlin DW, et al, eds. *Red Book: 2024–2027 Report of the Committee on Infectious Diseases*. 33rd ed. 2024:756–760
175. Kotloff KL, et al. *Lancet*. 2018;391(10122):801–812 PMID: 29254859
176. CDC. NARMS Now: Human Data. Accessed October 29, 2024. https://wwwn.cdc.gov/narmsnow
177. Rognrud K, et al. *Case Rep Infect Dis*. 2020;2020:7185834 PMID: 33101743
178. El Beaino M, et al. *Int J Infect Dis*. 2018;77:68–73 PMID: 30267938
179. AAP. Rat-bite fever. In: Kimberlin DW, et al, eds. *Red Book: 2024–2027 Report of the Committee on Infectious Diseases*. 33rd ed. 2024:711–713
180. Stevens DL, et al. *Clin Infect Dis*. 2014;59(2):e10–e52 PMID: 24973422

181. Sharma R, et al. *Curr Infect Dis Rep*. 2019;21(10):37 PMID: 31486979
182. Korczowski B, et al. *Pediatr Infect Dis J*. 2016;35(8):e239–e247 PMID: 27164462
183. Bradley J, et al. *Pediatrics*. 2017;139(3):e20162477 PMID: 28202770
184. Rybak MJ, et al. *Am J Health Syst Pharm*. 2020;77(11):835–864 PMID: 32191793
185. Arrieta AC, et al. *Pediatr Infect Dis J*. 2018;37(9):893–900 PMID: 29406465
186. Becker K, et al. *Expert Rev Anti Infect Ther*. 2020;18(4):349–366 PMID: 32056452
187. Sader HS, et al. *Diagn Microbiol Infect Dis*. 2016;85(1):80–84 PMID: 26971182
188. Mojica MF, et al. *JAC Antimicrob Resist*. 2022;4(3):dlac040 PMID: 35529051
189. Anđelković MV, et al. *J Chemother*. 2019;31(6):297–306 PMID: 31130079
190. Delgado-Valverde M, et al. *J Antimicrob Chemother*. 2020;75(7):1840–1849 PMID: 32277821
191. Edholm A, et al. *Clin Pract Cases Emerg Med*. 2021;5(4):407–411 PMID: 34813430
192. Gerber MA, et al. *Circulation*. 2009;119(11):1541–1551 PMID: 19246689
193. AAP. Group B streptococcal infections. In: Kimberlin DW, et al, eds. *Red Book: 2024–2027 Report of the Committee on Infectious Diseases*. 33rd ed. 2024:799–806
194. Faden H, et al. *Pediatr Infect Dis J*. 2017;36(11):1099–1100 PMID: 28640003
195. Furuichi M, et al. *J Infect Chemother*. 2018;24(2):99–102 PMID: 29050796
196. Faden HS. *Pediatr Infect Dis J*. 2016;35(9):1047–1048 PMID: 27294306
197. Otto WR, et al. *J Pediatric Infect Dis Soc*. 2021;10(3):309–316 PMID: 32955086
198. Baltimore RS, et al. *Circulation*. 2015;132(15):1487–1515 PMID: 26373317
199. Bradley JS, et al. *Clin Infect Dis*. 2011;53(7):e25–e76 PMID: 21880587
200. Mendes RE, et al. *Diagn Microbiol Infect Dis*. 2014;80(1):19–25 PMID: 24974272
201. Kaplan SL, et al. *Pediatrics*. 2019;144(3):e20190567 PMID: 31420369
202. AAP. Syphilis. In: Kimberlin DW, et al, eds. *Red Book: 2024–2027 Report of the Committee on Infectious Diseases*. 33rd ed. 2024:825–841
203. Viscardi RM, et al. *Arch Dis Child Fetal Neonatal Ed*. 2020;105(6):615–622 PMID: 32170033
204. CDC. Treating cholera. April 12, 2024. Accessed October 29, 2024. www.cdc.gov/cholera/treatment
205. Kanungo S, et al. *Lancet*. 2022;399(10333):1429–1440 PMID: 35397865
206. Trinh SA, et al. *Antimicrob Agents Chemother*. 2017;61(12):e01106-17 PMID: 28971862
207. Coerdt KM, et al. *Cutis*. 2021;107(2):E12–E17 PMID: 33891847
208. Leng F, et al. *Eur J Clin Microbiol Infect Dis*. 2019;38(11):1999–2004 PMID: 31325061
209. AAP. *Yersinia enterocolitica* and *Yersinia pseudotuberculosis* infections. In: Kimberlin DW, et al, eds. *Red Book: 2024–2027 Report of the Committee on Infectious Diseases*. 33rd ed. 2024:960–963
210. Kato H, et al. *Medicine (Baltimore)*. 2016;95(26):e3988 PMID: 27368001
211. Yang R. *J Clin Microbiol*. 2017;56(1):e01519-17 PMID: 29070654
212. Barbieri R, et al. *Clin Microbiol Rev*. 2020;34(1):e00044-19 PMID: 33298527
213. CDC. Clinical care of plague. May 15, 2024. Accessed November 18, 2023. www.cdc.gov/plague/hcp/clinical-care
214. Somova LM, et al. *Pathogens*. 2020;9(6):436 PMID: 32498317

Chapter 4

1. Bosheva M, et al. *Pediatr Infect Dis J*. 2021;40(6):e222–e229 PMID: 33480665
2. Cannavino CR, et al. *Pediatr Infect Dis J*. 2016;35(7):752–759 PMID: 27093162
3. Bhatt J, et al. *Cochrane Database Syst Rev*. 2019;(9):CD002009 PMID: 31483853
4. Kaye KS, et al. *Infect Dis Ther*. 2023(3):777–806 PMID: 36847998
5. Schmid H, et al. *Pediatr Infect Dis J*. 2024;43(8):772–776 PMID: 38564757
6. Chang CK, et al. *Front Pharmacol*. 2022;13:814333 PMID: 35387340
7. Wirth S, et al. *Pediatr Infect Dis J*. 2018;37(8):e207–e213 PMID: 29356761
8. Jackson MA, et al. *Pediatrics*. 2016;138(5):e20162706 PMID: 27940800
9. Bradley JS, et al. *Pediatrics*. 2014;134(1):e146–e153 PMID: 24918220

Chapter 5

1. Groll AH, et al. *Lancet Oncol*. 2014;15(8):e327–e340 PMID: 24988936
2. Wingard JR, et al. *Blood*. 2010;116(24):5111–5118 PMID: 20826719
3. Van Burik JA, et al. *Clin Infect Dis*. 2004;39(10):1407–1416 PMID: 15546073

4. Cornely OA, et al. *N Engl J Med.* 2007;356(4):348–359 PMID: 17251531
5. Kung HC, et al. *Cancer Med.* 2014;3(3):667–673 PMID: 24644249
6. Science M, et al. *Pediatr Blood Cancer.* 2014;61(3):393–400 PMID: 24424789
7. Bow EJ, et al. *BMC Infect Dis.* 2015;15:128 PMID: 25887385
8. Tacke D, et al. *Ann Hematol.* 2014;93(9):1449–1456 PMID: 24951122
9. Almyroudis NG, et al. *Curr Opin Infect Dis.* 2009;22(4):385–393 PMID: 19506476
10. Maschmeyer G. *J Antimicrob Chemother.* 2009;63(suppl 1):i27–i30 PMID: 19372178
11. Freifeld AG, et al. *Clin Infect Dis.* 2011;52(4):e56–e93 PMID: 21258094
12. Fisher BT. *JAMA.* 2019;322(17):1673–1681 PMID: 31688884
13. Dvorak CC, et al. *J Pediatric Infect Dis Soc.* 2021;10(4):417–425 PMID: 33136159
14. Kim BK, et al. *Children (Basel).* 2022;9(3):372 PMID: 35327744
15. De Pauw BE, et al. *N Engl J Med.* 2007;356(4):409–411 PMID: 17251538
16. Salavert M. *Int J Antimicrob Agents.* 2008;32(suppl 2):S149–S153 PMID: 19013340
17. Eschenauer GA, et al. *Liver Transpl.* 2009;15(8):842–858 PMID: 19642130
18. Winston DJ, et al. *Am J Transplant.* 2014;14(12):2758–2764 PMID: 25376267
19. Sun HY, et al. *Transplantation.* 2013;96(6):573–578 PMID: 23842191
20. Radack KP, et al. *Curr Infect Dis Rep.* 2009;11(6):427–434 PMID: 19857381
21. Patterson TF, et al. *Clin Infect Dis.* 2016;63(4):e1–e60 PMID: 27365388
22. Thomas L, et al. *Expert Rev Anti Infect Ther.* 2009;7(4):461–472 PMID: 19400765
23. Friberg LE, et al. *Antimicrob Agents Chemother.* 2012;56(6):3032–3042 PMID: 22430956
24. Burgos A, et al. *Pediatrics.* 2008;121(5):e1286–e1294 PMID: 18450871
25. Herbrecht R, et al. *N Engl J Med.* 2002;347(6):408–415 PMID: 12167683
26. Mousset S, et al. *Ann Hematol.* 2014;93(1):13–32 PMID: 24026426
27. Blyth CC, et al. *Intern Med J.* 2014;44(12b):1333–1349 PMID: 25482744
28. Denning DW, et al. *Eur Respir J.* 2016;47(1):45–68 PMID: 26699723
29. Cornely OA, et al. *Clin Infect Dis.* 2007;44(10):1289–1297 PMID: 17443465
30. Maertens JA, et al. *Lancet.* 2016;387(10020):760–769 PMID: 26684607
31. Tissot F, et al. *Haematologica.* 2017;102(3):433–444 PMID: 28011902
32. Ullmann AJ, et al. *Clin Microbiol Infect.* 2018;24(suppl 1):e1–e38 PMID: 29544767
33. Walsh TJ, et al. *Antimicrob Agents Chemother.* 2010;54(10):4116–4123 PMID: 20660687
34. Arrieta AC, et al. *Antimicrob Agents Chemother.* 2021;65(8):e0029021 PMID: 34031051
35. Maertens JA, et al. *Lancet.* 2021;397(10273):499–509 PMID: 33549194
36. Bartelink IH, et al. *Antimicrob Agents Chemother.* 2013;57(1):235–240 PMID: 23114771
37. Slavin MA, et al. *J Antimicrob Chemother.* 2022;77(1):16–23 PMID: 34508633
38. Marr KA, et al. *Ann Intern Med.* 2015;162(2):81–89 PMID: 25599346
39. Verweij PE, et al. *Drug Resist Updat.* 2015;21–22:30–40 PMID: 26282594
40. Kohno S, et al. *Eur J Clin Microbiol Infect Dis.* 2013;32(3):387–397 PMID: 23052987
41. Naggie S, et al. *Clin Chest Med.* 2009;30(2):337–353 PMID: 19375639
42. Revankar SG, et al. *Clin Microbiol Rev.* 2010;23(4):884–928 PMID: 20930077
43. Wong EH, et al. *Infect Dis Clin North Am.* 2016;30(1):165–178 PMID: 26897066
44. Revankar SG, et al. *Clin Infect Dis.* 2004;38(2):206–216 PMID: 14699452
45. Li DM, et al. *Lancet Infect Dis.* 2009;9(6):376–383 PMID: 19467477
46. Chowdhary A, et al. *Clin Microbiol Infect.* 2014;20(suppl 3):47–75 PMID: 24483780
47. McCarty TP, et al. *Med Mycol.* 2015;53(5):440–446 PMID: 25908651
48. Schieffelin JS, et al. *Transplant Infect Dis.* 2014;16(2):270–278 PMID: 24628809
49. Chapman SW, et al. *Clin Infect Dis.* 2008;46(12):1801–1812 PMID: 18462107
50. McKinnell JA, et al. *Clin Chest Med.* 2009;30(2):227–239 PMID: 19375630
51. Walsh CM, et al. *Pediatr Infect Dis J.* 2006;25(7):656–658 PMID: 16804444
52. Fanella S, et al. *Med Mycol.* 2011;49(6):627–632 PMID: 21208027
53. Smith JA, et al. *Proc Am Thorac Soc.* 2010;7(3):173–180 PMID: 20463245
54. Bariola JR, et al. *Clin Infect Dis.* 2010;50(6):797–804 PMID: 20166817
55. Limper AH, et al. *Am J Respir Crit Care Med.* 2011;183(1):96–128 PMID: 21193785
56. Thompson GR, et al. *Lancet Infect Dis.* 2021;21(12):e364–e374 PMID: 34364529
57. Pappas PG, et al. *Clin Infect Dis.* 2016;62(4):e1–e50 PMID: 26679628

58. Lortholary O, et al. *Clin Microbiol Infect.* 2012;18(suppl 7):68–77 PMID: 23137138
59. Ullman AJ, et al. *Clin Microbiol Infect.* 2012;18(suppl 7):53–67 PMID: 23137137
60. Hope WW, et al. *Clin Microbiol Infect.* 2012;18(suppl 7):38–52 PMID: 23137136
61. Cornely OA, et al. *Clin Microbiol Infect.* 2012;18(suppl 7):19–37 PMID: 23137135
62. Hope WW, et al. *Antimicrob Agents Chemother.* 2015;59(2):905–913 PMID: 25421470
63. Piper L, et al. *Pediatr Infect Dis J.* 2011;30(5):375–378 PMID: 21085048
64. Watt KM, et al. *Antimicrob Agents Chemother.* 2015;59(7):3935–3943 PMID: 25896706
65. Ascher SB, et al. *Pediatr Infect Dis J.* 2012;31(5):439–443 PMID: 22189522
66. Sobel JD. *Lancet.* 2007;369(9577):1961–1971 PMID: 17560449
67. Kim J, et al. *J Antimicrob Chemother.* 2020;75(1):215–220 PMID: 31586424
68. Almangour TA, et al. *Saudi Pharm J.* 2021;29(4):315–323 PMID: 33994826
69. Barnes KN, et al. *Ann Pharmacother.* 2023;57(1):99–106 PMID: 35502451
70. Martinez RL, et al. *Clin Dermatol.* 2007;25(2):188–194 PMID: 17350498
71. Ameen M. *Clin Exp Dermatol.* 2009;34(8):849–854 PMID: 19575735
72. Chowdhary A, et al. *Clin Microbiol Infect.* 2014;20(suppl 3):47–75 PMID: 24483780
73. Queiroz-Telles F. *Rev Inst Med Trop Sao Paulo.* 2015;57(suppl 19):46–50 PMID: 26465369
74. Queiroz-Telles F, et al. *Clin Microbiol Rev.* 2017;30(1):233–276 PMID: 27856522
75. Galgiani JN, et al. *Clin Infect Dis.* 2016;63(6):717–722 PMID: 27559032
76. Anstead GM, et al. *Infect Dis Clin North Am.* 2006;20(3):621–643 PMID: 16984872
77. Williams PL. *Ann N Y Acad Sci.* 2007;1111:377–384 PMID: 17363442
78. Homans JD, et al. *Pediatr Infect Dis J.* 2010;29(1):65–67 PMID: 19884875
79. Kauffman CA, et al. *Transplant Infectious Diseases.* 2014;16(2):213–224 PMID: 24589027
80. McCarty JM, et al. *Clin Infect Dis.* 2013;56(11):1579–1585 PMID: 23463637
81. Bravo R, et al. *J Pediatr Hematol Oncol.* 2012;34(5):389–394 PMID: 22510771
82. Catanzaro A, et al. *Clin Infect Dis.* 2007;45(5):562–568 PMID: 17682989
83. Thompson GR, et al. *Clin Infect Dis.* 2016;63(3):356–362 PMID: 27169478
84. Thompson GR III, et al. *Clin Infect Dis.* 2017;65(2):338–341 PMID: 28419259
85. Chayakulkeeree M, et al. *Infect Dis Clin North Am.* 2006;20(3):507–544 PMID: 16984867
86. Jarvis JN, et al. *Semin Respir Crit Care Med.* 2008;29(2):141–150 PMID: 18365996
87. Perfect JR, et al. *Clin Infect Dis.* 2010;50(3):291–322 PMID: 20047480
88. Joshi NS, et al. *Pediatr Infect Dis J.* 2010;29(12):e91–e95 PMID: 20935590
89. Day JN, et al. *N Engl J Med.* 2013;368(14):1291–1302 PMID: 23550668
90. Chang CC, et al. *Lancet Infect Dis.* 2024;24(8):e495–e512 PMID: 38346436
91. Jarvis JN, et al. *N Engl J Med.* 2022;386(12):1109–1120 PMID: 3532064
92. Cortez KJ, et al. *Clin Microbiol Rev.* 2008;21(1):157–197 PMID: 18202441
93. Tortorano AM, et al. *Clin Microbiol Infect.* 2014;20(suppl 3):27–46 PMID: 24548001
94. Horn DL, et al. *Mycoses.* 2014;57(11):652–658 PMID: 24943384
95. Muhammed M, et al. *Medicine (Baltimore).* 2013;92(6):305–316 PMID: 24145697
96. Rodriguez-Tudela JL, et al. *Med Mycol.* 2009;47(4):359–370 PMID: 19031336
97. Wheat LJ, et al. *Clin Infect Dis.* 2007;45(7):807–825 PMID: 17806045
98. Myint T, et al. *Medicine (Baltimore).* 2014;93(1):11–18 PMID: 24378739
99. Assi M, et al. *Clin Infect Dis.* 2013;57(11):1542–1549 PMID: 24046304
100. Chayakulkeeree M, et al. *Eur J Clin Microbiol Infect Dis.* 2006;25(4):215–229 PMID: 16568297
101. Spellberg B, et al. *Clin Infect Dis.* 2009;48(12):1743–1751 PMID: 19435437
102. Reed C, et al. *Clin Infect Dis.* 2008;47(3):364–371 PMID: 18558882
103. Cornely OA, et al. *Clin Microbiol Infect.* 2014;20(suppl 3):5–26 PMID: 24479848
104. Spellberg B, et al. *Clin Infect Dis.* 2012;54(suppl 1):S73–S78 PMID: 22247449
105. Chitasombat MN, et al. *Curr Opin Infect Dis.* 2016;29(4):340–345 PMID: 27191199
106. Pana ZD, et al. *BMC Infect Dis.* 2016;16(1):667 PMID: 27832748
107. Pagano L, et al. *Haematologica.* 2013;98(10):e127–e130 PMID: 23716556
108. Kyvernitakis A, et al. *Clin Microbiol Infect.* 2016;22(9):811.e1–811.e8 PMID: 27085727
109. Marty FM, et al. *Lancet Infect Dis.* 2016;16(7):828–837 PMID: 26969258
110. Cornely OA. *Lancet Infect Dis.* 2019;19(12):e405–e421 PMID: 31699664
111. Queiroz-Telles F, et al. *Clin Infect Dis.* 2007;45(11):1462–1469 PMID: 17990229

112. Menezes VM, et al. *Cochrane Database Syst Rev.* 2006;(2):CD004967 PMID: 16625617
113. Marques SA. *An Bras Dermatol.* 2013;88(5):700–711 PMID: 24173174
114. Borges SR, et al. *Med Mycol.* 2014;52(3):303–310 PMID: 24577007
115. Panel on Opportunistic Infections in Children With and Exposed to HIV. Guidelines for the prevention and treatment of opportunistic infections in children with and exposed to HIV. What's new in the guidelines? Updated July 3, 2024. Accessed October 29, 2024. https://clinicalinfo.hiv.gov/en/guidelines/hiv-clinical-guidelines-pediatric-opportunistic-infections/whats-new
116. Siberry GK, et al. *Pediatr Infect Dis J.* 2013;32(suppl 2):i–KK4 PMID: 24569199
117. Maschmeyer G, et al. *J Antimicrob Chemother.* 2016;71(9):2405–2413 PMID: 27550993
118. Kauffman CA, et al. *Clin Infect Dis.* 2007;45(10):1255–1265 PMID: 17968818
119. Aung AK, et al. *Med Mycol.* 2013;51(5):534–544 PMID: 23286352
120. Ali S, et al. *Pediatr Emerg Care.* 2007;23(9):662–668 PMID: 17876261
121. Shy R. *Pediatr Rev.* 2007;28(5):164–174 PMID: 17473121
122. Andrews MD, et al. *Am Fam Physician.* 2008;77(10):1415–1420 PMID: 18533375
123. Kakourou T, et al. *Pediatr Dermatol.* 2010;27(3):226–228 PMID: 20609140
124. Gupta AK, et al. *Pediatr Dermatol.* 2013;30(1):1–6 PMID: 22994156
125. Chen X, et al. *J Am Acad Dermatol.* 2017;76(2):368–374 PMID: 27816294
126. Gupta AK, et al. *Pediatr Dermatol.* 2020;37(6):1014–1022 PMID: 32897584
127. de Berker D. *N Engl J Med.* 2009;360(20):2108–2116 PMID: 19439745
128. Ameen M, et al. *Br J Dermatol.* 2014;171(5):937–958 PMID: 25409999
129. Gupta AK. *J Eur Acad Dermatol Venereol.* 2020;34(3):580–588 PMID: 31746067
130. Sprenger AB. *J Fungi (Basel).* 2019;5(3):82 PMID: 31487828
131. Pantazidou A, et al. *Arch Dis Child.* 2007;92(11):1040–1042 PMID: 17954488
132. Gupta AK, et al. *J Cutan Med Surg.* 2014;18(2):79–90 PMID: 24636433

Chapter 6

1. Cavassin FB, et al. *Paediatr Drugs.* 2022;24(5):513–528 PMID: 35849282
2. Cornely OA, et al. *Clin Infect Dis.* 2007;44(10):1289–1297 PMID: 17443465
3. Lestner JM, et al. *Antimicrob Agents Chemother.* 2016;60(12):7340–7346 PMID: 27697762
4. Seibel NL, et al. *Antimicrob Agents Chemother.* 2017;61(2):e01477-16 PMID: 27855062
5. Azoulay E, et al. *PLoS One.* 2017;12(5):e0177093 PMID: 28531175
6. Ascher SB, et al. *Pediatr Infect Dis J.* 2012;31(5):439–443 PMID: 22189522
7. Piper L, et al. *Pediatr Infect Dis J.* 2011;30(5):375–378 PMID: 21085048
8. Gerhart JG, et al. *CPT Pharmacometrics Syst Pharmacol.* 2019;8(7):500–510 PMID: 31087536
9. Watt KM, et al. *Antimicrob Agents Chemother.* 2015;59(7):3935–3943 PMID: 25896706
10. Watt KM, et al. *CPT Pharmacometrics Syst Pharmacol.* 2018;7(10):629–637 PMID: 30033691
11. Mathew JL, et al. *Indian J Pediatr.* 2023;90(7):708–717 PMID: 37264275
12. Agarwal R, et al. *Eur Respir J.* 2024;63(4):2400061 PMID: 38423624
13. Friberg LE, et al. *Antimicrob Agents Chemother.* 2012;56(6):3032–3042 PMID: 22430956
14. Schweiger JA, et al. *J Pediatr Hematol Oncol.* 2024;46(6):e419–e425 PMID: 38934583
15. Zembles TN, et al. *J Pediatr Pharmacol Ther.* 2023;28(3):247–254 PMID: 37303767
16. Zembles TN, et al. *Pharmacotherapy.* 2016;36(10):1102–1108 PMID: 27548272
17. Moriyama B, et al. *Clin Pharmacol Ther.* 2017;102(1):45–51 PMID: 27981572
18. McCann S, et al. *Clin Pharmacokinet.* 2023;62(7):997–1009 PMID: 37179512
19. Kane Z, et al. *Antimicrob Agents Chemother.* 2023;67(7):e0007723 PMID: 37260401
20. Arrieta AC, et al. *PLoS One.* 2019;14(3):e0212837 PMID: 30913226
21. Groll AH, et al. *Int J Antimicrob Agents.* 2020;56(3):106084 PMID: 32682946
22. Winchell G, et al. *Antimicrob Agents Chemother.* 2024;68(4):e0119723 PMID: 38376229
23. Bernardo V, et al. *Pediatr Transplant.* 2020;24(6):e13777 PMID: 32639095
24. Maertens JA, et al. *Lancet.* 2016;387(10020):760–769 PMID: 26684607
25. Marty FM, et al. *Lancet Infect Dis.* 2016;16(7):828–837 PMID: 26969258
26. Cornely OA, et al. *Lancet Infect Dis.* 2019;19(12):e405–e421 PMID: 31699664
27. Arrieta AC, et al. *Antimicrob Agents Chemother.* 2021;65(8):e0029021 PMID: 34031051
28. Furfaro E, et al. *J Antimicrob Chemother.* 2019;74(8):2341–2346 PMID: 31119272

29. Fisher BT, et al. *JAMA*. 2019;322(17):1673–1681 PMID: 31688884
30. Dvorak CC, et al. *J Pediatric Infect Dis Soc*. 2021;10(4):417–425 PMID: 33136159
31. Niu CH, et al. *Front Pharmacol*. 2020;11:184 PMID: 32194415
32. Du B, et al. *J Antimicrob Chemother*. 2024;79(10):2678–2687 PMID: 39119901
33. Smith PB, et al. *Pediatr Infect Dis J*. 2009;28(5):412–415 PMID: 19319022
34. Hope WW, et al. *Antimicrob Agents Chemother*. 2010;54(6):2633–2637 PMID: 20308367
35. Benjamin DK Jr, et al. *Clin Pharmacol Ther*. 2010;87(1):93–99 PMID: 19890251
36. Auriti C, et al. *Antimicrob Agents Chemother*. 2021;65(4):e02494-20 PMID: 33558294
37. Bury D, et al. *Int J Antimicrob Agents*. 2024;63(1):107058 PMID: 38081549
38. Kim BK, et al. *Children (Basel)*. 2022;9(3):372 PMID: 35327744
39. Cohen-Wolkowiez M, et al. *Clin Pharmacol Ther*. 2011;89(5):702–707 PMID: 21412233
40. Roilides E, et al. *Pediatr Infect Dis J*. 2019;38(3):275–279 PMID: 30418357
41. Roilides E, et al. *Pediatr Infect Dis J*. 2020;39(4):305–309 PMID: 32032174
42. Thompson GR, et al. *Lancet*. 2023;401(10370):49–59 PMID: 36442484
43. Spec A, et al. *J Antimicrob Chemother*. 2019;74(10):3056–3062 PMID: 31304536

Chapter 7

1. Lenaerts L, et al. *Rev Med Virol*. 2008;18(6):357–374 PMID: 18655013
2. Michaels MG. *Expert Rev Anti Infect Ther*. 2007;5(3):441–448 PMID: 17547508
3. Biron KK. *Antiviral Res*. 2006;71(2–3):154–163 PMID: 16765457
4. Boeckh M, et al. *Blood*. 2009;113(23):5711–5719 PMID: 19299333
5. Vaudry W, et al. *Am J Transplant*. 2009;9(3):636–643 PMID: 19260840
6. Emanuel D, et al. *Ann Intern Med*. 1988;109(10):777–782 PMID: 2847609
7. Reed EC, et al. *Ann Intern Med*. 1988;109(10):783–788 PMID: 2847610
8. Studies of Ocular Complications of AIDS Research Group in collaboration with the AIDS Clinical Trials Group. *Ophthalmology*. 1994;101(7):1250–1261 PMID: 8035989
9. Singh N, et al. *JAMA*. 2020;323(14):1378–1387 PMID: 32286644
10. Martin DF, et al. *N Engl J Med*. 2002;346(15):1119–1126 PMID: 11948271
11. Kempen JH, et al. *Arch Ophthalmol*. 2003;121(4):466–476 PMID: 12695243
12. Studies of Ocular Complications of AIDS Research Group. The AIDS Clinical Trials Group. *Am J Ophthalmol*. 2001;131(4):457–467 PMID: 11292409
13. Dieterich DT, et al. *J Infect Dis*. 1993;167(2):278–282 PMID: 8380610
14. Gerna G, et al. *Antiviral Res*. 1997;34(1):39–51 PMID: 9107384
15. Markham A, et al. *Drugs*. 1994;48(3):455–484 PMID: 7527763
16. Kimberlin DW, et al. *J Infect Dis*. 2008;197(6):836–845 PMID: 18279073
17. Kimberlin DW, et al. *N Engl J Med*. 2015;372(10):933–943 PMID: 25738669
18. Griffiths P, et al. *Herpes*. 2008;15(1):4–12 PMID: 18983762
19. Panel on Opportunistic Infections in Children With and Exposed to HIV. Guidelines for the prevention and treatment of opportunistic infections in children with and exposed to HIV. What's new in the guidelines? Updated July 3, 2024. Accessed October 29, 2024. https://clinicalinfo.hiv.gov/en/guidelines/hiv-clinical-guidelines-pediatric-opportunistic-infections/whats-new
20. Marty FM, et al. *N Engl J Med*. 2017;377(25):2433–2444 PMID: 29211658
21. Abzug MJ, et al. *J Pediatric Infect Dis Soc*. 2016;5(1):53–62 PMID: 26407253
22. Biebl A, et al. *Nat Clin Pract Neurol*. 2009;5(3):171–174 PMID: 19262593
23. Chadaide Z, et al. *J Med Virol*. 2008;80(11):1930–1932 PMID: 18814244
24. AAP. Epstein-Barr virus infections. In: Kimberlin DW, et al, eds. *Red Book: 2024–2027 Report of the Committee on Infectious Diseases*. 33rd ed. 2024:372–376
25. Gross TG. *Herpes*. 2009;15(3):64–67 PMID: 19306606
26. Styczynski J, et al. *Bone Marrow Transplant*. 2009;43(10):757–770 PMID: 19043458
27. Jonas MM, et al. *Hepatology*. 2016;63(2):377–387 PMID: 26223345
28. Marcellin P, et al. *Gastroenterology*. 2016;150(1):134–144.e10 PMID: 26453773
29. Chen HL, et al. *Hepatology*. 2015;62(2):375–386 PMID: 25851052
30. Wu Q, et al. *Clin Gastroenterol Hepatol*. 2015;13(6):1170–1176 PMID: 25251571

31. Hou JL, et al. *J Viral Hepat*. 2015;22(2):85–93 PMID: 25243325
32. Kurbegov AC, et al. *Expert Rev Gastroenterol Hepatol*. 2009;3(1):39–49 PMID: 19210112
33. Jonas MM, et al. *Hepatology*. 2008;47(6):1863–1871 PMID: 18433023
34. Lai CL, et al. *Gastroenterology*. 2002;123(6):1831–1838 PMID: 12454840
35. Honkoop P, et al. *Expert Opin Investig Drugs*. 2003;12(4):683–688 PMID: 12665423
36. Shaw T, et al. *Expert Rev Anti Infect Ther*. 2004;2(6):853–871 PMID: 15566330
37. Elisofon SA, et al. *Clin Liver Dis*. 2006;10(1):133–148 PMID: 16376798
38. Jonas MM, et al. *Hepatology*. 2010;52(6):2192–2205 PMID: 20890947
39. Haber BA, et al. *Pediatrics*. 2009;124(5):e1007–e1013 PMID: 19805457
40. Shneider BL, et al. *Hepatology*. 2006;44(5):1344–1354 PMID: 17058223
41. Jain MK, et al. *J Viral Hepat*. 2007;14(3):176–182 PMID: 17305883
42. Sokal EM, et al. *Gastroenterology*. 1998;114(5):988–995 PMID: 9558288
43. Jonas MM, et al. *N Engl J Med*. 2002;346(22):1706–1713 PMID: 12037150
44. Chang TT, et al. *N Engl J Med*. 2006;354(10):1001–1010 PMID: 16525137
45. Liaw YF, et al. *Gastroenterology*. 2009;136(2):486–495 PMID: 19027013
46. Terrault NA, et al. *Hepatology*. 2018;67(4):1560–1599 PMID: 29405329
47. Keam SJ, et al. *Drugs*. 2008;68(9):1273–1317 PMID: 18547135
48. Marcellin P, et al. *Gastroenterology*. 2011;140(2):459–468 PMID: 21034744
49. Poordad F, et al. *N Engl J Med*. 2011;364(13):1195–1206 PMID: 21449783
50. Schwarz KB, et al. *Gastroenterology*. 2011;140(2):450–458 PMID: 21036173
51. Nelson DR. *Liver Int*. 2011;31(suppl 1):53–57 PMID: 21205138
52. Strader DB, et al. *Hepatology*. 2004;39(4):1147–1171 PMID: 15057920
53. Soriano V, et al. *AIDS*. 2007;21(9):1073–1089 PMID: 17502718
54. Murray KF, et al. *Hepatology*. 2018;68(6):2158–2166 PMID: 30070726
55. Feld JJ, et al. *N Engl J Med*. 2014;370(17):1594–1603 PMID: 24720703
56. Zeuzem S, et al. *N Engl J Med*. 2014;370(17):1604–1614 PMID: 24720679
57. Andreone P, et al. *Gastroenterology*. 2014;147(2):359–365.e1 PMID: 24818763
58. Ferenci P, et al. *N Engl J Med*. 2014;370(21):1983–1992 PMID: 24795200
59. Poordad F, et al. *N Engl J Med*. 2014;370(21):1973–1982 PMID: 24725237
60. Jacobson IM, et al. *Lancet*. 2014;384(9941):403–413 PMID: 24907225
61. Manns M, et al. *Lancet*. 2014;384(9941):414–426 PMID: 24907224
62. Forns X, et al. *Gastroenterology*. 2014;146(7):1669–1679.e3 PMID: 24602923
63. Zeuzem S, et al. *Gastroenterology*. 2014;146(2):430–441.e6 PMID: 24184810
64. Lawitz E, et al. *Lancet*. 2014;384(9956):1756–1765 PMID: 25078309
65. Afdhal N, et al. *N Engl J Med*. 2014;370(20):1889–1898 PMID: 24725239
66. Afdhal N, et al. *N Engl J Med*. 2014;370(16):1483–1493 PMID: 24725238
67. Kowdley KV, et al. *N Engl J Med*. 2014;370(20):1879–1888 PMID: 24720702
68. Lawitz E, et al. *N Engl J Med*. 2013;368(20):1878–1887 PMID: 23607594
69. Jacobson IM, et al. *N Engl J Med*. 2013;368(20):1867–1877 PMID: 23607593
70. Zeuzem S, et al. *N Engl J Med*. 2014;370(21):1993–2001 PMID: 24795201
71. American Association for the Study of Liver Diseases, Infectious Diseases Society of America. HCV in children. Updated October 24, 2022. Accessed October 29, 2024. www.hcvguidelines.org/unique-populations/children
72. Hollier LM, et al. *Cochrane Database Syst Rev*. 2008;(1):CD004946 PMID: 18254066
73. Pinninti SG, et al. *J Pediatr*. 2012;161(1):134–138 PMID: 22336576
74. ACOG. *Obstet Gynecol*. 2020;135(5):e193–e202 PMID: 32332414
75. Kimberlin DW, et al. *Clin Infect Dis*. 2010;50(2):221–228 PMID: 20014952
76. Mofenson LM, et al. *MMWR Recomm Rep*. 2009;58(RR-11):1–166 PMID: 19730409
77. Kuhar DT, et al. *Infect Control Hosp Epidemiol*. 2013;34(9):875–892 PMID: 23917901
78. Abdel Massih RC, et al. *World J Gastroenterol*. 2009;15(21):2561–2569 PMID: 19496184
79. Acosta EP, et al. *J Infect Dis*. 2010;202(4):563–566 PMID: 20594104
80. Kimberlin DW, et al. *J Infect Dis*. 2013;207(5):709–720 PMID: 23230059
81. McPherson C, et al. *J Infect Dis*. 2012;206(6):847–850 PMID: 22807525

82. Bradley JS, et al. *Pediatrics*. 2017;140(5):e20162727 PMID: 29051331
83. AAP. Measles. In: Kimberlin DW, et al, eds. *Red Book: 2024–2027 Report of the Committee on Infectious Diseases*. 33rd ed. 2024:570–585
84. AAP Committee on Infectious Diseases and Bronchiolitis Guidelines Committee. *Pediatrics*. 2014;134(2):415–420 PMID: 25070315
85. AAP Committee on Infectious Diseases and Bronchiolitis Guidelines Committee. *Pediatrics*. 2014;134(2):e620–e638 PMID: 25070304
86. Whitley RJ. *Adv Exp Med Biol*. 2008;609:216–232 PMID: 18193668

Chapter 9

1. Gonzales MLM, et al. *Cochrane Database Syst Rev*. 2019;(1):CD006085 PMID: 30624763
2. Haque R, et al. *N Engl J Med*. 2003;348(16):1565–1573 PMID: 1270037
3. Rossignol JF, et al. *Trans R Soc Trop Med Hyg*. 2007;101(10):1025–1031 PMID: 17658567
4. Mackey-Lawrence NM, et al. *BMJ Clin Evid*. 2011;2011:0918 PMID: 21477391
5. Fox LM, et al. *Clin Infect Dis*. 2005;40(8):1173–1180 PMID: 15791519
6. Cope JR, et al. *Clin Infect Dis*. 2016;62(6):774–776 PMID: 26679626
7. Vargas-Zepeda J, et al. *Arch Med Res*. 2005;36(1):83–86 PMID: 15900627
8. Linam WM, et al. *Pediatrics*. 2015;135(3):e744–e748 PMID: 25667249
9. Visvesvara GS, et al. *FEMS Immunol Med Microbiol*. 2007;50(1):1–26 PMID: 17428307
10. Martínez DY, et al. *Clin Infect Dis*. 2010;51(2):e7–e11 PMID: 20550438
11. Chotmongkol V, et al. *Am J Trop Med Hyg*. 2009;81(3):443–445 PMID: 19706911
12. Lo Re V III, et al. *Am J Med*. 2003;114(3):217–223 PMID: 12637136
13. Jitpimolmard S, et al. *Parasitol Res*. 2007;100(6):1293–1296 PMID: 17177056
14. Checkley AM, et al. *J Infect*. 2010;60(1):1–20 PMID: 19931558
15. Bethony J, et al. *Lancet*. 2006;367(9521):1521–1532 PMID: 16679166
16. Krause PJ, et al. *N Engl J Med*. 2000;343(20):1454–1458 PMID: 11078770
17. Vannier E, et al. *Infect Dis Clin North Am*. 2008;22(3):469–488 PMID: 18755385
18. Krause PJ, et al. *Clin Infect Dis*. 2021;72(2):185–189 PMID: 33501959
19. Sanchez E, et al. *JAMA*. 2016;315(16):1767–1777 PMID: 27115378
20. Kletsova EA, et al. *Ann Clin Microbiol Antimicrob*. 2017;16(1):26 PMID: 28399851
21. Schuster FL, et al. *Clin Microbiol Rev*. 2008;21(4):626–638 PMID: 18854484
22. Murray WJ, et al. *Clin Infect Dis*. 2004;39(10):1484–1492 PMID: 15546085
23. Sircar AD, et al. *MMWR Morb Mortal Wkly Rep*. 2016;65(35):930–933 PMID: 27608169
24. Malik K, et al. Albendazole. In: StatPearls. StatPearls Publishing; 2024 PMID: 31971723
25. Rossignol JF, et al. *Clin Gastroenterol Hepatol*. 2005;3(10):987–991 PMID: 16234044
26. Nigro L, et al. *J Travel Med*. 2003;10(2):128–130 PMID: 12650658
27. Bern C, et al. *JAMA*. 2007;298(18):2171–2181 PMID: 18000201
28. Salvador F, et al. *Clin Infect Dis*. 2015;61(11):1688–1694 PMID: 26265500
29. Miller DA, et al. *Clin Infect Dis*. 2015;60(8):1237–1240 PMID: 25601454
30. Smith HV, et al. *Curr Opin Infect Dis*. 2004;17(6):557–564 PMID: 15640710
31. Davies AP, et al. *BMJ*. 2009;339:b4168 PMID: 19841008
32. Krause I, et al. *Pediatr Infect Dis J*. 2012;31(11):1135–1138 PMID: 22810017
33. Abubakar I, et al. *Cochrane Database Syst Rev*. 2007;(1):CD004932 PMID: 17253532
34. Jelinek T, et al. *Clin Infect Dis*. 1994;19(6):1062–1066 PMID: 7534125
35. Schuster A, et al. *Clin Infect Dis*. 2013;57(8):1155–1157 PMID: 23811416
36. Hoge CW, et al. *Lancet*. 1995;345(8951):691–693 PMID: 7885125
37. Ortega YR, et al. *Clin Microbiol Rev*. 2010;23(1):218–234 PMID: 20065331
38. Steffen R, et al. *J Travel Med*. 2018;25(1):tay116 PMID: 30462260
39. Nash TE, et al. *Neurology*. 2006;67(7):1120–1127 PMID: 17030744
40. Garcia HH, et al. *Lancet Neurol*. 2014;13(12):1202–1215 PMID: 25453460
41. Lillie P, et al. *J Infect*. 2010;60(5):403–404 PMID: 20153773
42. White AC Jr, et al. *Clin Infect Dis*. 2018;66(8):1159–1163 PMID: 29617787
43. Verdier RI, et al. *Ann Intern Med*. 2000;132(11):885–888 PMID: 10836915

44. Stark DJ, et al. *Trends Parasitol.* 2006;22(2):92–96 PMID: 16380293
45. Röser D, et al. *Clin Infect Dis.* 2014;58(12):1692–1699 PMID: 24647023
46. Smego RA Jr, et al. *Clin Infect Dis.* 2003;37(8):1073–1083 PMID: 14523772
47. Brunetti E, et al. *Acta Trop.* 2010;114(1):1–16 PMID: 19931502
48. Fernando SD, et al. *J Trop Med.* 2011;2011:175941 PMID: 21234244
49. Walker M, et al. *Clin Infect Dis.* 2015;60(8):1199–2017 PMID: 25537873
50. Debrah AY, et al. *Clin Infect Dis.* 2015;61(4):517–526 PMID: 25948064
51. Mand S, et al. *Clin Infect Dis.* 2012;55(5):621–630 PMID: 22610930
52. Ottesen EA, et al. *Annu Rev Med.* 1992;43:417–424 PMID: 1580599
53. Jong EC, et al. *J Infect Dis.* 1985;152(3):637–640 PMID: 3897401
54. Sayasone S, et al. *Clin Infect Dis.* 2017;64(4):451–458 PMID: 28174906
55. Calvopina M, et al. *Trans R Soc Trop Med Hyg.* 1998;92(5):566–569 PMID: 9861383
56. Johnson RJ, et al. *Rev Infect Dis.* 1985;7(2):200–206 PMID: 4001715
57. Graham CS, et al. *Clin Infect Dis.* 2001;33(1):1–5 PMID: 11389487
58. Granados CE, et al. *Cochrane Database Syst Rev.* 2012;(12):CD007787 PMID: 23235648
59. Ross AG, et al. *N Engl J Med.* 2013;368(19):1817–1825 PMID: 23656647
60. Requena-Mendez A, et al. *J Infect Dis.* 2017;215(6):946–953 PMID: 28453841
61. Hotez PJ, et al. *N Engl J Med.* 2004;351(8):799–807 PMID: 15317893
62. Keiser J, et al. *JAMA.* 2008;299(16):1937–1948 PMID: 18430913
63. Steinmann P, et al. *PLoS One.* 2011;6(9):e25003 PMID: 21980373
64. Aronson N, et al. *Clin Infect Dis.* 2016;63(12):e202–e264 PMID: 27941151
65. Control of the leishmaniases: report of a meeting of the WHO Expert Committee on the Control of Leishmaniases, Geneva, 22–26 March 2010. 2010. Accessed October 29, 2024. https://apps.who.int/iris/handle/10665/44412
66. Alrajhi AA, et al. *N Engl J Med.* 2002;346(12):891–895 PMID: 11907288
67. Bern C, et al. *Clin Infect Dis.* 2006;43(7):917–924 PMID: 16941377
68. Ritmeijer K, et al. *Clin Infect Dis.* 2006;43(3):357–364 PMID: 16804852
69. Monge-Maillo B, et al. *Clin Infect Dis.* 2015;60(9):1398–1404 PMID: 25601455
70. Sundar S, et al. *N Engl J Med.* 2002;347(22):1739–1746 PMID: 12456849
71. Sundar S, et al. *N Engl J Med.* 2007;356(25):2571–2581 PMID: 17582067
72. Pinart M, et al. *Cochrane Database Syst Rev.* 2020;(8):CD004834 PMID: 32853410
73. Drugs for head lice. *JAMA.* 2017;317(19):2010–2011 PMID: 28510677
74. Nolt D, et al. *Pediatrics.* 2022;150(4):e2022059282 PMID: 36156158
75. Ashley EA, et al. *Lancet Child Adolesc Health.* 2020;4(10):775–789 PMID: 32946831
76. *CDC Yellow Book: Health Information for International Travel.* 2024. Reviewed August 14, 2023. Accessed November 18, 2024. https://wwwnc.cdc.gov/travel/page/yellowbook-home
77. Haghiri A, et al. *Clin Pharmacol Ther.* 2023;114(6):1304–1312 PMID: 37666798
78. Usha V, et al. *J Am Acad Dermatol.* 2000;42(2, pt 1):236–240 PMID: 10642678
79. Brodine SK, et al. *Am J Trop Med Hyg.* 2009;80(3):425–430 PMID: 19270293
80. Doenhoff MJ, et al. *Expert Rev Anti Infect Ther.* 2006;4(2):199–210 PMID: 16597202
81. Fenwick A, et al. *Curr Opin Infect Dis.* 2006;19(6):577–582 PMID: 17075334
82. Marti H, et al. *Am J Trop Med Hyg.* 1996;55(5):477–481 PMID: 8940976
83. Segarra-Newnham M. *Ann Pharmacother.* 2007;41(12):1992–2001 PMID: 17940124
84. Barisani-Asenbauer T, et al. *J Ocul Pharmacol Ther.* 2001;17(3):287–294 PMID: 11436948
85. McAuley JB. *Pediatr Infect Dis J.* 2008;27(2):161–162 PMID: 18227714
86. Maldonado YA, et al. *Pediatrics.* 2017;139(2):e20163860 PMID: 28138010
87. de-la-Torre A, et al. *Ocul Immunol Inflamm.* 2011;19(5):314–320 PMID: 21970662
88. Shane AL, et al. *Clin Infect Dis.* 2017;65(12):e45–e80 PMID: 29053792
89. DuPont HL. *Clin Infect Dis.* 2007;45(suppl 1):S78–S84 PMID: 17582576
90. Riddle MS, et al. *J Travel Med.* 2017;24(suppl 1):S57–S74 PMID: 28521004
91. Gottstein B, et al. *Clin Microbiol Rev.* 2009;22(1):127–145 PMID: 19136437
92. Workowski KA, et al. *MMWR Recomm Rep.* 2015;64(RR-03):1–137 PMID: 26042815
93. Fairlamb AH. *Trends Parasitol.* 2003;19(11):488–494 PMID: 14580959

94. Schmid C, et al. *Lancet*. 2004;364(9436):789–790 PMID: 15337407
95. Bisser S, et al. *J Infect Dis*. 2007;195(3):322–329 PMID: 17205469
96. Priotto G, et al. *Lancet*. 2009;374(9683):56–64 PMID: 19559476
97. Buscher P, et al. *Lancet*. 2017;390(10110):2397–2409 PMID: 28673422
98. Control and surveillance of human African trypanosomiasis: report of a WHO expert committee. 2013. Accessed October 29, 2024. https://apps.who.int/iris/handle/10665/95732

Chapter 10

1. Mergenhagen KA, et al. *Antimicrob Agents Chemother*. 2020;64(3):e02167-19 PMID: 31871085

Chapter 12

1. Wu W, et al. *Clin Microbiol Rev*. 2019;32(2):e00115-18 PMID: 30700432
2. Hultén KG, et al. *Pediatr Infect Dis J*. 2018;37(3):235–241 PMID: 28859018
3. Acree ME, et al. *Infect Control Hosp Epidemiol*. 2017;38(10):1226–1234 PMID: 28903801
4. Liu C, et al. *Clin Infect Dis*. 2011;52(3):e18–e55 PMID: 21208910
5. Korczowski B, et al. *Pediatr Infect Dis J*. 2016;35(8):e239–e247 PMID: 27164462
6. Cannavino CR, et al. *Pediatr Infect Dis J*. 2016;35(7):752–759 PMID: 27093162
7. Blumer JL, et al. *Pediatr Infect Dis J*. 2016;35(7):760–766 PMID: 27078119
8. Bradley JS. *Pediatr Infect Dis J*. 2020;39(5):411–418 PMID: 32091493
9. Rybak MJ. *Am J Health Syst Pharm*. 2020;77(11):835–864 PMID: 32191793
10. Le J, et al. *Pediatr Infect Dis J*. 2013;32(4):e155–e163 PMID: 23340565
11. McNeil JC, et al. *Pediatr Infect Dis J*. 2016;35(3):263–268 PMID: 26646549
12. Sader HS, et al. *Antimicrob Agents Chemother*. 2017;61(9):e01043-17 PMID: 28630196
13. Depardieu F, et al. *Clin Microbiol Rev*. 2007;20(1):79–114 PMID: 17223624
14. Miller LG, et al. *N Engl J Med*. 2015;372(12):1093–1103 PMID: 25785967
15. Bradley J, et al. *Pediatrics*. 2017;139(3):e20162477 PMID: 28202770
16. Arrieta AC, et al. *Pediatr Infect Dis J*. 2018;37(9):890–900 PMID: 29406465
17. Bradley JS, et al. *Pediatr Infect Dis J*. 2020;39(9):814–823 PMID: 32639465
18. Huang JT, et al. *Pediatrics*. 2009;123(5):e808–e814 PMID: 19403473
19. Finnell SM, et al. *Clin Pediatr (Phila)*. 2015;54(5):445–450 PMID: 25385929
20. Kaplan SL, et al. *Clin Infect Dis*. 2014;58(5):679–682 PMID: 24265356
21. McNeil JC, et al. *Curr Infect Dis Rep*. 2019;21(4):12 PMID: 30859379

Chapter 14

1. Nelson JD. *J Pediatr*. 1978;92(1):175–176 PMID: 619073
2. Nelson JD, et al. *J Pediatr*. 1978;92(1):131–134 PMID: 619055
3. Tetzlaff TR, et al. *J Pediatr*. 1978;92(3):485–490 PMID: 632997
4. Ballock RT, et al. *J Pediatr Orthop*. 2009;29(6):636–642 PMID: 19700997
5. Peltola H, et al. *N Engl J Med*. 2014;370(4):352–360 PMID: 24450893
6. Bradley JS, et al. *Pediatrics*. 2011;128(4):e1034–e1045 PMID: 21949152
7. Rice HE, et al. *Arch Surg*. 2001;136(12):1391–1395 PMID: 11735866
8. Fraser JD, et al. *J Pediatr Surg*. 2010;45(6):1198–1202 PMID: 20620320
9. Strohmeier Y, et al. *Cochrane Database Syst Rev*. 2014;(7):CD003772 PMID: 25066627
10. Tingsgård S, et al. *JAMA Netw Open*. 2024;7(1):e2352314 PMID: 38261322
11. Omrani AS, et al. *Clin Microbiol Infect*. 2024;30(4):492–498 PMID: 37858867
12. Drusano GL, et al. *J Infect Dis*. 2024;210(8):1319–1324 PMID: 24760199
13. Arnold JC, et al. *Pediatrics*. 2012;130(4):e821–e828 PMID: 22966033
14. Zaoutis T, et al. *Pediatrics*. 2009;123(2):636–642 PMID: 19171632
15. Keren R, et al. *JAMA Pediatr*. 2015;169(2):120–128 PMID: 25506733
16. Gunter SG, et al. *Pharmacy (Basel)*. 2022;10(1):16 PMID: 35076616
17. Desai AA, et al. *J Pediatr Surg*. 2015;50(6):912–914 PMID: 25812441
18. Marino NE, et al. *Surg Infect (Larchmt)*. 2017;18(8):894–903 PMID: 29064344
19. Haynes AS, et al. *Antimicrob Agents Chemother*. 2024;68(5):e0018224 PMID: 38597672

20. Liu C, et al. *Clin Infect Dis.* 2011;52(3):e18–e55 PMID: 21208910
21. Syrogiannopoulos GA, et al. *Lancet.* 1988;1(8575–8576):37–40 PMID: 2891899

Chapter 15

1. Oehler RL, et al. *Lancet Infect Dis.* 2009;9(7):439–447 PMID: 19555903
2. Bula-Rudas FJ, et al. *Pediatr Rev.* 2018;39(10):490–500 PMID: 30275032
3. Elcock KL, et al. *Injury.* 2022;53(2):227–236 PMID: 34838260
4. Talan DA, et al. *Clin Infect Dis.* 2003;37(11):1481–1489 PMID: 14614671
5. Aziz H, et al. *J Trauma Acute Care Surg.* 2015;78(3):641–648 PMID: 25710440
6. CDC. Clinical overview of rabies. June 20, 2024. Accessed November 18, 2024. www.cdc.gov/rabies/hcp/clinical-overview
7. AAP. Tetanus. In: Kimberlin DW, et al, eds. *Red Book: 2024–2027 Report of the Committee on Infectious Diseases.* 33rd ed. 2024:848–854
8. Wilson WR, et al. *Circulation.* 2021;143(20):e963–e978 PMID: 33853363
9. Baltimore RS, et al. *Circulation.* 2015;132(15):1487–1515 PMID: 26373317
10. Williams ML, et al. *Ther Adv Cardiovasc Dis.* 2021;15:17539447211002687 PMID: 33784909
11. Gupta S, et al. *Congenit Heart Dis.* 2017;12(2):196–201 PMID: 27885814
12. Cahill TJ, et al. *Heart.* 2017;103(12):937–944 PMID: 28213367
13. Dayer M, et al. *J Infect Chemother.* 2018;24(1):18–24 PMID: 29107651
14. AAP. Lyme disease. In: Kimberlin DW, et al, eds. *Red Book: 2024–2027 Report of the Committee on Infectious Diseases.* 33rd ed. 2024:549–556
15. McNamara LA, et al. Meningococcal disease. In: *Manual for the Surveillance of Vaccine-Preventable Diseases.* 2019. October 30, 2024. Accessed November 18, 2024. www.cdc.gov/surv-manual/php/table-of-contents/chapter-8-meningococcal-disease.html
16. McNamara LA, et al. *Lancet Infect Dis.* 2018;18(9):e272–e281 PMID: 29858150
17. AAP. Pertussis. In: Kimberlin DW, et al, eds. *Red Book: 2024–2027 Report of the Committee on Infectious Diseases.* 33rd ed. 2024:656–667
18. CDC. Whooping cough (pertussis). Postexposure antimicrobial prophylaxis. April 2, 2024. Accessed October 29, 2024. www.cdc.gov/pertussis/php/postexposure-prophylaxis
19. CDC. Clinical overview of tetanus. August 15, 2024. Accessed October 29, 2024. www.cdc.gov/tetanus/hcp/clinical-overview
20. CDC. Tuberculosis (TB). Treatment regimens for latent TB infection. Reviewed February 13, 2020. Accessed October 29, 2024. www.cdc.gov/tb/topic/treatment/ltbi.htm
21. AAP. Tuberculosis. In: Kimberlin DW, et al, eds. *Red Book: 2024–2027 Report of the Committee on Infectious Diseases.* 33rd ed. 2024:888–920
22. Sterling TR, et al. *MMWR Recomm Rep.* 2020;69(1):1–11 PMID: 32053584
23. ACOG. *Obstet Gynecol.* 2020;135(5):e193–e202 PMID: 32332414
24. Pinninti SG, et al. *Semin Perinatol.* 2018;42(3):168–175 PMID: 29544668
25. AAP. Herpes simplex. In: Kimberlin DW, et al, eds. *Red Book: 2024–2027 Report of the Committee on Infectious Diseases.* 33rd ed. 2024:467–478
26. AAP Committee on Infectious Diseases. *Pediatrics.* 2020;146(4):e2020024588 PMID: 32900875
27. Kimberlin DW, et al. *J Infect Dis.* 2013;207(5):709–720 PMID: 23230059
28. AAP. Rabies. In: Kimberlin DW, et al, eds. *Red Book: 2024–2027 Report of the Committee on Infectious Diseases.* 33rd ed. 2024:702–711
29. AAP. Varicella-zoster virus infections. In: Kimberlin DW, et al, eds. *Red Book: 2024–2027 Report of the Committee on Infectious Diseases.* 33rd ed. 2024:938–951
30. Leach AJ, et al. *Cochrane Database Syst Rev.* 2006;(4):CD004401 PMID: 17054203
31. Lieberthal AS, et al. *Pediatrics.* 2013;131(3):e964–e999 PMID: 23439909
32. Williams G, et al. *Cochrane Database Syst Rev.* 2023;(4):CD001321 PMID: 37068952
33. Marsh MC, et al. *Pediatr Rev.* 2024;45(5):260–270 PMID: 38689106
34. RIVUR Trial Investigators, et al. *N Engl J Med.* 2014;370(25):2367–2376 PMID: 24795142
35. AAP Subcommittee on Urinary Tract Infection and Steering Committee on Quality Improvement and Management. *Pediatrics.* 2011;128(3):595–610 PMID: 21873693

36. Craig JC. *J Pediatr.* 2015;166(3):778 PMID: 25722276
37. National Institute for Health and Care Excellence. Urinary tract infection (recurrent): antimicrobial prescribing; treatment for children and young people under 16 years with recurrent UTI. October 31, 2018. Accessed October 29, 2024. www.nice.org.uk/guidance/ng112/chapter/Recommendations#treatment-for-children-and-young-people-under-16-years-with-recurrent-uti
38. Williams G, et al. *Cochrane Database Syst Rev.* 2019;(4):CD001534 PMID: 30932167
39. AAP. *Pneumocystis jirovecii* infections. In: Kimberlin DW, et al, eds. *Red Book: 2024–2027 Report of the Committee on Infectious Diseases.* 33rd ed. 2024:676–682
40. Caselli D, et al. *J Pediatr.* 2014;164(2):389–392.e1 PMID: 24252793
41. Proudfoot R, et al. *J Pediatr Hematol Oncol.* 2017;39(3):194–202 PMID: 28267082
42. Stern A, et al. *Cochrane Database Syst Rev.* 2014;(10):CD005590 PMID: 25269391
43. Delaplain PT, et al. *Surg Infect (Larchmt).* 2022;23(3):232–247 PMID: 35196154
44. UpToDate. Antimicrobial prophylaxis for prevention of surgical site infection in adults. Updated October 18, 2022. Accessed October 29, 2024. www.uptodate.com/contents/antimicrobial-prophylaxis-for-prevention-of-surgical-site-infection-in-adults#H852308389
45. Paruk F, et al. *Int J Antimicrob Agents.* 2017;49(4):395–402 PMID: 28254373
46. Branch-Elliman W, et al. *JAMA Surg.* 2019;154(7):590–598 PMID: 31017647
47. Berríos-Torres SI, et al. *JAMA Surg.* 2017;152(8):784–791 PMID: 28467526
48. Calderwood MS, et al. *Infect Control Hosp Epidemiol.* 2023;44(5):695–720 PMID: 37137483
49. PREP-IT Investigators, et al. *N Engl J Med.* 2024;390(5):409–420 PMID: 38294973
50. Darouiche RO, et al. *N Engl J Med.* 2010;362(1):18–26 PMID: 20054046
51. de Tymowski C, et al. *Antibiotics (Basel).* 2023;12(1):85 PMID: 36671286
52. De Cock PA, et al. *J Antimicrob Chemother.* 2017;72(3):791–800 PMID: 27999040
53. Marino NE, et al. *Surg Infect (Larchmt).* 2017;18(8):894–903 PMID: 29064344
54. Andersen BR, et al. *Cochrane Database Syst Rev.* 2005;(3):CD001439 PMID: 16034862

Chapter 16

1. Broyles AD, et al. *J Allergy Clin Immunol Pract.* 2020;8(9)(suppl):S16–S116 PMID: 33039007
2. Bergmann MM, et al. *Pediatr Allergy Immunol.* 2023;34(12):e14058 PMID: 38146108
3. Delli Colli L, et al. *J Allergy Clin Immunol Pract.* 2021;9(2):916–921 PMID: 32898711
4. Copaescu AM, et al. *JAMA Netw Open.* 2022;5(9):e2233703 PMID: 36121658
5. Khan DA, et al. *J Allergy Clin Immunol.* 2022;150(6):1333–1393 PMID: 36122788
6. Ponvert C, et al. *Allergy.* 2007;62(1):42–46 PMID: 17156340

Chapter 17

1. Merriam-Webster. Stewardship. Accessed October 29, 2024. www.merriam-webster.com/dictionary/stewardship
2. CDC. Infection control. Guidelines and guidance library. April 8, 2024. Accessed November 18, 2024. www.cdc.gov/infection-control/hcp/guidance/index.html
3. Farnaes L, et al. *Diagn Microbiol Infect Dis.* 2019;94(2):188–191 PMID: 30819624

Index

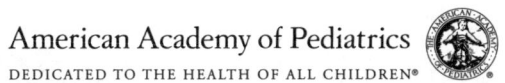
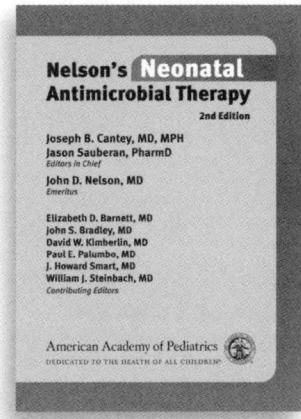
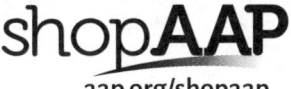